ADVANCES IN SURGICAL PATHOLOGY

BRAIN CANCER

ADVANCES IN SURGICAL PATHOLOGY
BRAIN CANCER

Andreana Rivera, MD
Staff Neuropathologist
Department of Pathology and Genomic Medicine
Houston Methodist Hospital
Houston, Texas

Hidehiro Takei, MD
Associate Professor
Department of Pathology and Laboratory Medicine
Weill Medical College of Cornell University
New York, New York
Pathologist
Department of Pathology and Genomic Medicine
Houston Methodist Hospital
Houston, Texas

SERIES EDITORS

Philip T. Cagle, MD
Professor of Pathology and Laboratory Medicine
Weill Medical College of Cornell University
New York, New York
Director, Pulmonary Pathology
Houston Methodist Hospital
Houston, Texas

Timothy Craig Allen, MD, JD
Professor, Department of Pathology
Director of Anatomic Pathology
The University of Texas Medical Branch
Galveston, Texas

Wolters Kluwer

Philadelphia • Baltimore • New York • London
Buenos Aires • Hong Kong • Sydney • Tokyo

Acquisitions Editor: Ryan Shaw
Product Development Editor: Kate Marshall
Production Project Manager: Bridgett Dougherty
Design Coordinator: Stephen Druding
Manufacturing Coordinator: Beth Welsh
Prepress Vendor: SPi Global

9 8 7 6 5 4 3 2 1

Printed in China

Library of Congress Cataloging-in-Publication Data
Advances in surgical pathology. Brain cancer / [edited by] Andreana Rivera, Hidehiro Takei.
p. ; cm. — (Advances in surgical pathology series)
Brain cancer
Includes bibliographical references and index.
ISBN 978-1-4511-9091-5
I. Rivera, Andreana, editor. II. Takei, Hidehiro, editor. III. Title: Brain cancer. IV. Series: Advances in surgical pathology series.
[DNLM: 1. Central Nervous System Neoplasms—physiopathology. 2. Central Nervous System Neoplasms—diagnosis. 3. Central Nervous System Neoplasms—therapy. WL 358]
RD663
616.99'481059—dc23
2014045572

LWW.com

RRS1503

Series Overview

Expectations for the pathologist practicing today exceed those for pathologists in practice only a few years ago. In addition to the rapid growth of knowledge and new technologies in the field of pathology, recent years have seen the emergence of many trends that significantly impact the traditional practice of pathology including the subspecialized multidisciplinary approach to patient care, personalized therapeutics including targeted molecular therapies, and imaging techniques such as endoscopic microscopy, molecular radiology, and imaging multimodality theranostics that compete with conventional light microscopy. In order to remain a viable member of the patient care team, the pathologist must keep up with growing knowledge in traditional subjects as well as in new areas of expertise such as molecular testing. Additionally, the pathologist is subject to an increasing number of credentialing requirements and, for those now completing training, Self-Assessment Modules for Maintenance of Certification, which require the pathologist to be examined on the recent advances in pathology in order to sustain their qualifications to practice.

Each volume in the series *Advances in Surgical Pathology* focuses on a specific subject in pathology that has undergone recent advancement in terms of knowledge, technical procedures, application, and/or integration as part of current trends in pathology and medicine. This series of books not only updates the pathologist on recently acquired knowledge but emphasizes the new uses of that knowledge within the context of the changing landscape of pathology practice in the 21st century. Rather than information in a vacuum, the pathologist is educated on how to apply the new knowledge as part of a subspecialized multidisciplinary team and for purposes of personalized patient therapy.

Each volume in the series will be divided into the following sections: (1) Overview—updates the pathologist on the general topic, including epidemiology, bringing the pathologist generally up to date on a topic as a basis for the more specialized sections that follow. (2) Histopathology—reviews histopathology and specific recent changes that warrant more description and more illustration, for example, recently described entities and recent revisions in classifications. This will also emphasize histopathology figures to illustrate recently described entities and to demonstrate the basis for classification changes so that the pathologist is able to understand and recognize these changes. (3) Imaging—reviews the impact of imaging techniques on histopathologic diagnosis and on the practice of pathology. An example of the former is the use of increasingly sensitive high-resolution CT scan in the diagnosis of interstitial lung diseases. An example of the latter is the use of multimodality theranostics rather than traditional histopathology for the diagnosis and treatment of lung cancer. Figures linking the radiologic images to the histopathology will be emphasized. (4) Molecular Pathology—a review and update on specific molecular pathology as it applies to specific diseases for the practicing pathologist in regard to molecular diagnostics and molecular therapeutics. An example of the former is the identification of a specific fusion gene to diagnose synovial sarcoma. An example of the latter is the identification of specific EGFR mutations in pulmonary adenocarcinoma and its relationship to treatment with EGFR antagonists. (5) For those volumes dealing with cancers (Lung Cancer, Breast Cancer, Prostate Cancer, Colon Cancer, etc.), additional sections will include Preneoplastic and Preinvasive Lesions, which will emphasize histopathologic figures and staging, particularly emphasizing the new staging systems and to illustrate specific problems in staging.

These books will assist the pathologist in daily practice in the modern setting and provide a basis for interacting with other physicians in patient care. They will also provide the timely updates in knowledge that are necessary for daily practice, for current credentialing and for Maintenance of Certification. As such, this series is invaluable to pathologists in practice at all levels of experience who need to keep up with advances for their daily performance and their periodic credentialing and to pathologists-in-training who will apply this knowledge to their boards and their future practice. In the latter case, this series will serve as a useful library for pathology training programs.

Contributors

Adekunle M. Adesina, MD, PhD, FCAP, FMCPath
Professor of Pathology, Immunology and Pediatrics-Hematology/Oncology
Medical Director, Neuropathology and Molecular Neuropathology
Texas Children's Hospital
Baylor College of Medicine
Houston, Texas

Wamidh Adwar, MD
Resident
Department of Pathology and Laboratory Medicine
Henry Ford Health System
Detroit, Michigan

Junjeong Choi, MD
Assistant Professor
Department of Pathology
Yonsei University
Wonju College of Medicine
Wonju, South Korea

Matthew Daniel Cykowski, MD
Fellow in Neuropathology
Department of Pathology and Genomic Medicine
Houston Methodist Hospital
Houston, Texas

Steve Huntz Fung, MD
Assistant Professor of Radiology
Weill Cornell Medical College
Staff Neuroradiologist
Houston Methodist Hospital Physician Organization
Medical Director of MRI Research
Departments of Neuroradiology, Radiology
Houston Methodist Hospital Research Institute
Houston, Texas

Tamio Ito, MD
Neurosurgeon
Nakamura Memorial Hospital
Sapporo, Japan

Hiromi Kanno, MD
Pathologist
Department of Surgical Pathology
Hokkaido University Hospital
Sapporo, Japan

Fumi Kawakami, MD, PhD
Visiting Scientist
Department of Translational Molecular Pathology
The University of Texas MD Anderson Cancer Center
Houston, Texas

Yvonne Kew, MD, PhD
Neuro-Oncologist
Department of Neurosurgery
Houston Methodist Hospital
Assistant Member
Houston Methodist Research Institute
Assistant Professor
Department of Neurology
Baylor College of Medicine
Houston, Texas

Se Hoon Kim, MD, PhD
Professor
Department of Pathology
Yonsei University
College of Medicine
Severance Hospital
Seoul, Korea

Takashi Komori, MD, PhD
Neuropathologist, Head of Department
Department of Laboratory Medicine and Pathology (Neuropathology)
Tokyo Metropolitan Neurological Hospital
Tokyo, Japan

Jian Yi Li, MD, PhD
Associate Professor
Department of Pathology and Laboratory Medicine
North Shore-Long Island Jewish Health System
Hofstra North Shore-LIJ School of Medicine
Lake Success, New York

Abir Mukherjee, MD
Assistant Professor
Department of Pathology and Laboratory Medicine
Temple University Hospital and Medical School
Philadelphia, Pennsylvania

Adriana Olar, MD
Fellow
Department of Pathology
The University of Texas MD Anderson Cancer Center
Houston, Texas

Jo Elle G. Peterson, MD
Assistant Professor
Department of Pathology
University of Oklahoma Health Sciences Center
Oklahoma City, Oklahoma

Aditya Raghunathan, MD, MPH
Assistant Professor
Division of Anatomic Pathology
Department of Laboratory Medicine and Pathology
Mayo Clinic
Rochester, Minnesota

Andreana Rivera, MD
Staff Neuropathologist
Department of Pathology and Genomic Medicine
Houston Methodist Hospital
Houston, Texas

Sanjay K. Singh, MD
Assistant Professor of Radiology
Department of Radiology
Weill Cornell Medical College
Houston Methodist Hospital
Houston, Texas

Yasuo Sugita, MD
Professor
Department of Pathology
Kurume University School of Medicine
Kurume, Fukuoka, Japan

Yeon-Lim Suh, MD, PhD
Professor
Department of Pathology
Samsung Medical Center
Sungkyunkwan University, School of Medicine
Seoul, Republic of Korea

Hidehiro Takei, MD
Associate Professor
Department of Pathology and Laboratory Medicine
Weill Medical College of Cornell University
New York, New York
Pathologist
Department of Pathology and Genomic Medicine
Houston Methodist Hospital
Houston, Texas

Shinya Tanaka, MD, PhD
Professor
Department of Cancer Pathology
Hokkaido University Graduate School of Medicine
Sapporo, Japan

Nishant Tiwari, MD, MS
Resident
Department of Pathology and Immunology
Baylor College of Medicine
Houston, Texas

Qun-Fang Wan
Research Scientist
Methodist Hospital Research Institute
Houston, Texas

Xinmin Zhang, MD
Assistant Professor
Department of Pathology and Laboratory Medicine
Hofstra North Shore-LIJ School of Medicine
Lake Success, New York

Preface

Although rare, a diagnosis of a primary brain tumor is associated with significant morbidity and high mortality, despite advances in the development of new therapeutic and imaging approaches. Consequently, although they represent only 1 to 2% of all new cancer cases in the United States, primary brain cancers exert a devastating impact not only on patients, who fall within a wide range of ages, but also on their families and caregivers.

As with other cancer types, an accurate pathologic diagnosis of brain tumors serves as a cornerstone of optimal treatment and improved prognosis. However, the diagnosis is often not straightforward because brain tumors are highly heterogeneous neoplasms that can originate from cells within the brain parenchyma, meninges, or nerves. Subsequently, the current WHO classification identifies over 130 histologic brain tumor entities. In addition, the biologic behavior of brain tumors ranges from benign to highly malignant, and even benign tumors can be lethal due to their location in the brain, their ability to infiltrate locally, and their propensity to undergo malignant transformation. Moreover, each tumor entity is associated with its own biology, treatment, and prognosis. Combined, these unique features make brain cancer pathologic diagnosis and treatment very challenging.

The past decade has brought a rapid expansion in knowledge and new technologies in the field of molecular neurooncology, which led to identification of key genetic markers behind brain tumor genesis, proliferation, and resistance to therapy. For instance, increased clinical utilization of next-generation sequencing technology has enabled an integrative high-throughput genetic analysis of brain tumors. However, additional analyses aimed at identification of the genetic neurooncology makers that are unique to a particular diagnosis, capable of predicting response to certain therapies, and those that help determine patient prognosis, are still critically needed. An integrated approach to diagnosis that incorporates clinical information, neurosurgical findings, radiologic features, and molecular alterations is required.

This book is intended to assist practicing surgical pathologists, neuropathologists, and pathologists-in-training by establishing the basis for an integrated approach to brain tumor diagnosis. The 19 chapters detail clinicoradiologic and pathologic findings of all brain tumor entities listed in the current WHO classification, including separate chapters that provide an overview of molecular neuropathology of glial and nonglial tumors. In addition, unique to this book are separate chapters for basic neuroradiology and medical neurooncology, knowledge of which is becoming increasingly important for an integrated diagnostic approach.

Finally, we were delighted to work with many outstanding contributors, and with the highly experienced and supportive staff at Wolters Kluwer Health and Houston Methodist Hospital. We hope this book will serve as a practical guide for pathologists of all experience levels that can be used in their daily practice.

Hidehiro Takei, MD
Andreana Rivera, MD
Department of Pathology and Genomic Medicine
Houston Methodist Hospital
Houston, Texas

Contents

Series Overview v
Contributors vii
Preface ix

SECTION I. Overview

1 Normal Histology 3

SECTION II. Histopathology

2 Diffuse (Infiltrating) Gliomas 13
3 Circumscribed Astrocytomas (Pilocytic Astrocytoma, Pilomyxoid Astrocytoma, Pleomorphic Xanthoastrocytoma, and Subependymal Giant Cell Astrocytoma) 30
4 Ependymomas 37
5 Other Neuroepithelial Tumors (Chordoid Glioma, Astroblastoma, Angiocentric Glioma) 51
6 Neuronal/Mixed Glioneuronal Tumors 58
7 Embryonal Tumors 74
8 Choroid Plexus Tumors (Choroid Plexus Papilloma, Atypical Choroid Plexus Papilloma, Choroid Plexus Carcinoma, Xanthogranuloma of the Choroid Plexus, and Metastasis) 91
9 Pineal Region Tumors 101
10 Sellar and Suprasellar Region Tumors 112
11 Meningeal Tumors 123
12 Hereditary Syndromes 142
13 Tumors of Cranial and Peripheral Nerves and Other Tumors 157
14 Hematolymphoid and Histiocytic Tumors 173
15 Central Nervous System Metastasis 189

SECTION III. Imaging

16 Correlation of Imaging with Pathology 199

SECTION IV. Molecular Pathology

17 Glial Tumors 211

18 Nonglial Tumors 219

SECTION V. Current Therapy and Prognosis

19 Brain Cancer Treatment 229

Index 251

ADVANCES IN SURGICAL PATHOLOGY

BRAIN CANCER

SECTION

I

Overview

▶ CHAPTER 1: Normal Histology

Normal Histology

1

Andreana Rivera

INTRODUCTION

The nervous system is unique in its variation of form and structure. The central nervous system is made of simple constituents (neurons, astrocytes, oligodendrocytes, ependyma, meningothelial cells) artfully arranged in complex structures that vary as much in appearance as they do in function. Distinguishing a neoplastic process from nonneoplastic tissue can be tricky if not familiar with the underlying normal histology. The purpose of this chapter is to provide a brief familiarization of the normal histologic features.

ANATOMY AND HISTOLOGY

Meninges

The meninges provide covering for the central nervous system. They can be broken down into two basic layers: the dura (the thicker fibrous layer) and the pia–arachnoid (the thin delicate layer, also referred to as the leptomeninges). The leptomeninges intimately line the surface of the brain and spinal cord (Figure 1-1A). Meningothelial cells are round to ovoid and normally found in a thin layer but can form small nests (Figure 1-1B). Intranuclear pseudoinclusions, whorls, and psammoma bodies are found in normal meningothelial tissue as well as their neoplastic counterparts. Meningeal melanocytes can also be seen as a normal leptomeningeal constituent particularly over the brainstem and spinal cord.

Gray and White Matter

The cerebral cortex (cortical gray matter) contains six neuronal layers. The most apparent of these is the hypocellular molecular layer adjacent to the leptomeninges (Figure 1-2). This layering pattern helps to distinguish the cortical gray from other gray matter structures such as the basal ganglia, thalamus, and amygdala where layering is not present. Gray matter is composed of neurons and supporting glia (Figure 1-3). Neurons are classically identified by their large cell body, prominent nucleoli, and presence of Nissl substance. However, there is wide variation in neuronal size and appearance. Astrocytes can be found anywhere in the central nervous system but are perhaps most easily identified in gray matter. Astrocytes can vary greatly in appearance but in a normal resting state have ovoid hyperchromatic nuclei with processes that are often indistinguishable from the background neuropil (Figure 1-3).

White matter is largely composed of axons and their associated oligodendroglia. It can be found in large areas (subcortical white matter), in small islands (pencil fibers in the putamen), or in linear tracts (corpus callosum). There is often a sharp demarcation between white matter and adjacent gray matter (Figure 1-4). Oligodendroglia are the myelinating cells of the central nervous system. These cells wrap their processes around neuronal axons and can sometimes be seen in linear orientation lined up along axons in the white matter. Oligodendrocytes have small round hyperchromatic nuclei (Figure 1-5) and may have perinuclear clearing.

FIGURE 1-1: Leptomeninges covering the surface of the cortices and extending into the sulcus (**A**). Arachnoid nest. Similar to their neoplastic counterparts, intranuclear pseudoinclusions seen here are a feature of meningothelial cells (**B**).

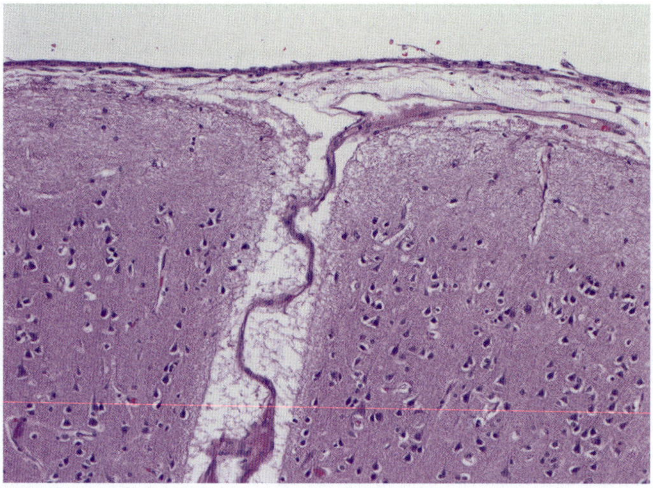

A

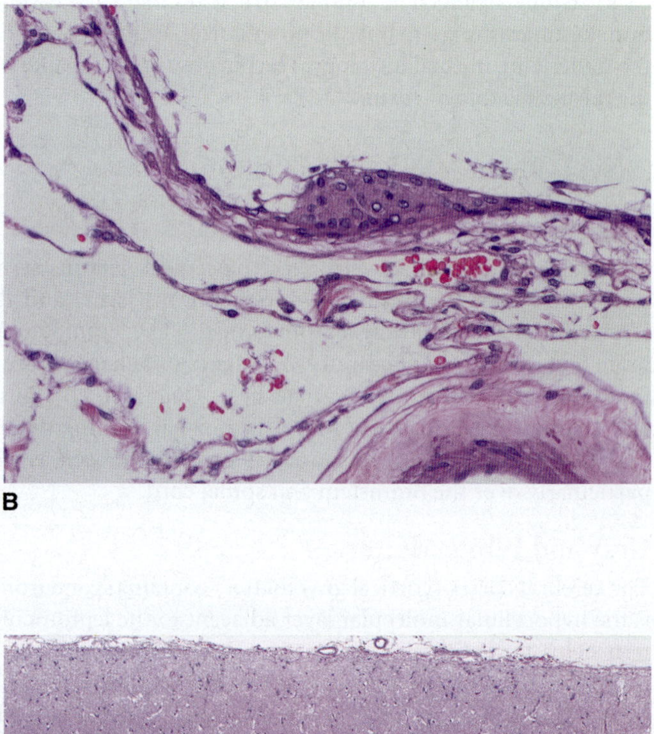

B

FIGURE 1-2: Cerebral cortex (cortical gray matter). Note the normal cellularity and neuronal layering.

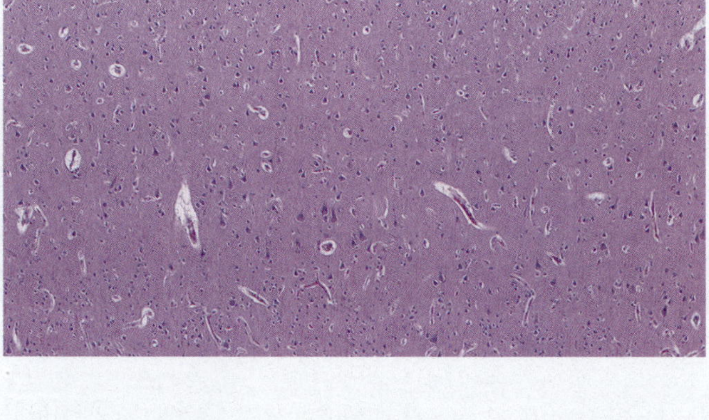

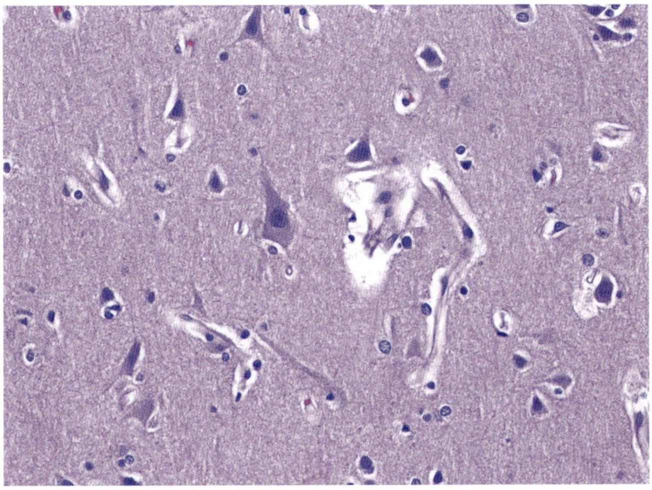

FIGURE 1-3: Gray matter. The *center* of the image shows a neuron with large cell body, prominent nucleolus, and dendritic processes. Adjacent to the neuron is a perineuronal oligodendrocyte; "satellitosis" is a feature of both normal and neoplastic oligodendroglia. Scattered resting astrocytes are also present.

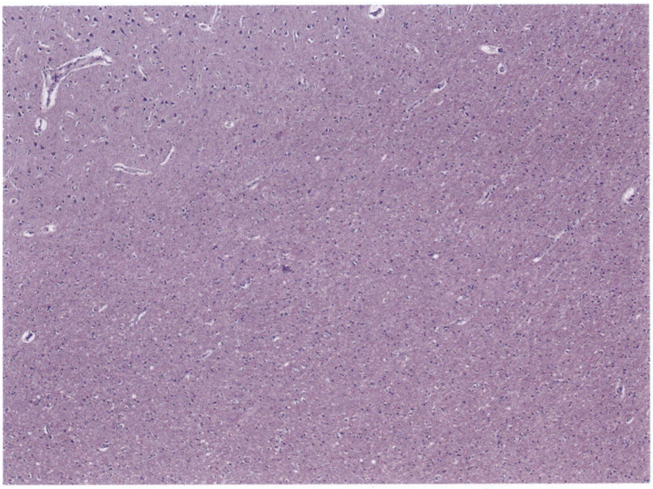

FIGURE 1-4: Gray–white junction. The sharp distinction between the gray matter (*top left*) and subcortical gray. Some larger neurons can be seen among the small round oligodendria at the gray–white interface.

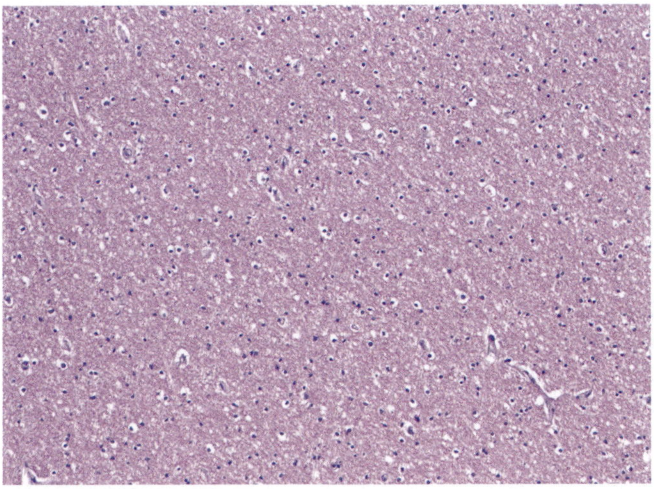

FIGURE 1-5: White matter. Perineuronal clearing ("fried egg" appearance) can be seen around some of the normal oligodendroglia. Note the cellularity and distribution of the normal oligodendroglia.

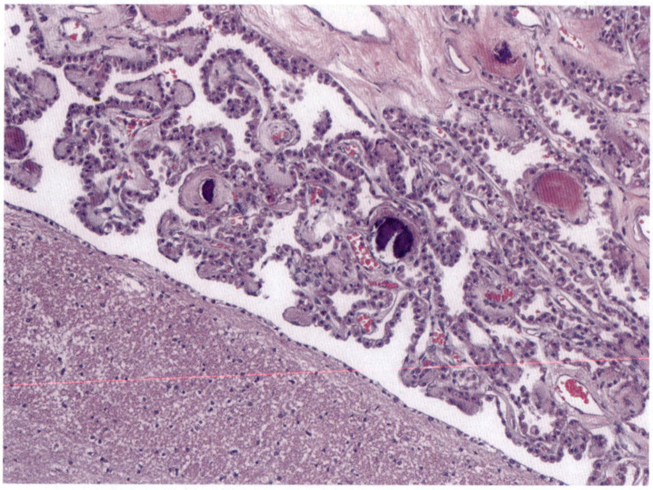

FIGURE 1-6: Ependyma and choroid plexus. The *bottom left* of the image shows periventricular neuropil lined by simple cuboidal cells. While prominent in children, ependymal cilia are often not easily seen on light microscopy in adults. The *top right* of the image shows papillary fibrovascular structure of the choroid plexus. The cores are lined by nonciliated simple cuboidal cells with a "hobnail" appearance. Calcifications, as those seen in the center of the image, are common with age.

This perinuclear clearing or "fried egg" appearance is often associated with their neoplastic counterparts and is the result of cytoplasmic vacuolation.

Ventricles

The ventricular system is lined throughout by ependyma, a ciliated cuboidal to columnar cell (Figure 1-6). The appearance of the ependymal lining can vary with age and location. For example, cilia are pronounced in children and are almost unidentifiable by light microscopy in older adults. Small nests of normal ependyma can be seen within the neuropil adjacent to ventricles and do not represent a diagnostic abnormality.

Choroid plexus is a specialized structure found within the ventricular system, specifically the atrium, body, and temporal horns of the lateral ventricles, foramina of Monro, roof of the third ventricle, roof of the fourth ventricle, and foramina of Luschka. It is responsible for the production of cerebrospinal fluid. The choroid plexus is composed of a single layer of cuboidal cells with a "hobnail" appearance overlying a papillary fibrovascular core (Figure 1-6). Meningothelial tissue can be present within the choroid plexus fibrovascular stroma due to the invagination of this tissue during development. This accounts for the occurrence of intraventricular meningiomas particularly in the atrium of the lateral ventricle where meningothelial rests are more common. Calcifications within the choroid plexus are often present and increase with age.

Cerebellum

The cerebellum has one of the most distinct appearances of any region of the brain, both grossly and microscopically. The cerebellar cortex has three layers (from outer to innermost): molecular layer, Purkinje cell layer, and internal granular cell layer (Figure 1-7). The molecular layer is histologically similar to that seen in the cerebral cortex. What makes the cerebellar cortex distinct is the layering of a single row of large Purkinje cells with their large cell bodies, prominent nucleoli, and tree-like dendritic processes and adjacent hypercellular internal granular cell layer with its small hyperchromatic neurons highlighting the extreme variability of neuronal morphology. Also seen in the Purkinje cell layer are cerebellar astrocytes called Bergmann glia. In small surgical specimens, the hypercellular granular cells may be mistaken for a small cell neoplasm or lymphocytic process.

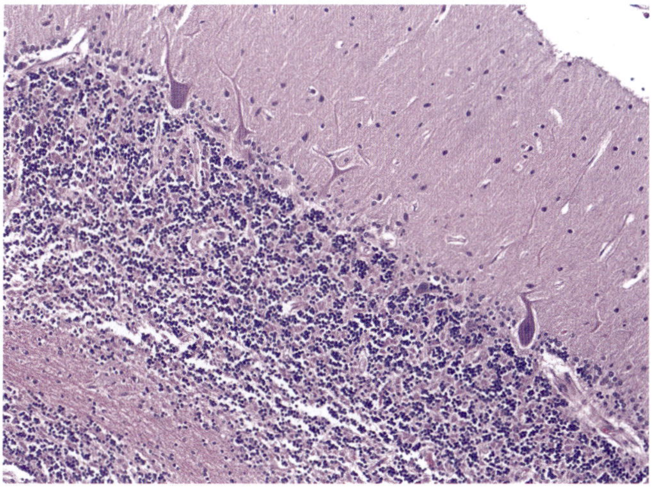

FIGURE 1-7: Cerebellar cortex. The cerebellar cortex is composed of three layers (from *top* to *bottom*): the molecular layer, Purkinje layer, and internal granular cell layer. Note the difference in morphology of the large Purkinje cells with impressive dendritic processes and much smaller granular cell neurons below highlighting the variation of neuronal size in the nervous system.

The cerebellum, like the cerebrum, contains subcortical white matter in the folia and large tracts of white matter forming the cerebellar peduncles.

Pituitary and Pineal Glands

The pituitary is a specialized organ involved in both secreting and storing hormones and is composed of an anterior lobe (adenohypophysis) and posterior lobe (neurohypophysis). The anterior pituitary embryologically arises from Rathke pouch and Rathke remnants can be seen as small ciliated columnar lined cysts. On hematoxylin and eosin stains, the anterior pituitary is composed of three basic cell types: acidophils, basophils, and chromophobes. These cells are arranged in acinar structures often with different cell types within a single acinus (Figure 1-8). Distribution of the cell types can vary by region of the gland.

The posterior pituitary arises from the floor of the diencephalon. Its histologic appearance is strikingly different from the anterior lobe due to its neuroectodermal origin. The posterior pituitary is composed of unmyelinated axons and specialized glial cells called pituicytes that have

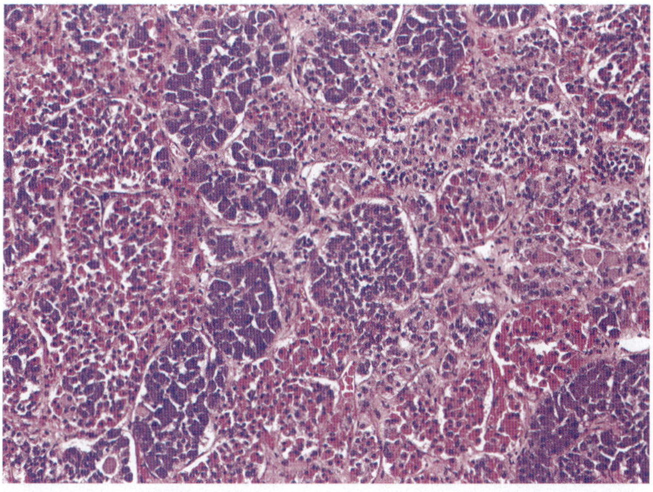

FIGURE 1-8: Anterior pituitary (adenohypophysis). The acinar architecture and different cell types are the hallmark of the anterior pituitary. Note the mixture of cell types even within individual acini.

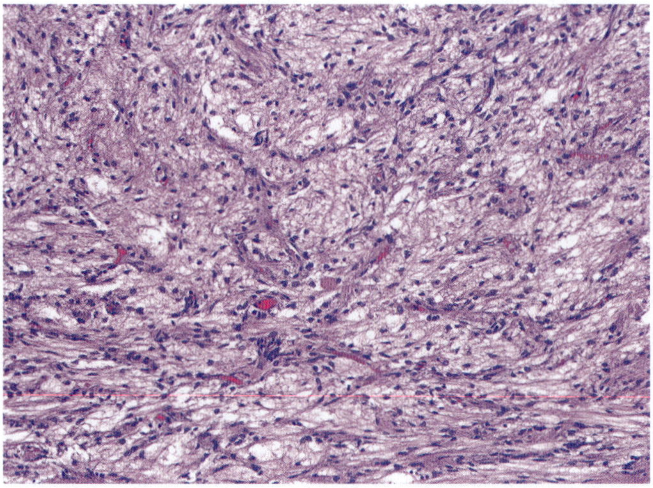

FIGURE 1-9: Posterior pituitary (neurohypophysis). Composed primarily of pituicytes (glia) and unmyelinated axons, the posterior pituitary can be mistaken for a glioma. Herring bodies (axonal swellings) like the ovoid eosinophilic structure in the center of the image can aid in identifying this as neurohypophysis.

ovoid nuclei and elongated processes. The posterior pituitary is responsible for storing and releasing hypothalamic hormones. This structure can be mistaken for a glioma if not familiar with its appearance. A helpful clue in identifying neurohypophysis is the presence of axonal swellings called Herring bodies (Figure 1-9).

The pineal gland is a rarely sampled region of the brain. It is a midline structure in close relationship to the tectum of the midbrain and posterior aspect of the third ventricle. The pineal gland is lobulated and composed of nests of neurosecretory cells called pineocytes surrounded by pineal astrocytes. Pineocytic rosettes, rings of nuclei around an acellular zone, are a feature of normal pineal gland as well as pineal parenchymal tumors. Calcifications (corpora arenacea) are a common finding in normal pineal gland, and their presence increases with age (Figure 1-10). Another normal histologic finding that increases with age is the presence of pineal cysts. The cysts are typically benign but can be large with surrounding gliosis.

This chapter is a brief look at the normal histology of the central nervous system to help familiarize readers with the various cell types of the neoplastic processes reviewed in this book. Several selected readings are referenced below for those interested in more in-depth discussion. Enjoy.

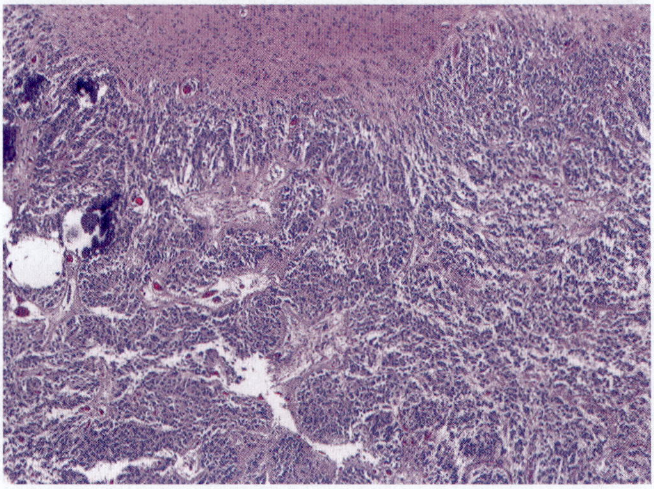

FIGURE 1-10: Pineal gland. The pineal gland is composed of lobules of small neurosecretory cells encompassed by astrocytes. Small neurocytic rosettes can be seen within some of the lobules. Calcifications can be present and increase with age. The *top* of the image shows the gliotic wall of an adjacent pineal cyst.

Suggested Readings

Fuller GN, Burger PC. Central nervous system. In: Mills SE, ed. *Histology for Pathologists*. 4th ed. Philadelphia, PA: Wolters Kluwer Health/Lippincott Williams & Wilkins; 2012:295–342.

Burger PC, Scheithauer BW. *Tumors of the Central Nervous System*. 4th series, AFIP Fascicle 7. Washington, DC: American Registry of Pathology (ARP) Press; 2007:5–31. Chapter 2.

Lopes MBS, Pernicone PJ, Scheithauer BW, et al. Pituitary and sellar region. In: Mills SE, ed. *Histology for Pathologists*. 4th ed. Philadelphia, PA: Wolters Kluwer Health/Lippincott Williams & Wilkins; 2012:343–374.

Carpenter MB. *Core Text of Neuroanatomy*. 3rd ed. Baltimore, MD: Williams & Wilkins; 1985.

Crosby EC; National Institute on Drug Abuse, Addiction Research Center (U.S.). *Correlative Anatomy of the Nervous System*. New York: MacMillan; 1962.

Haines DE. *Neuroanatomy: An Atlas of Structures, Sections, and Systems*. 7th ed. Philadelphia, PA: Wolters Kluwer Health/Lippincott Williams & Wilkins; 2008.

Mai JK, Paxinos G. *The Human Nervous System*. 3rd ed. Amsterdam, The Netherlands/Boston, MA: Elsevier Academic Press; 2012.

SECTION

II

Histopathology

- CHAPTER 2: Diffuse (Infiltrating) Gliomas
- CHAPTER 3: Circumscribed Astrocytomas (Pilocytic Astrocytoma, Pilomyxoid Astrocytoma, Pleomorphic Xanthoastrocytoma, and Subependymal Giant Cell Astrocytoma)
- CHAPTER 4: Ependymomas
- CHAPTER 5: Other Neuroepithelial Tumors (Chordoid Glioma, Astroblastoma, Angiocentric Glioma)
- CHAPTER 6: Neuronal/Mixed Glioneuronal Tumors
- CHAPTER 7: Embryonal Tumors
- CHAPTER 8: Choroid Plexus Tumors (Choroid Plexus Papilloma, Atypical Choroid Plexus Papilloma, Choroid Plexus Carcinoma, Xanthogranuloma of the Choroid Plexus, and Metastasis)
- CHAPTER 9: Pineal Region Tumors
- CHAPTER 10: Sellar and Suprasellar Region Tumors
- CHAPTER 11: Meningeal Tumors
- CHAPTER 12: Hereditary Syndromes
- CHAPTER 13: Tumors of Cranial and Peripheral Nerves and Other Tumors
- CHAPTER 14: Hematolymphoid and Histiocytic Tumors
- CHAPTER 15: Central Nervous System Metastasis

Diffuse (Infiltrating) Gliomas

2

- Matthew Daniel Cykowski
- Andreana Rivera
- Hidehiro Takei

INTRODUCTION

This chapter provides an overview of the clinical, radiologic, pathologic, and molecular features of the diffuse (infiltrating) gliomas. The two major aims of the chapter are to provide an introduction to key concepts involved in the diagnosis of these tumors and to describe the implications of these diagnoses for the patient.

The diffuse gliomas discussed in this chapter represent a heterogeneous group of glial neoplasms with diverse molecular underpinnings and prognostic associations. Despite their unique identifying features, two important features unite these neoplasms: their infiltration of normal brain and their status as malignant tumors. The first of these points is implicit in the title of this chapter though it bears repeating. Diffuse gliomas *invade* into normal brain structures in both subtle ways and in forms that render the native architecture unrecognizable. In this way, diffuse gliomas differ from *circumscribed* gliomas. The circumscribed gliomas include tumors like pleomorphic xanthoastrocytoma, ependymoma, pilocytic astrocytoma, and angiocentric glioma. These circumscribed tumors may have focally infiltrative borders but, unlike the infiltrating gliomas, do not typically recur after gross total resection. The second commonality in each of the entities discussed is that these tumors are all *malignant*. In other words, any diffuse glioma, regardless of tumor grade, is a pathologic diagnosis associated with significant morbidity and mortality. For the diagnosis of glioblastoma (GBM), or any of its histologic variants, this point is self-evident. However, this principle may be less evident for a diagnosis of oligodendroglioma, World Health Organization (WHO) grade II, with codeletion of chromosome arms 1p and 19q. Such tumors may appear as nonenhancing masses in young patients, show no evident mitotic activity, necrosis, or microvascular proliferation, and have a very low Ki-67 proliferation index (<2%). For these tumors, the patient may have a 10-year interval or more before the tumor undergoes anaplastic progression to WHO grade III anaplastic oligodendroglioma. In many cases, prior to this histologic progression, these patients may have received chemotherapy and/or radiation therapy, which are associated with their own toxicities. Anaplastic progression eventually ensues, heralded by a large and enhancing focus of tumor at the site of prior low-grade tumor. With radiation therapy and chemotherapy, including procarbazine, lomustine, and vincristine (PCV) or temozolomide, median survival in 1p/19q codeleted *anaplastic* oligodendroglioma is relatively favorable among high-grade gliomas with a median survival exceeding 8 years.[1] Even in this "best case" scenario, however, these tumors will result in the death of most patients.

The diffuse gliomas reviewed in this chapter may have histologic grades of II, III, or IV, according to the 2007 WHO classification system for central nervous system (CNS) tumors.[2] These entities include diffuse astrocytoma, WHO grade II; anaplastic astrocytoma, WHO grade III; glioblastoma, WHO grade IV; oligodendroglioma, WHO grade II; and anaplastic oligodendroglioma, WHO grade III, all of which are discussed here. In addition, diffuse gliomas recognized in the WHO include oligoastrocytoma, WHO grade II, and anaplastic oligoastrocytoma, WHO grade III.

The concept of mixed gliomas is only briefly covered here as it is currently unclear as to whether these mixed gliomas have a definitive molecular "signature." This chapter also covers gemistocytic astrocytoma (under the category of diffuse astrocytoma) and gliomatosis cerebri (GC).

OLIGODENDROGLIOMA AND ANAPLASTIC OLIGODENDROGLIOMA

Oligodendroglioma is the prototypical infiltrating glioma, often demonstrating many of the "secondary structures" that help to define diffuse gliomas architecturally. As originally defined, the "secondary structures" assumed the "primary" structures were the cytologic and histogenetic classification system of Bailey and Cushing proposed in 1926.[3] These "secondary structures" represented the interaction of tumor cells with native brain architecture to generate *perineural* (now "perineuronal") and *surface* (now "subpial") growth in the cortex, perivascular growth, and perifascicular or intrafascicular growth between or within nerve bundles, respectively.[3] Preferential intracortical or white matter growth constitute two additional "structures." Scherer noted that the combination of perineuronal, perivascular, and subpial growth was the most common pattern among these.[3]

Oligodendroglioma also provides one of the best examples in neuropathology of how genetic analyses of brain tumors provide diagnostic, prognostic, and predictive information. This defining molecular feature of these tumors is the allelic loss of genetic material on chromosomes 1p and 19q. This genetic loss is the result of an unbalanced translocation [der(1;19)(p10;q10)] in which only the reciprocal derivative chromosome is retained (with 1q and 19p).[4] The combined allelic losses at 1p and 19q are associated with mutations in *CIC* (on 19q) and *FUBP1* (on 1p). Oligodendrogliomas may therefore arise via a loss-of-heterozygosity mechanism with an alteration in the residual *CIC* and *FUBP1* genes, which act as possible tumor suppressors.[5] 1p/19q codeletion also commonly occurs with mutations in isocitrate dehydrogenase (IDH) 1 or 2 (*IDH1/IDH2*).[6] These changes are often mutually exclusive with *TP53* mutations associated with low-grade diffuse astrocytoma and predict improved survival as well as improved response to PCV chemotherapy.[7]

Clinical and Radiologic Features

Oligodendrogliomas most often occur in middle-aged patients with a peak incidence between 40 and 45 years of age.[8] Presentations in children and teenagers are very uncommon. These childhood tumors also lack 1p/19q codeletion in many cases, suggesting they may not be equivalent to their adult counterparts.[4] Clinical presentations may include headache, new-onset seizures, and changes in mental status. None of the well-characterized familial tumor syndromes appear to predispose to this tumor type, possibly because the tumorigenic alterations are so unique.

On magnetic resonance imaging (MRI), WHO grade II oligodendroglioma is often a superficially located, *nonenhancing* tumor involving the subcortical white matter and cortex. There is often significant peritumoral edema, reflected by hyperintensity on T2/fluid-attenuated inversion recovery (T2/FLAIR) MRI sequences (see Figure 2-1). There are some WHO grade II tumors that demonstrate vague, faint enhancement following gadolinium administration. However, this finding is not common, and ring-like enhancement is much more characteristic of WHO grade III anaplastic oligodendroglioma.[9] Solid, nodular enhancement on gadolinium-administered T1-weighted MRI is also strongly suggestive of a WHO grade III tumor. The histologic correlate of this enhancement on preoperative MRI is microvascular proliferation, which allow gadolinium uptake in the region of tumor. Currently, however, the diagnosis of anaplastic progression to WHO grade III anaplastic oligodendroglioma requires the presence of tissue demonstrating microvascular proliferation, brisk mitotic activity, and/or necrosis.

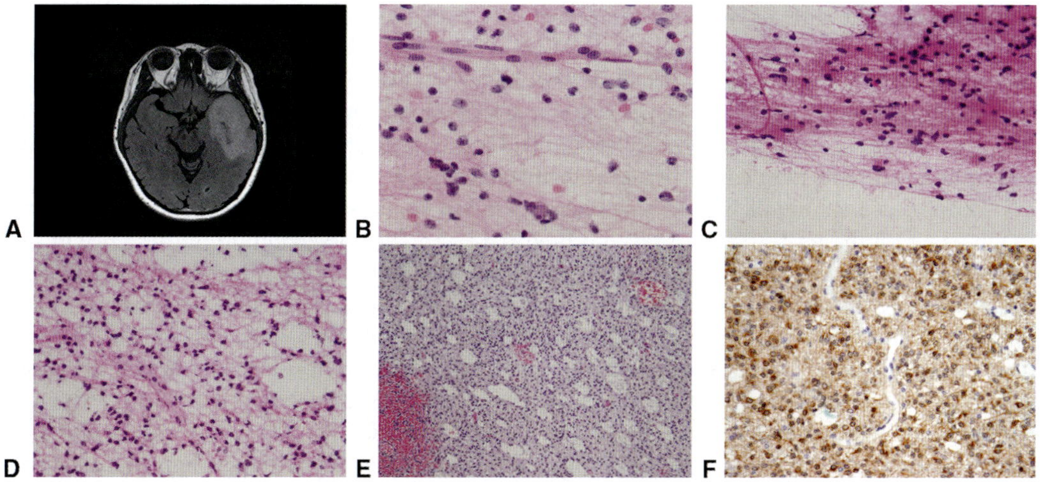

FIGURE 2-1: Oligodendroglioma. MRI studies of WHO grade II oligodendroglioma typically demonstrate a nonenhancing, T2/FLAIR hyperintense mass lesion in the cerebrum (**A**). Note that the T2/FLAIR hyperintensity extends to the pial surface of the left temporal lobe, which is something not seen in vasogenic edema. Characteristic monomorphic cytologic features of oligodendroglioma replete with thin-walled capillaries and perineuronal satellitosis (*bottom* and *center of image*) (**B, C**). Frozen section of oligodendroglioma can introduce misleading nuclear pleomorphism (**D**) such that "diffuse glioma, favor low grade" is a sufficient diagnosis for the frozen section shown. Low-power appearance of oligodendroglioma is critical to the diagnosis (**E**). Note the hemorrhage (*lower left corner*), microcysts, and monomorphism of the lesion. The characteristic molecular features are codeletion of 1p and 19q, as well as *IDH1* or *IDH2* mutation. Here, cells demonstrate granular, cytoplasmic staining for IDH1 R132H mutant protein (**F**) (note the endothelial cells serve as an internal negative control).

Histologic and Immunohistochemical Features

The most characteristic aspect of oligodendroglioma is the cytologic appearance (see Figure 2-1). On cytologic preparations (squash/smear, touch, or drag preparations), these tumor cells are monotonous, having a round nucleus with crisp nuclear membranes, finely granular chromatin, and inconspicuous or small nucleoli. As the name of the tumor implies, cells have few dendritic processes[10] and lack the elongate, fibrillary processes of astrocytic or ependymal tumors. Smear preparations may also contain slightly basophilic mucoid material, which correlates to the mucin-filled microcysts seen on frozen and permanent sections.

Another helpful feature of oligodendroglioma is that tumor cells often disperse in a single-cell pattern on cytologic preparations. This feature is not unique to oligodendroglioma and is also seen in metastatic melanoma and primary CNS lymphoma (PCNSL). "Minigemistocytes" are also commonly seen on intraoperative cytologic preparations of oligodendroglial tumors.[11] These cells have eccentrically located nuclei and small bellies of densely eosinophilic cytoplasm. Unlike larger gemistocytes (described further under "Gemistocytic Astrocytoma" below), minigemistocytes have nuclei that resemble classic oligodendroglial tumor cells. Additional cytologic clues to the diagnosis include the presence of thin-walled capillaries and calcifications. If mitoses are easily noted on cytologic preparations of an otherwise conventional-appearing oligodendroglioma, this may be a hint to look carefully for evidence of histologic anaplasia on permanent sections.

Frozen section of oligodendroglioma brings together all of these features (cortical infiltration, microcysts, calcifications) except for perhaps the most critical one—cellular monomorphism. The process of tissue freezing often significantly alters the cytologic appearance on frozen section. As a result, tumor cells become angulated and hyperchromatic and lose their characteristic monomorphism. Further, these cells lack perinuclear halos since this is an artifact that requires fixation in formalin in order to be manifest. As a result, the error of classifying these tumors intraoperative as astrocytoma accounts for about one-fifth of frozen/permanent section discrepancies in CNS tumors.[12] This emphasizes the importance of quality cytologic preparations and caution at the time of frozen section diagnosis. A diagnosis of these tumors as "glioma" or "diffuse glioma" is sufficient. Even "diffuse glioma, favor low grade" is acceptable in the absence of worrisome histologic features or definitive enhancement on preoperative MRI. This information is accurate enough to allow the neurosurgeon to complete their procedure appropriately. For low-grade gliomas, once diagnosed as such, the surgical approach is more likely to depend on anatomic constraints than concerns about histogenesis.

Permanent sections of "classic" oligodendroglioma demonstrate characteristic features that in tandem with the nuclear monotony and predict 1p and 19q codeletion on fluorescence in situ hybridization (FISH) in up to 86% of tumors.[4] The best recognized of these features are perinuclear halos, resulting from shrinkage of cell cytoplasm in the interval between tissue devitalization and formalin fixation. As a result, oligodendrogliomas without a substantial delay to fixation may not have these artifactual halos. Likewise, when present, this feature is nonspecific and may also been seen in tumors as varied as dysembryoplastic neuroepithelial tumor (DNET), central and extraventricular neurocytoma, diffuse astrocytoma, and PCNSL. Rare pilocytic astrocytomas may also have extensive oligodendroglial-like cytomorphology, which raises the differential of oligodendroglioma. Nuclear features of oligodendroglioma on cytologic preparations in tandem with architectural proof of parenchymal infiltration are therefore critical in recognizing the entity. Equally well recognized in oligodendroglioma is the presence of a delicate capillary network. This fine capillary network insinuates between nests of oligodendroglial tumor cells, which at low-power magnification gives the tumor a regular and geometric arrangement likened to chicken wire. Other salient architectural features, best identified on low-power examination, include a nodular arrangement of tumor cells, infiltration of the cortex with perineuronal satellitosis and subpial spread, and mucoid-filled microcysts. Again, none of these alterations is specific to oligodendroglioma. When these architectural features are present in tandem with the appropriate cytologic features, they are usually diagnostic.

Minigemistocytes may be very prominent on permanent sections of oligodendroglioma and perhaps a predominant feature. Their bellies of eosinophilic cytoplasm are strongly positive on GFAP, which corresponds to abundant intracytoplasmic intermediate filament.[8] Minigemistocytes may be confused and overlap with conventional gemistocytes of diffuse and gemistocytic astrocytomas (also seen in GBM). The main differentiating feature is that gemistocytes have more cytoplasmic volume and larger nuclei, which are hyperchromatic and irregular.

Some "astrocytic"-appearing cells may be present in tumors with 1p/19q codeletion. If present in sufficient numbers, these cells raise the possibility of a mixed glioma or oligoastrocytoma. Currently, however, the major determinants of prognosis and treatment are histologic grade and genetic features. It may not be critical to distinguish WHO grade II oligodendroglioma with 1p/19q codeletion from WHO grade II oligoastrocytoma with 1p/19q codeletion. Grade for grade, the categorizations that matter most at this time are (a) 1p/19q codeletion, IDH mutated, (b) 1p/19q intact, IDH mutated, and (c) 1p/19q intact, IDH wild type.[13] This raises the question as to whether the concept of "mixed" glioma will be supported in future editions of the WHO Classification of Tumors of the CNS. A safe (and reproducible) approach is to integrate molecular findings into the final diagnosis for these most challenging cases. This presumes that 1p/19q codeletion is the molecular hallmark of the "oligodendroglial" phenotype.[7] That is, tumors with a mixed population of oligodendroglial-appearing and astrocytic-appearing tumor cells, but with 1p/19 codeletion, *IDH1* mutation, and no histologic features of anaplasia, are categorized as oligodendroglioma, WHO grade II. Likewise, similar tumors with a "mixed glioma" or indeterminate phenotype, but without 1p and 19q codeletion, are categorized as diffuse astrocytoma, WHO grade II, or perhaps diffuse glioma, WHO grade II. The next WHO classification of central nervous system tumors is anticipated to provide further clarification as to the histologic and molecular bases (or lack thereof) for the diagnosis of "mixed glioma."

Grading

The principle of grading in oligodendroglioma is that the prototypical tumor described above is a WHO grade II malignancy and that anaplastic progression is possible to WHO grade III but no further. In principle, WHO grade II oligodendroglioma *does not progress to a secondary*

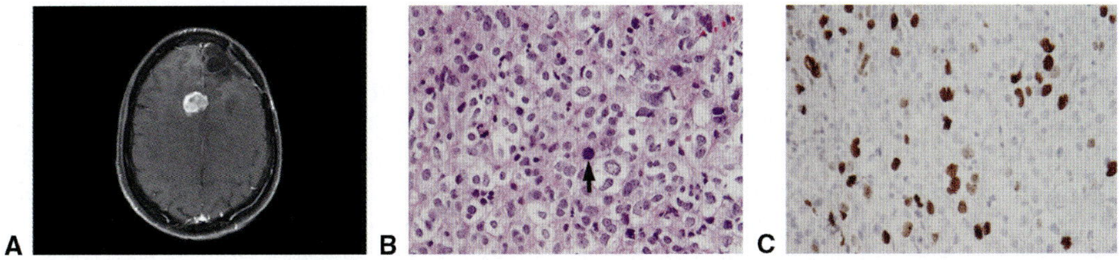

FIGURE 2-2: Anaplastic oligodendroglioma. Anaplastic progression in oligodendroglioma characteristically presents with nodular and solid enhancement on MRI, which is shown in the right frontal/cingulate region of this patient (**A**). Note the surgical resection site in the left frontal lobe as a hypointense, nonenhancing cavity. As at any body site, this prior specimen should be reviewed if available. In this patient, it demonstrated WHO grade II oligodendroglioma. Characteristics of anaplastic transformation in these tumors are increased cellularity, nuclear pleomorphism, and mitotic activity (*arrow*), as well as microvascular proliferation and/or necrosis (not shown) (**B**). The Ki-67 labeling index is correspondingly elevated in this patient (**C**).

glioblastoma, WHO grade IV, with oligodendroglial features, or "GBM-O." GBM-O is a term created for GBMs in relatively young patients (median age of 50 years), typically arising as a secondary GBM that has progressed from a lower-grade glioma that often has p53 overexpression, *IDH1* mutation, and in one-third, 1p/19q codeletion.[14] Presumably, these tumors represent a form of WHO grade IV oligoastrocytoma. Survival analyses of "GBM-O" with *IDH1* mutations and 1p/19q codeletion raises the question as to whether some or all of these represent anaplastic oligodendroglioma, WHO grade III. Not surprisingly then, the concept of GBM-O remains controversial.[15]

Anaplastic oligodendroglioma, WHO grade III, is more widely accepted. The reproducible histologic determinants for a WHO grade III designation are high cellularity, mitotic activity (see Figure 2-2), endothelial hypertrophy and endothelial proliferation, and necrosis.[16] Small nodules of hypercellularity are common in these tumors and may be a clue at low power. The significant vascular changes are usually apparent and are defined as plump, single-layered endothelium and plump vessel walls (endothelial hypertrophy) versus two or more endothelial cell layers (endothelial proliferation)—both appear to be significant grading determinants in oligodendroglioma.[16] Regarding mitotic activity, as with other gliomas (e.g., ependymomas and astrocytomas), there is not a strict threshold for what level of proliferative activity defines anaplasia in this setting. Ki-67 (MIB-1) labeling indices do correlate with grade and outcome, with 5-year survival rates of 35%, 30%, and 14% in oligodendrogliomas with labeling indices of less than 10%, 10% to 20%, and greater than 20%, respectively.[17] In the same study, survival in patients with 1 to 4 mitoses per 10 high-power fields and greater than or equal to 5 per 10 high-power fields did not significantly differ.[17]

Further, there is not a requirement that mitotic activity, microvascular proliferation, and necrosis all come together in one tumor to render a diagnosis of anaplastic oligodendroglioma. For example, a moderately hypercellular oligodendroglioma with 1p/19q codeletion and brisk mitotic activity (e.g., 7 per 10 high-power fields) may qualify for anaplastic oligodendroglioma, WHO grade III, even without microvascular proliferation or necrosis (see Figure 2-2). Also, significant, solid or ring-like contrast enhancement on T1-weighted MRI with gadolinium requires careful scrutiny of tissue sections for microvascular proliferation.

Molecular Features and Prognosis

The most important determinants of behavior and treatment that pathologic examination can provide are the histologic grade, 1p/19q codeletion status, *IDH1/IDH2* mutation status, and O^6-methyl-guanine-DNA methyltransferase (*MGMT*) promoter methylation status. These three molecular alterations are strongly associated with 1p/19q codeletion, *IDH1/IDH2* mutation, and a methylated *MGMT* promoter all conferring survival benefit.[7] Some authors go so far as to state that essentially all codeleted tumors harbor an *IDH1* or *IDH2* mutation. Other studies have found rare examples of 1p/19q codeleted oligodendrogliomas without *IDH1/IDH2* mutations on sensitive pyrosequencing assays, however.[6]

For 1p/19q, the presence of *codeletion* is critical and is not equivalent to partial loss (e.g., loss of 1p with intact 19q and vice versa), which may be seen in other tumors, such as "GBM-O."[14] Patients with 1p deleted/19q intact tumors may still have a better response to PCV therapy than 1p/19q intact patients,[18] although overall survival is still worse than in codeleted tumors. Whole arm codeletion is also not equivalent to interstitial or terminal deletions on 1p and 19q. These types of deletions may also be seen even in non-oligodendroglial tumors.[4]

The presence of codeletion of 1p and 19q in oligodendroglioma is associated with a longer median survival and improved response to PCV chemotherapy.[7] This data also allows neurooncologists to put off radiation therapy to later in the patient's course in favor of early use of PCV or temozolomide. This delays the possibility of radiation-associated toxicity in patients who will have a relatively long survival among the diffuse glioma groups.[18]

Differential Diagnosis

The differential diagnosis with oligodendroglioma includes a variety of "clear cell" tumors, including central neurocytoma, extraventricular neurocytoma, DNET, and clear cell ependymoma. The list also includes infiltrating tumors with prominent perinuclear clearing (due to delay in formalin fixation), which can include diffuse astrocytoma and PCNSL. Pilocytic astrocytomas may also contain focal or extensive oligodendroglial-like cytomorphology. In the majority of cases, histologic findings suggestive of pilocytic astrocytoma will be present, including "dense" fascicular areas, Rosenthal fibers and eosinophilic granular bodies, and glomeruloid endothelial hyperplasia. In those cases where these features are not present, particularly within the posterior fossa, it is reasonable to perform FISH testing for *BRAF-KIAA1549* fusion (diagnostic of pilocytic astrocytoma), as well as 1p and 19q status.

Neurocytoma, whether extraventricular or central, consists of cells with neurocytic (not glial) differentiation. Therefore, the first clue in separating these tumors from oligodendroglioma comes from cytologic and frozen section preparations. Neurocytoma tumor cells have round nuclei and discrete nucleoli, are set in fine neuropil matrix, and may demonstrate ganglion cell differentiation.[19] On permanent sections, neurocytomas may strongly resemble oligodendroglioma, with clear cells, a fine capillary network, and even calcifications. Unlike oligodendroglioma, however, neurocytomas are *not* infiltrative tumors, and therefore infiltration into brain parenchyma calls this diagnosis into question. On immunohistochemical studies, neurocytomas characteristically demonstrate synaptophysin expression and have Ki-67 proliferation indices that are very low (typically <2%). On radiologic studies, an important distinction is that neurocytomas often have some degree of postcontrast enhancement, a finding that is uncommon in WHO grade II oligodendroglioma.

DNET is an important entity in this differential, and in fact, many of these tumors were recognized as oligodendrogliomas prior to their original description.[20] Typically, these are cortically based neoplasms in the mesial temporal lobes of young patients with a history of intractable seizures. The imaging features are distinctive and demonstrate a nonenhancing, nodular and cortically based neoplasm that is T2/FLAIR hyperintense. Cytologically, they consist of oligodendroglial-like cells (OLCs), and satellitosis around neurons is common. Permanent sections characteristically demonstrate columns of OLCs aligning about thin capillaries and axons. Like oligodendrogliomas, these tumors may have mucin-filled microcysts within which are "floating" neurons (this feature is not specific to DNET, nor may it be seen in all DNETs). Immunohistochemical studies demonstrate variable positivity for markers of neuronal lineage, including synaptophysin, CD34, and calbindin.[21] Neu-N and GFAP are less likely to be positive in these tumor cells. Recent studies have identified *BRAF* V600E mutant protein in DNET (approximately one-third of tumors) although this needs further study.[22] FISH testing for 1p19q codeletion and/or testing for *IDH1* and *IDH2* mutations are helpful in cases that raise the differential diagnosis of glioma versus DNET and lack prototypical clinical, radiologic, and histologic features of DNET.

Clear cell ependymoma typically arises as a cerebral hemispheric mass in a patient younger than the prototypical oligodendroglioma patient. On MRI, these tumors also demonstrate post-contrast enhancement. Cytologically, these tumors have "ependymal" nuclear features, which consist of hyperchromatic nuclei with granular chromatin and inconspicuous nucleoli and aggregation of tumor cells about blood vessels in smear preparations. On permanent sections, these tumors may have an organoid arrangement (much like a neuroendocrine tumor), as well as brisk mitotic activity, necrosis, and microvascular proliferation. At least focal perivascular rosettes are present in these tumors, and epithelial membrane antigen and GFAP reactivity are common.[23] Unlike diffuse gliomas, these tumors are circumscribed. Even in these noninfiltrative tumors, however, the Ki-67 proliferation index may be very high. These are aggressive tumors and may recur with frank anaplastic and/or small blue cell tumor histologic features.

Diffuse astrocytoma and PCNSL both can mimic infiltrating oligodendrogliomas due to the extent of perinuclear clearing. PCNSL, however, has cytologic features characteristic of high-grade B-cell lymphoma, including irregular nuclear contours and prominent nucleoli in many cases, which are not characteristic of oligodendroglioma. Mitotic figures and apoptotic bodies, as well as angiocentric growth, are also characteristic. Radiologically, these are solidly enhancing tumors, often multifocal and in a periventricular position, which further helps to distinguish them. A panel of lymphoid markers, including CD20 and CD79a, would help to identify difficult cases resembling high-grade infiltrating glioma, including anaplastic oligodendroglioma. Diffuse astrocytomas, in contrast, can look convincingly oligodendroglial. For this reason, some laboratories run 1p19q FISH analyses on all low-grade gliomas, regardless of their cytologic phenotype.

DIFFUSE ASTROCYTOMA AND ANAPLASTIC ASTROCYTOMA

Diffuse astrocytomas, like oligodendroglioma, are *malignant* diffuse gliomas that invade brain parenchyma. Traditionally, these tumors have an astrocytic phenotype, which is defined cytologically. The secondary structures seen in oligodendroglioma as previously discussed may be seen in the entire spectrum of astrocytomas, including WHO grade IV GBM. Perinuclear halos may also be present to a variable extent in diffuse astrocytomas, and there are tumors with unequivocal, mixed cytologic features. As discussed above, while H&E-based classification schemes are useful, the molecular features and grade of these tumors are of most relevance to determine prognosis and treatment. In this context, the molecular signature of oligodendroglioma is 1p/19q codeletion (except in children). Whether tumors without this molecular signature are called "oligoastrocytoma" or "astrocytoma" is probably less relevant.[7]

Clinical and Radiologic Features

Diffuse astrocytoma is a tumor of younger adults (peak incidence of 30 to 40 years), whereas anaplastic astrocytoma is a tumor of middle-aged adults (40 to 50 years).[24,25] The clinical presentations of oligodendroglioma (see preceding section) and astrocytoma overlap significantly with seizures being common to both.

Radiologically, WHO grade II diffuse astrocytomas often appear as a nonenhancing, T2/FLAIR hyperintense tumor. Often, the abnormal T2/FLAIR signal frequently extends into the cortex with signal changes extending up through the cortex and to the pial surface (see Figure 2-3). This pattern contrasts with vasogenic edema, the hyperintense T2 signal of which stops abruptly at the junction of cortical and subcortical white matter. Peritumoral or intratumoral contrast enhancement in this radiologic setting should raise the possibility of anaplastic astrocytoma, WHO grade III, or glioblastoma, WHO grade IV.

Anaplastic astrocytoma also presents as a T2/FLAIR hyperintensity with no contrast enhancement (or faint enhancement at most). Undersampled GBMs, with ring-like enhancement and necrosis radiologically, may appear to be anaplastic astrocytomas histologically. A possible solution to these discrepant radiologic and pathologic features is to issue a diagnosis of "diffuse glioma, minimum WHO grade III." An appropriate comment can be made regarding the absence of GBM histology.

Histologic and Immunohistochemical Features

The architectural features described previously for oligodendroglioma (parenchymal/cortical infiltration, microcyst formation, and microcalcifications) all can apply in diffuse astrocytoma. On cytologic preparations, however, the nuclei of these cells are typically larger than oligodendroglioma cells or normal glia. These cells are also hyperchromatic, lack the discrete and small nucleoli of oligodendroglioma, and frequently have irregular nuclear membranes. Astrocytic tumor cells also contain fibrillary cytoplasmic processes although cytologic preparations can reveal "naked" nuclei with the aforementioned nuclear features and no processes. Minigemistocytes and gemistocytes can also be identified on cytologic preparations. A background of necrotic debris or multilayered vessels with a haphazard arrangement of endothelial cells, in tandem with astrocytic cytology, usually excludes diffuse or anaplastic astrocytoma and indicates GBM.[11] Frozen sections of diffuse astrocytomas demonstrate an infiltrating astrocytic tumor with microcysts and infiltration of native neuropil and, often, cortex.

On permanent sections, an important feature of WHO grade II diffuse astrocytoma is that the tumor cells can be quite pleomorphic and there may be moderately hypercellular foci (see Figure 2-3). In a diffuse astrocytoma without mitotic activity, necrosis, or microvascular proliferation, these worrisome features do not alter the grade. Unlike conventional oligodendrogliomas, diffuse astrocytomas typically demonstrate diffuse, strong GFAP immunoreactivity on immunostains. This reflects the abundant intermediate (glial) filaments in their cytoplasm and cytoplasmic processes. These tumors are also frequently positive for p53 protein. The p53 positivity in most cases reflects an increased half-life of mutant p53 protein and therefore a possible *TP53* mutation. This is especially true of cases with diffuse and strong immunoreactivity, which is not uncommon. However, this immunostain is not a proxy for an underlying *TP53* mutation, as some p53 protein expression can be present in glial tumors that lack a *TP53* mutation. Likewise, p53 protein expression may be absent in *TP53*-mutated tumors with proximal frameshift mutations resulting in a truncated protein.[26] In contrast, *strong, granular, and cytoplasmic immunoreactivity for IDH1 R132H mutant protein is thought to indicate an underlying mutation* in *IDH1*.

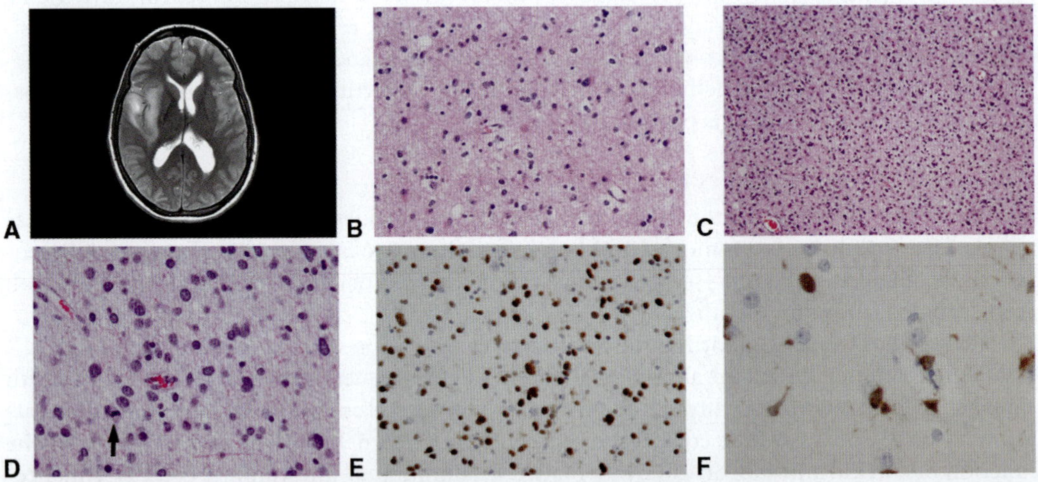

FIGURE 2-3: Diffuse Astrocytoma, WHO grade II and Anaplastic Astrocytoma, WHO grade III. As with oligodendroglioma (see MR image in Figure 2-1), this T2-weighted image of diffuse astrocytoma demonstrates hyperintense signal involving the anterior right temporal lobe and insula and extending to the pial surface (**A**). Low- and medium-power examination of diffuse (**B**) and anaplastic (**C**) oligodendroglioma shows pleomorphic, infiltrating tumor cells with rarefaction of overrun neuropil. Mitotic activity (*arrow*) and increased cellularity are present in anaplastic astrocytoma, but not microvascular proliferation or necrosis (**D**). Diffuse nuclear immunoreactivity for p53 is characteristic of diffuse astrocytomas (**E**). Immunostains for IDH1 R132H mutant protein often reveal infiltrating tumor cells that are not apparent on H&E stain (note the IDH1-negative neurons) (**F**).

Grading

For diffuse astrocytomas, *current WHO grading criteria do not formally utilize nuclear pleomorphism, cellularity, or MRI features to grade oligodendroglial or astrocytic tumors.* The determinants of grade are instead mitotic activity (for WHO grade III) and microvascular proliferation and/or necrosis (for WHO grade IV GBM). These other variables are likely to exert some subjective influence on the grading process, including features such as the density of tumor cells, cytologic atypia and multinucleation, the frequency of apoptotic bodies, and the presence of "faint" or "wispy" contrast enhancement on MRI.

The number of mitoses required to reach a WHO grade III designation is not specified by current (2007) WHO classification system, and this is not likely to change. A common sense approach is to allow for a diagnosis of WHO grade III when *even one mitotic figure is identified in a stereotactic biopsy. For larger excisions,* sometimes as large anterior temporal lobectomies exceeding 5 cm, *a single mitosis is insufficient* for an anaplastic designation. Some authors have proposed quantification of pHH3-stained mitotic figures per 1,000 cells, finding that ≥3 to 4 immunopositive mitoses/1,000 cells stratifies patients into groups corresponding closely to WHO grades II and III, respectively.[27] Ki-67 labeling indices likewise provide additional data to support these distinctions and have been shown to significantly and strongly correlate with mitotic count.[27] Still, the WHO does not provide formal cutoffs for these proliferative indices, and there is no single method suggested for their analysis.

Differential Diagnosis

Among the key differentials for diffuse and anaplastic astrocytoma are tumors of the oligodendroglioma group (discussed in the preceding section). An additional, critical differential diagnosis with low-grade diffuse astrocytoma is reactive gliosis. In reactive gliosis, brain parenchyma may be mildly hypercellular and nuclear atypia may be present. It is even possible to find rare mitoses although this is usually limited to reactive cells such as macrophages. Further, immunoreactivity in gliotic parenchyma with either p53 or Ki-67 is not indicative of tumor as staining for both may be present in nonneoplastic, reactive brain tissue.

An important tool in this regard is the demonstration of an *IDH* mutation by immunohistochemical or molecular methods. The most common *IDH1* mutation results from a guanine to adenine change at nucleotide position 395 of codon 132 in the *IDH1* gene, leading to replacement of arginine by histidine (R132H).[28] Expression of mutant IDH1 R132H protein, detected by immunohistochemical methods, is therefore diagnostic of glioma. Even when present in rare tumor cells (e.g., superficial biopsy largely consisting of cortex), this distinguishes glioma from gliosis.[29] In the event the immunostain is negative, sequence analysis can be performed for noncanonical *IDH1* and *IDH2* mutations (~10% of all IDH mutant tumors). Sensitive methods, such as pyrosequencing, can detect these noncanonical mutations at thresholds as low as 5% and 10% mutant DNA for *IDH1* and *IDH2*, respectively.[6]

GEMISTOCYTIC ASTROCYTOMA

Gemistocytic astrocytoma is a *variant* of WHO grade II diffuse astrocytoma, and therefore the clinical and radiologic presentation is similar. The histologic hallmark of this variant is the presence of "gemistocytes," which are tumor cells with eccentrically located nuclei and densely eosinophilic cytoplasm. Often, these cells are in a nonspecific, sheet-like arrangement and are accompanied by perivascular mononuclear inflammatory cells (see Figure 2-4). GFAP and vimentin immunostains demonstrate strong and diffuse staining of these tumor cells since their cytoplasmic bellies are filed with intermediate (glial) filaments. Current WHO criteria state that at least 20% of tumor cells should be gemistocytic to qualify for this designation.[25]

A well-known and challenging feature in the grading of gemistocytic astrocytoma is the discordance between proliferative activity and tumor behavior. Frequently, mitoses are difficult to identify,

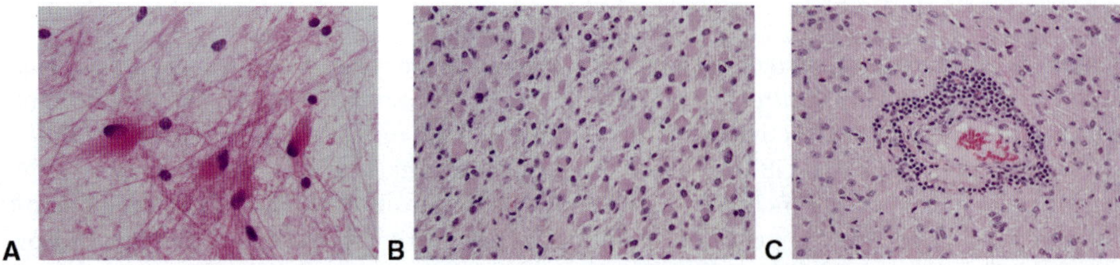

FIGURE 2-4: Gemistocytic astrocytoma. On cytologic preparations, these tumor cells have bellies of densely eosinophilic cytoplasm, eccentrically located and hyperchromatic nuclei, and fibrillary cytoplasmic processes. Note the presence of "naked tumor cell nuclei" as well, which often forms the proliferative component of these tumors (**A**). Characteristic gemistocytic cells on permanent section with perivascular mononuclear infiltrate (**B, C**).

and the Ki-67 labeling index may be low.[25] Strong, diffuse immunoreactivity for p53 is often present, consistent with an "astrocytic" phenotype. In spite of this, these lesions often behave aggressively, recurring as increasingly anaplastic tumors on their way to GBM. As such, any *bona fide* gemistocytic tumor with preoperative postcontrast enhancement on MRI should be treated with caution, and evidence of microvascular proliferation should be carefully sought. Further, high-power examination of "lower-grade" gemistocytic tumors often demonstrates scattered small, hyperchromatic, nongemistocytic cells, which may go unnoticed on initial examination. In recurrent tumors, these forms may come to predominate. As discussed under oligodendrogliomas, gemistocytes may be distinguished from "minigemistocytes" based on cell size and nuclear features. The latter cell type, also strongly GFAP positive, is more commonly encountered in oligodendroglioma and anaplastic oligodendroglioma than in astrocytoma and can be conspicuous in other glial tumors (e.g., ependymomas).

OLIGOASTROCYTOMA/"MIXED" GLIOMA

Tumors harboring both oligodendroglial and astrocytic cytologic features are not uncommon. This problem, including potential solutions that integrate molecular features into the final interpretation, is discussed in the preceding section on oligodendrogliomas. The chief issue with this category is that the definitions are solely histologic at this time. For that reason, some experts find the concept of mixed glioma/oligoastrocytoma to be a poorly reproducible diagnosis with no objective/molecular criteria available to support it.[7] As data from large-scale sequencing analyses of low-grade gliomas becomes available, such as that of The Cancer Genome Atlas Research Network,[30] the category of mixed glioma is likely to come under further scrutiny. In the next edition of the WHO classification of central nervous system tumors, it is not clear whether the diagnoses of oligoastrocytoma, anaplastic oligoastrocytoma, or GBM-O (essentially anaplastic oligoastrocytoma with necrosis) will continue to be supported.

For infiltrating gliomas with mixed oligodendroglial and astrocytic features, our understanding of histogenesis and tumorigenesis continues to evolve. At the time of this writing, neuropathology as a field is between a 2007 WHO edition that provides explicit descriptions of mixed gliomas and increasing evidence that these tumors lack a defining molecular signature. This does not mean that morphology is not relevant to tumor behavior (across identical grades and genotypes). It is also impossible to predict whether new discoveries will be made that prompt reconsideration of the concept of mixed gliomas. Until that time, a solution to this problem is to describe the presence of mixed oligodendroglial and astrocytic cytologic features in a comment while integrating tumor grade and molecular features to guide the final diagnosis.

GLIOBLASTOMA

Glioblastoma is a WHO grade IV diffuse *astrocytoma*, traditionally been divided into "primary" GBMs that arise *de novo* and "secondary" GBMs that arise from lower-grade diffuse astrocytomas. The historical term "glioblastoma multiforme," or "GBM," has been replaced in the most recent

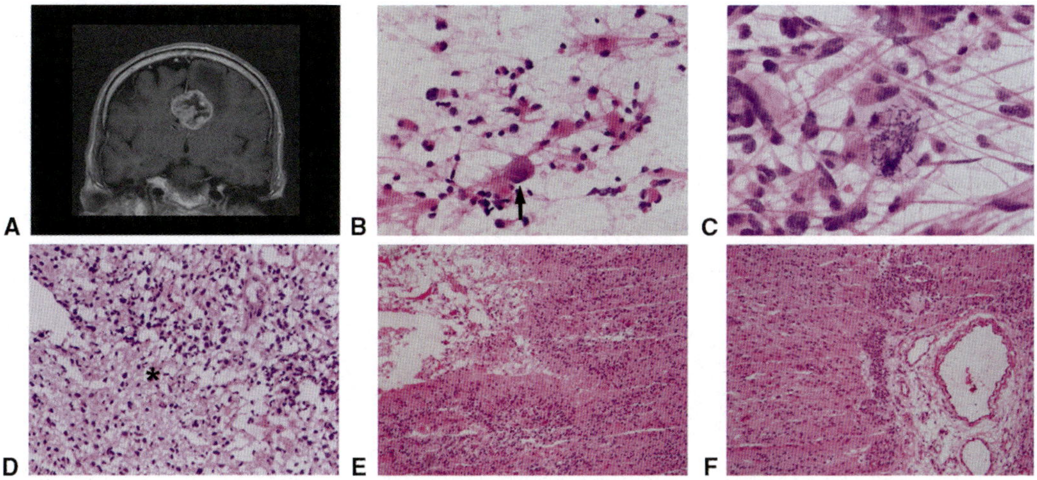

FIGURE 2-5: Glioblastoma, features at intraoperative consultation. The hallmark MRI feature of glioblastoma is ring or rim enhancement on T1-weighted MRI with gadolinium. Note the irregular contour of the enhancing rim and the significant mass effect exerted on adjacent brain (**A**). Cytologic preparations demonstrate pleomorphic tumor cells having fibrillary process, scattered gemistocytic cells, and neurons (*arrow*), indicative of cortical involvement and biopsy site (**B**). Granular mitoses are also common (**C**). Necrosis may be subtle on frozen section (*asterisk*, **D**). Apoptotic material within the focus is a helpful confirmatory feature as is "fracturing" of the tissue along the planes of necrosis (**E**). Microvascular proliferation (**F**), seen as a small arcade of vessels adjacent to ectatic and benign veins, is diagnostic of glioblastoma in the setting of an infiltrating glioma.

edition of the WHO classification scheme with the simpler term "glioblastoma," recognizing that some tumors are monomorphic (e.g., small cell GBM). Nonetheless, the abbreviation "GBM" is retained in current practice and is therefore used below.

Clinical and Radiologic Features

GBMs occur in older patients than diffuse and anaplastic astrocytoma with a mean age of approximately 61 years.[31] Unlike lower-grade gliomas, patients with GBM typically have a shorter course of symptoms. Radiologically, GBM demonstrates the signal abnormalities of lower-grade gliomas (T2/FLAIR hyperintensity, mass effect with midline shift and compression, edema) as well as avid contrast enhancement. This last feature is due to breakdown of the blood–brain barrier in foci of microvascular proliferation (see Figure 2-5). Other features that are seen include crossing of the midline/corpus callosum as a "butterfly" lesion, central necrosis, and cyst formation.[31] Less commonly, GBMs may occur as multiple distinct masses within the same or contralateral hemisphere, which typically raises the radiologic differential of metastases and PCNSL. Such tumors are referred to as *multicentric* when there is no evidence of infiltrating glioma between the enhancing foci (e.g., as evaluated on T2/FLAIR MRI). In contrast, *multifocal* GBMs can be demonstrated on MRI to be one continuous tumor cell population with multiple, separate foci of enhancement.

Histologic Features

GBM can show all of the histologic features discussed previously, including seemingly "indolent" features such as microcalcifications. The diagnostic features of GBM though are the presence of either coagulative tumor necrosis or microvascular proliferation in the setting of an infiltrating glial neoplasm (see Figure 2-5). Moderate to marked cytologic atypia and mitotic activity are also typically present, and these are evident on cytologic preparations. Corresponding elevations of the Ki-67 proliferation index are seen, usually to a degree far beyond diffuse and anaplastic astrocytomas. Importantly, a diagnosis of GBM can also be rendered in the setting of microvascular proliferation in an infiltrating glial neoplasm. On occasion, such tumors will have little evidence of mitotic activity on routine stains and/or not demonstrate evident tumor necrosis. A diagnosis of GBM is also possible when necrosis is present in an infiltrating

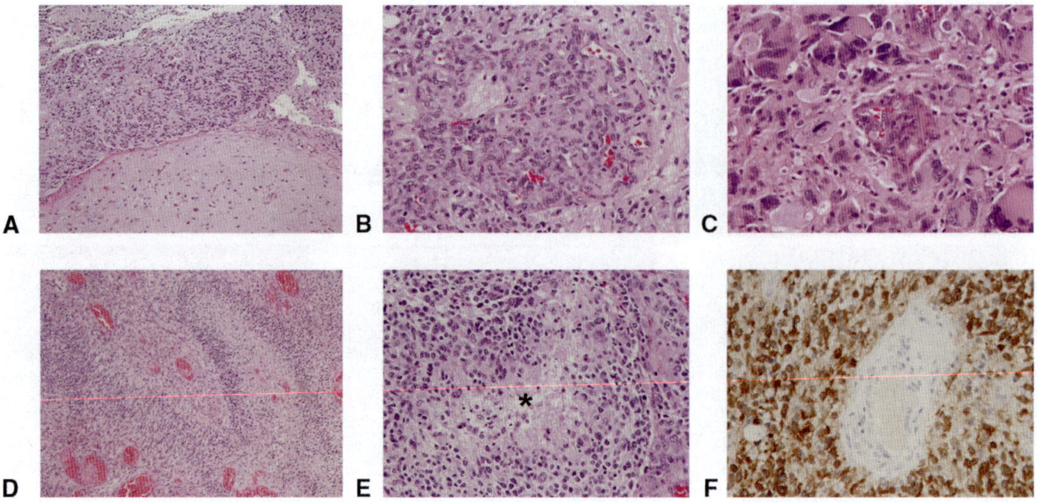

FIGURE 2-6: Glioblastoma, features on permanent section. Astrocytic tumors may demonstrate dense cortical infiltration and subpial spread, just as do oligodendrogliomas. Note the crest of a gyrus far less involved by tumor in the bottom half of the image (**A**). Microvascular proliferation is diagnostic and accounts for the avid enhancement of these tumors on MRI (**B,C**). Necrosis in any form is sufficient for diagnosis, although classic pseudopalisading necrosis is easily recognized (**D**). Fibrin thrombi are also common (**D,** *lower left*). The presence of apoptotic material (**E**, indicated by an asterisk), as seen on frozen section, is confirmatory that the tissue is necrotic. Positivity for IDH1 R132H mutant protein in this GBM serves two purposes: to indicate a prognostically favorable form of "secondary" GBM that has progressed from low-grade glioma and to highlight an immunonegative focus of microvascular proliferation (*center of image*) (**F**).

astrocytic neoplasm, even in the absence of microvascular proliferation (see Figure 2-6). Rarely, in GBMs with extensive gemistocytic cytologic features, it may be difficult to appreciate mitotic activity. Nonetheless, if microvascular proliferation and/or necrosis are present, the diagnosis of GBM is still appropriate. In both settings, however, it is important to ensure that the radiologic features are appropriate.

Histologic Types and Variants

GBMs may take on several unusual histologic appearances, often having one or more per individual tumor. *Whether there is any prognostic or therapeutic significance of subclassifying GBMs by histologic variant is not clear*, beyond the obvious point that patients with "secondary" GBMs having *IDH1* mutations and *MGMT* promoter methylation fare better.[32] Therefore, the major importance of discussing and recognizing these entities is to make sure these are distinguished from other histologically overlapping entities.

Giant cell GBM, formerly termed "monstrocellular sarcoma," is a specific clinical and pathologic variant. Clinically, patients are younger, having a median age of 41 years, and radiologically, these are *circumscribed* tumors in subcortical white matter.[31] Given their sharp radiologic borders, these may be mistaken as circumscribed gliomas, PCNSL, or metastases. On microscopic examination, the diagnostic feature is the presence of very large, mono- to multinucleated tumor cells with abundant eosinophilic cytoplasm (see Figure 2-7). These cells are GFAP positive and have a pericellular reticulin network. As with gemistocytic astrocytoma, there are often less conspicuous, small- to medium-sized tumor cells, which may be proliferative. Paradoxically, these tumors typically lack the *EGFR* amplification of "primary" GBM yet have *PTEN* mutations and *TP53* mutations (frequently, these tumors are p53 immunoreactive as well).[31]

Small cell GBM is another clinicopathologic variant of GBM that should be recognized as such. Radiologically, these tumors may be nonenhancing at presentation even though they behave like "primary" GBMs and rapidly progress to culminate in the patient's death (often <1 year after diagnosis).[33] Due to their hypercellularity, macroscopic examination of sectioned tumor may reveal fleshy pink-tan tissue that is more reminiscent of lymphoma than

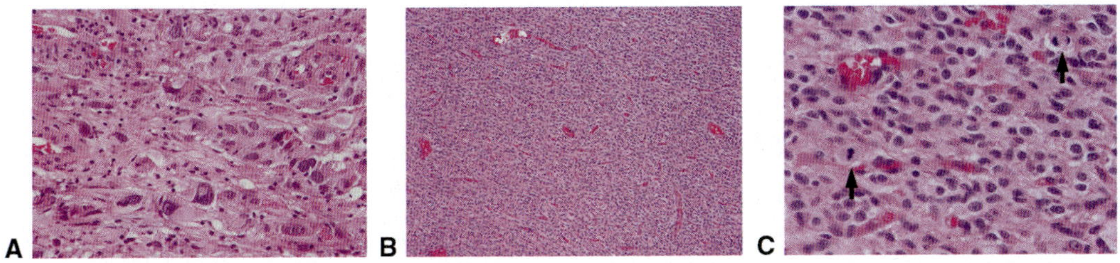

FIGURE 2-7: Glioblastoma, histologic variants. There are many histologic variants of GBM, which are important for their diagnostic if not prognostic importance. Giant cell glioblastoma may closely resemble pleomorphic xanthoastrocytoma, both in histologic appearance and in its typical presentation as a superficially located, enhancing tumor (**A**). Mitotic activity is the first clue to the correct diagnosis. Small cell glioblastoma may closely resemble oligodendroglioma on low-power examination (**B**). High-power examination, however, demonstrates brisk mitotic activity (*arrows*), which is an important clue (**C**). These tumors are negative for 1p/19q codeletion and often demonstrate features of other "primary" GBMs, such as *EGFR* amplification.

a glioma. This macroscopic feature contrasts with the homogeneous, mucoid tan cut surface of oligodendroglioma or the dense and rubbery cut surface of diffuse astrocytoma. Microscopic examination of these tumors at low power reveals a tumor that strongly resembles anaplastic oligodendroglioma, WHO grade III. However, on intermediate- and high-power microscopic examination, two features distinguish small cell GBM from oligodendroglioma. First, tumor cells in the former are ovoid to elongated with irregular nuclear contours, hyperchromatism, and more coarse chromatin than is expected for oligodendroglial tumor cells. Second, mitotic activity is markedly elevated, such that one or more mitotic figures per high-power microscopic field are not uncommon (see Figure 2-7). Therefore, extensive and conspicuous mitotic activity in what otherwise appears to be a conventional anaplastic oligodendroglioma should be among the first morphologic clues to the diagnosis of small cell GBM. Molecular confirmation of the diagnosis may come through demonstration of *EGFR* amplification (via fluorescence *in situ* hybridization or immunohistochemistry with monoclonal antibody 528), 10q (*PTEN*) deletions, and a lack of 1p/19q codeletion.[33]

Gliosarcoma, once thought to be a prognostically significant form of GBM, is now thought to have the same implications for patient outcome as conventional, "primary" GBM. These tumors are recognized by the combination of unequivocal features of GBM with a high-grade component having sarcomatoid differentiation. The soft tissue counterparts of the latter include leiomyosarcoma, fibrosarcoma, osteosarcoma, and chondrosarcoma. Current WHO criteria require that a biphasic appearance with both glial and mesenchymal differentiation be demonstrated. Typically, this is apparent on low-power H&E examination. The most efficient means to confirm the impression of glial/mesenchymal differentiation is via the application of GFAP and S100 protein immunostains, as well as reticulin special stain (see Figure 2-8). The glial component will be strongly positive on GFAP and S100 protein immunostains, whereas the mesenchymal component will be negative. Further, in the mesenchymal component, particularly in spindled cells, there will be pericellular distribution of reticulin. This reflects the presence of a basal lamina in the mesenchymal component. Molecular studies have demonstrated largely overlapping features between gliosarcoma and "primary" GBM, including *PTEN* mutation/deletion and $p16^{INK4a}$ deletion, although *EGFR* amplification is less common.[31]

GBM with Primitive Neuroectodermal Tumor-Like Foci

As originally described, these tumors are malignant gliomas, recognizable as such, with sharply demarcated nodules of small blue tumor cells strongly resembling PNET. In addition to the sharp demarcation between PNET-like foci and conventional GBM, the small blue cell component has a higher mitotic rate, histologic anaplasia, and a significantly higher Ki-67 proliferation index.[34] Like PNET/medulloblastoma, these tumors may also show Homer Wright rosettes, which consist of a circumferential palisade of small blue tumor cells about a solid fibrillary core (no lumen is

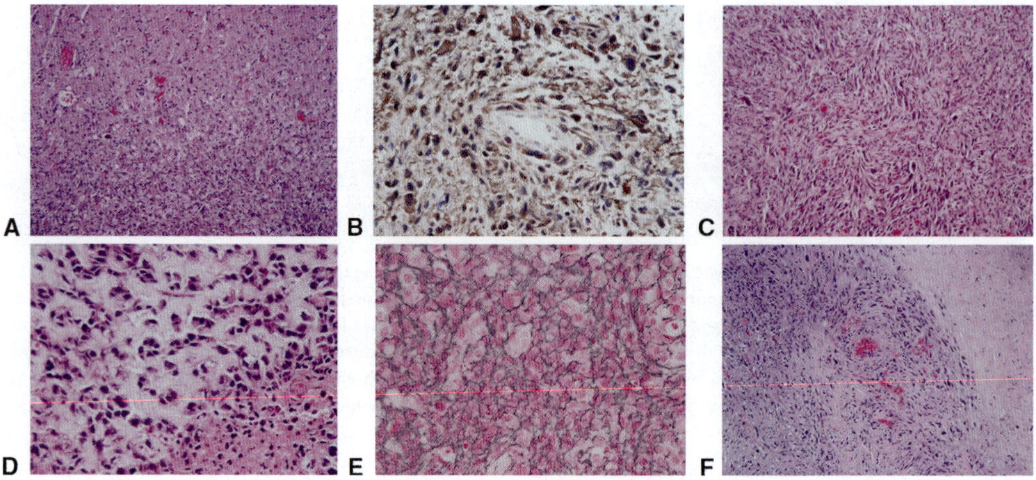

FIGURE 2-8: Gliosarcoma. These tumors are GBMs with sarcomatoid differentiation and have the same poor prognosis of any *IDH* wild-type GBM. This example demonstrates a glial component infiltrating cortex (**A**, *top of image*) and strong GFAP positivity (**B**). Also present are mesenchymal-appearing foci with a fascicular to storiform arrangement (**C**) as well as foci with a chondroid appearance (**D**). Pericellular reticulin staining (**E**) with loss of GFAP is characteristic in foci of sarcomatoid differentiation. The sarcomatoid differentiation of gliosarcoma may be closely mimicked by recurrent (and conventional) GBM involving dura (**F**), as well as anaplastic meningioma (not shown).

present, unlike true ependymal rosettes and Flexner-Wintersteiner rosettes). In addition, these small blue tumor cell foci may lose GFAP expression, demonstrate increased synaptophysin expression, and demonstrate *N-myc* or *c-myc* amplification.[34] An additional histologic feature is the presence of lower-grade foci, suggesting anaplastic progression to GBM with PNET-like features from a WHO grade II or III tumor. These tumors are associated with more frequent seeding of the CSF than is seen with other GBMs, which does suggest an important clinical correlate of this variant.[34]

Grading

All GBMs, including the histologic variants discussed, currently receive a WHO grade of IV.

Molecular Features

Relevant molecular features of primary GBMs are 10q loss, *PTEN* deletion/mutation, *EGFR* amplification (and/or polysomy of chromosome 7 on FISH analyses), and *p16* deletion. The most critical alterations identified in the more prognostically favorable secondary GBM category include *IDH1/IDH2* mutation, *MGMT* promoter methylation, and *TP53* mutation. These are further discussed in the preceding chapter under the sections of oligodendroglioma, diffuse astrocytoma, and histologic variants of GBM.

GLIOMATOSIS CEREBRI

GC is *not a specific histologic diagnosis* as the histologic features may range from WHO grade II oligodendroglioma to WHO grade IV GBM. However, GC is a clinical and radiologic entity so pathologists should be familiar with its unique clinical and radiologic features. By definition, GC is an infiltrating glioma, regardless of grade, that involves three or more lobes of the cerebral hemisphere. The WHO recognizes two clinicoradiologic forms, including type 1 GC and type 2 GC.[31] Type 1 GC, or "classical GC," consists of diffusely infiltrating, occasionally enhancing tumor without formation of a discrete mass. Type 2 GC, in contrast, has the radiologic features of type 1 GC as well as a discrete mass. Many GC patients, however, have an underlying WHO grade III tumor although this is not absolute.

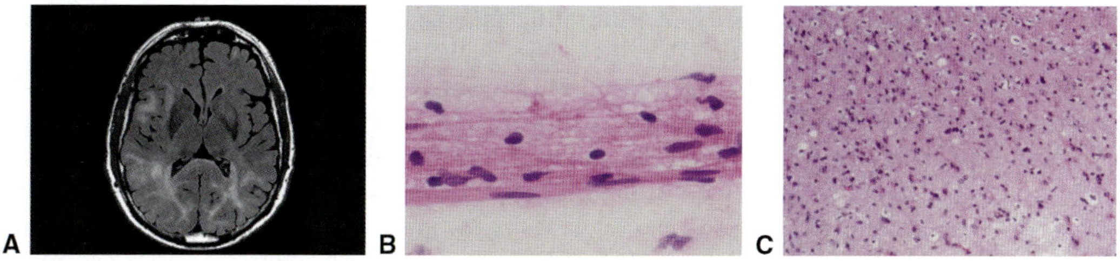

FIGURE 2-9: Gliomatosis cerebri. These tumors demonstrate diffuse signal abnormalities on T2/FLAIR that involves three or more cerebral lobes (**A**) and that may involve the subcortical nuclei, brainstem, and cerebellum, and rarely, spinal cord. The cytologic and permanent section preparations in this case are indistinguishable from diffuse astrocytoma (**B, C**). This is an example of type I gliomatosis cerebri, in which there is not a predominant mass lesion. Type II gliomatosis cerebri, in contrast, shows radiologic and histologic features of GBM (see text and Figures 2-5, 2-6, and 2-7) with similarly abnormal and diffuse T2/FLAIR signal indicative of multilobar spread.

Clinical and Radiologic Features

The clinical presentation in GC is varied and depends on the brain regions affected and whether there is a dominant mass lesion. Patients are typically in the fifth decade of life[31] although pediatric presentations are not uncommon. Commonly, these patients experience mental status changes with symptoms such as confusion and forgetfulness. If sensorimotor cortices or tracts are involved, the patients may also have corresponding motor or sensory deficits.

Radiologically, GC presents as diffusely abnormal T2/FLAIR signal involving three or more lobes of the brain (see Figure 2-9). Typically, the signal abnormalities are bilateral and involve subcortical structures and brainstem. There may be faint contrast enhancement in type 1 GC (without a mass lesion). In type 2 GC, there is a mass, which may have rim or solid enhancement, consistent with GBM.

Histologic Features and Grading

Histopathologic analyses may demonstrate mildly atypical cells with little increase in cellularity over background neuroglial tissue in GC. Conversely, there can be densely hypercellular foci of tumor with frequent mitoses and even pseudopalisading necrosis, diagnostic of a WHO grade IV tumor. Those arising as type 2 GC (i.e., GC with a predominant mass) may originally present as localized tumors resembling diffuse astrocytoma or GBM. Rare cases of gliomatosis with predominant oligodendroglial cytology have also been described.[35]

Molecular Features and Prognosis

There is no specific genetic alteration in GC, but a particularly common alteration is *TP53* mutation, which is a common alteration in low-grade diffuse glioma more generally.[36] Rare cases with *IDH1* mutations have been found, but only in those with a predominant mass (type 2 GC).[37] Therefore, the GC pattern of spread does not exclude the presence of this prognostically favorable mutation. The more important question perhaps, which is why these tumor cells can have such an exaggerated pattern of infiltration, remains unanswered.[36]

Differential Diagnosis

The obvious differential diagnosis for GC is diffuse glioma (without the GC pattern of spread). This distinction cannot be made without expert neuroradiology input (see also the preceding comment on type 2 GC). In most centers, prior to frozen section, the neurosurgery and/or neuroradiology staff will suspect a diagnosis of GC from the combination of radiologic features and the clinical presentation. It is imperative that pathologists also review the MRI data, if feasible, to make their own assessment. This also allows the pathology report to mention potential discrepancies, such as the presence of WHO grade II histology in the light of enhancing foci of GC. An additional histologic abnormality in the differential diagnosis is the presence of diffuse microglial activation. The majority of infiltrating gliomas contain CD68-positive microglia, however, which may appear ramified or histiocytic, depending on the grade of the tumor and presence of necrosis.[38] The role of microglia in this setting is not clear, and this complicates this particular differential. Both helpful roles of microglia, with antigen presentation to lymphocytes and immunoactivation against tumor cells, and harmful roles, with microglia recruited by tumor cell-produced chemoattractants, have been postulated.[38] Whatever their role, the immunohistochemical demonstration of abundant microglia is *not* incompatible with the diagnosis of either low- or high-grade glioma and should not be used in isolation as evidence against a neoplastic process.

References

1. Minniti G, Arcella A, Scaringi C, et al. Chemoradiation for anaplastic oligodendrogliomas: clinical outcomes and prognostic value of molecular markers. *J Neurooncol* 2014;116:275–282.
2. Louis DN, Ohgaki H, Wiestler OD, et al. The 2007 WHO classification of tumours of the central nervous system. *Acta Neuropathol* 2007;114:97–109.
3. Scherer HJ. Structural development in gliomas. *Cancer Res* 1938;34:333.
4. Horbinski C, Miller CR, Perry A. Gone FISHing: clinical lessons learned in brain tumor molecular diagnostics over the last decade. *Brain Pathol* 2011;21:57–73.
5. Sahm F, Koelsche C, Meyer J, et al. CIC and FUBP1 mutations in oligodendrogliomas, oligoastrocytomas and astrocytomas. *Acta Neuropathol* 2012;123:853–860.
6. Cykowski MD, Allen RA, Fung KM, et al. Pyrosequencing of IDH1 and IDH2 mutations in brain tumors and non-neoplastic conditions. *Diagn Mol Pathol* 2012;21:214–220.
7. Theeler BJ, Yung WK, Fuller GN, et al. Moving toward molecular classification of diffuse gliomas in adults. *Neurology* 2012;79:1917–1926.
8. Reifenberger G, Kros JM, Louis DN, et al. Oligodendroglioma. In: Louis DN, Ohgaki H, Wiestler OD, et al., eds. *WHO Classification of Tumors of the Central Nervous System*. Lyon, France: IARC; 2007.
9. Fellah S, Caudal D, De Paula AM, et al. Multimodal MR imaging (diffusion, perfusion, and spectroscopy): is it possible to distinguish oligodendroglial tumor grade and 1p/19q codeletion in the pretherapeutic diagnosis? *AJNR Am J Neuroradiol* 2013;34:1326–1333.
10. Earnest F III, Kernohan JW, Craig WM. Oligodendrogliomas; a review of 200 cases. *Arch Neurol Psychiatry* 1950;63:964–976.
11. Powell SZ. Intraoperative consultation, cytologic preparations, and frozen section in the central nervous system. *Arch Pathol Lab Med* 2005;129:1635–1652.
12. Plesec TP, Prayson RA. Frozen section discrepancy in the evaluation of central nervous system tumors. *Arch Pathol Lab Med* 2007;131:1532–1540.
13. Komori T, Hirose T, Shibuya M, et al. Controversies over the diagnosis of oligodendroglioma: a report from the satellite workshop at the 4th international symposium of brain tumor pathology, Nagoya Congress Center, May 23, 2012. *Brain Tumor Pathol* 2013;30:253–261.
14. Appin CL, Gao J, Chisolm C, et al. Glioblastoma with oligodendroglioma component (GBM-O): molecular genetic and clinical characteristics. *Brain Pathol* 2013;23:454–461.
15. Scheithauer BW, Fuller GN, VandenBerg SR. The 2007 WHO classification of tumors of the nervous system: controversies in surgical neuropathology. *Brain Pathol* 2008;18:307–316.
16. Giannini C, Scheithauer BW, Weaver AL, et al. Oligodendrogliomas: reproducibility and prognostic value of histologic diagnosis and grading. *J Neuropathol Exp Neurol* 2001;60:248–262.
17. Kros JM, Hop WC, Godschalk JJ, et al. Prognostic value of the proliferation-related antigen Ki-67 in oligodendrogliomas. *Cancer* 1996;78:1107–1113.
18. Yip S, Iafrate AJ, Louis DN. Molecular diagnostic testing in malignant gliomas: a practical update on predictive markers. *J Neuropathol Exp Neurol* 2008;67:1–15.
19. Brat DJ, Scheithauer BW, Eberhart CG, et al. Extraventricular neurocytomas: pathologic features and clinical outcome. *Am J Surg Pathol* 2001;25:1252–1260.
20. Daumas-Duport C, Scheithauer BW, Chodkiewicz JP, et al. Dysembryoplastic neuroepithelial tumor: a surgically curable tumor of young patients with intractable partial seizures. Report of thirty-nine cases. *Neurosurgery* 1988;23:545–556.

21. Thom M, Toma A, An S, et al. One hundred and one dysembryoplastic neuroepithelial tumors: an adult epilepsy series with immunohistochemical, molecular genetic, and clinical correlations and a review of the literature. *J Neuropathol Exp Neurol* 2011;70:859–878.
22. Prabowo AS, Iyer AM, Veersema TJ, et al. BRAF V600E mutation is associated with mTOR signaling activation in glioneuronal tumors. *Brain Pathol* 2014;24:52–66.
23. Fouladi M, Helton K, Dalton J, et al. Clear cell ependymoma: a clinicopathologic and radiographic analysis of 10 patients. *Cancer* 2003;98:2232–2244.
24. Kleihues P, Burger PC, Rosenblum MK, et al. Anaplastic astrocytoma. In: Louis DN, Ohgaki H, Wiestler OD, et al., eds. *WHO Classification of Tumors of the Central Nervous System*. Lyon, France: IARC; 2007.
25. von Deimling A, Burger PC, Nakazato Y, et al. Diffuse astrocytoma. In: Louis DN, Ohgaki H, Wiestler OD, et al., eds. *WHO Classification of Tumors of the Central Nervous System*. Lyon, France: IARC; 2007.
26. Cykowski MD, Allen RA, Kanaly AC, et al. The differential diagnosis of pilocytic astrocytoma with atypical features and malignant glioma: an analysis of 16 cases with emphasis on distinguishing molecular features. *J Neurooncol* 2013;115:477–486.
27. Colman H, Giannini C, Huang L, et al. Assessment and prognostic significance of mitotic index using the mitosis marker phospho-histone H3 in low and intermediate-grade infiltrating astrocytomas. *Am J Surg Pathol* 2006;30:657–664.
28. Yan H, Parsons DW, Jin G, et al. IDH1 and IDH2 mutations in gliomas. *N Engl J Med* 2009;360:765–773.
29. Camelo-Piragua S, Jansen M, Ganguly A, et al. Mutant IDH1-specific immunohistochemistry distinguishes diffuse astrocytoma from astrocytosis. *Acta Neuropathol* 2010;119:509–511.
30. Weinstein JN, Collisson EA, Mills GB, et al. The Cancer Genome Atlas Pan-Cancer analysis project. *Nat Genet* 2013;45:1113–1120.
31. Fuller GN, Kros JM. Gliomatosis cerebri. In: Louis DN, Ohgaki H, Wiestler OD, et al., eds. *WHO Classification of Tumors of the Central Nervous System*. Lyon, France: IARC; 2007.
32. Hartmann C, Hentschel B, Wick W, et al. Patients with IDH1 wild type anaplastic astrocytomas exhibit worse prognosis than IDH1-mutated glioblastomas, and IDH1 mutation status accounts for the unfavorable prognostic effect of higher age: implications for classification of gliomas. *Acta Neuropathol* 2010;120:707–718.
33. Perry A, Aldape KD, George DH, et al. Small cell astrocytoma: an aggressive variant that is clinicopathologically and genetically distinct from anaplastic oligodendroglioma. *Cancer* 2004;101:2318–2326.
34. Perry A, Miller CR, Gujrati M, et al. Malignant gliomas with primitive neuroectodermal tumor-like components: a clinicopathologic and genetic study of 53 cases. *Brain Pathol* 2009;19:81–90.
35. Miller DC. *Modern Surgical Neuropathology*. Cambridge, New York: Cambridge University Press; 2009.
36. Mawrin C. Molecular genetic alterations in gliomatosis cerebri: what can we learn about the origin and course of the disease? *Acta Neuropathol* 2005;110:527–536.
37. Seiz M, Tuettenberg J, Meyer J, et al. Detection of IDH1 mutations in gliomatosis cerebri, but only in tumors with additional solid component: evidence for molecular subtypes. *Acta Neuropathol* 2010;120:261–267.
38. Graeber MB, Scheithauer BW, Kreutzberg GW. Microglia in brain tumors. *Glia* 2002;40:252–259.

3 Circumscribed Astrocytomas (Pilocytic Astrocytoma, Pilomyxoid Astrocytoma, Pleomorphic Xanthoastrocytoma, and Subependymal Giant Cell Astrocytoma)

Jo Elle G. Peterson

PILOCYTIC ASTROCYTOMA

Pilocytic astrocytomas (PAs) are well-circumscribed gliomas arising most often in children and young adults, without a gender predilection.[1] PAs are the most common glioma in children,[2] occurring most often in the cerebellum. While they may arise at any point along the neuraxis, the most common extracerebellar sites are the hypothalamus and optic pathway.[3] Tumors in this location, sometimes referred to as optic nerve gliomas, are frequently associated with neurofibromatosis type 1 (NF1).[4,5] PAs of the spinal cord tend to be seen in older patients.[6]

The clinical presentation is dependent upon tumor location and may include signs of increased intracranial pressure, neurologic deficits and, in the case of optic gliomas, vision loss. Imaging studies show a well-circumscribed mass that is variably contrast enhancing.[7–9] PAs are frequently cystic, a feature that can be helpful in differentiating it radiologically from other gliomas. A cyst with an enhancing mural nodule is a common appearance (Table 3-1).

PAs are characteristically biphasic tumors composed of dense, fibrillar regions and looser areas often with microcysts. The cells have monotonous nuclei with a bipolar appearance and long hair-like processes (Figure 3-1C). These long processes are best seen on intraoperative cytologic preparations (Figure 3-1B). Multinucleated cells may be seen and are often referred to as "pennies on a plate" as the nuclei line up along the periphery of the cell. A sign of chronicity, Rosenthal fibers and eosinophilic granular bodies (EGBs) are frequently present and may be abundant (Figures 3-1A, D, and F). Tumor cells and Rosenthal fibers are both strongly immunoreactive for glial fibrillary acidic protein (GFAP). Rosenthal fibers and EGBs are also strongly positive for periodic acid-Schiff (PAS) (Figure 3-1E). Degenerative changes such as degenerative nuclear atypia are not infrequent. PAs may contain microvascular proliferation, owing to their enhancing nature on MRI, and tumor necrosis may be seen. Mitotic activity is rare, and MIB-1 labeling indices are low. Oligodendroglioma-like regions may be present and may present a diagnostic challenge in small samples. In addition, leptomeningeal and subarachnoid space invasion is frequent in PAs but is not a sign of cerebrospinal fluid (CSF) dissemination or the potential for aggressive behavior.[10]

PAs are classified by the WHO as a grade I tumor. Gross total resection is the treatment of choice. Even in cases of subtotal resection, however, 20-year survival rates of up to 80% have

Table 3-1	Differential Diagnosis of Cyst with Mural Nodule
Pilocytic astrocytoma	
Ganglioglioma	
Pleomorphic xanthoastrocytoma	
Hemangioblastoma	

been reported.[11] NF1-associated optic gliomas often remain stable[12] and may be less aggressive than nonsyndromic lesions.[13] Chemotherapy may be reserved for use in individuals with multiple recurrences and/or in cases where surgical resection is not possible and the patient is symptomatic.

PILOMYXOID ASTROCYTOMA

Previously considered to be a histologic subtype of PA, the pilomyxoid pattern was first described in 1996 in an abstract by Cottingham et al.[14] as an infantile variant of PA. The term pilomyxoid astrocytoma was first used by Tihan et al.[15] in 1999 and, since then, has been shown to be an entity distinct from PAs, with a worse outcome, shorter progression-free survival, and a higher incidence of leptomeningeal dissemination.

Pilomyxoid astrocytomas (PMAs) may arise anywhere along the neuraxis but have a predilection for the hypothalamic/chiasmatic and suprasellar spaces. Cases arising from the basal ganglia, thalamus, pineal gland, cerebellum, brainstem, and spinal cord have all been reported.[16–20] The clinical presentation is largely dependent on the location of the tumor. Symptoms may include failure to thrive, developmental delays, altered mental status, and other signs of increased intracranial pressure.[21] When arising in the spinal cord, scoliosis, back pain, and neurologic deficits may be seen.[19] The reported appearance of PMAs on MRI is variable. Most cases are described as solid, circumscribed masses. When compared to PAs, these lesions are less frequently cystic. Mass

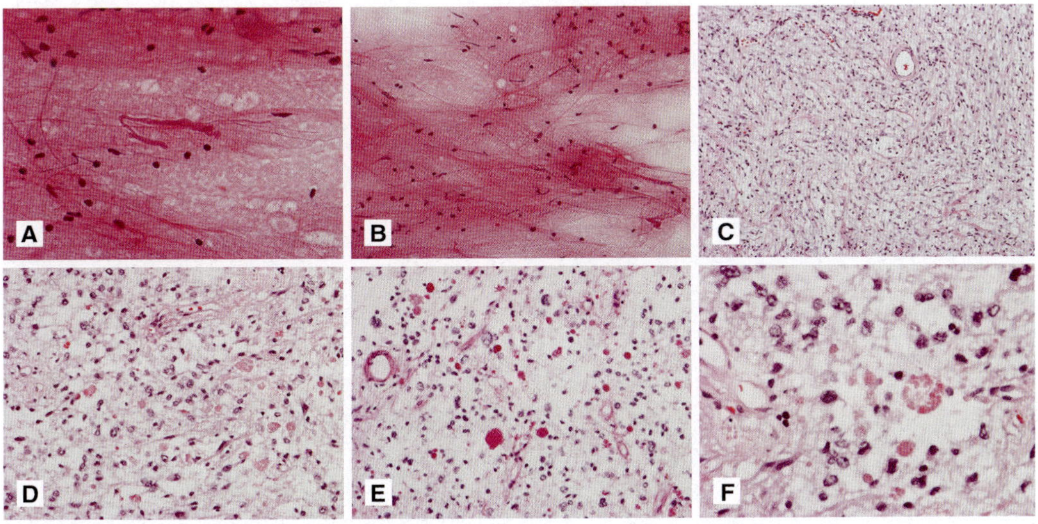

FIGURE 3-1: High-power H&E image of a squash preparation of a PA with an eosinophilic Rosenthal fiber (**A**). High-power H&E image of a squash preparation demonstrating hair-like, or piloid, cytoplasmic processes (**B**). Medium-power H&E image of a dense fibrillar region of a PA (**C**). Medium-power H&E image of abundant EGBs (**D**). Medium-power PAS image of abundant EGBs showing strong PAS-positivity (**E**). High-power H&E image of EGBs in a PA (**F**).

effect is common.[22] In two separate case series by Linscott et al.[23] and Komotar et al.,[22] the majority of cases are described as hyperintense on both T1 and T2 MRI sequences. Enhancement patterns were variable and included nonenhancing, rim-enhancing, heterogeneous enhancement with rim enhancement, and homogeneously enhancing. Lee et al.,[24] however, found PMAs to be hypointense on T1, hyperintense on T2, and uniformly nonenhancing following contrast administration. The presence of peritumoral edema is infrequent and, when present, minimal.[23] Diffusion-weighted imaging does not show diffusion restriction.[22,23] Intratumoral hemorrhage may be seen.[23]

PMAs occur predominantly in children. Tihan et al.[15] reported a median age at presentation of 10 months (range 3 to 84 months). Case reports of PMAs arising in older children and adults as old as 72 years have been published.[17,18] Multiple cases of PMAs arising in NF1 patients have been reported,[23] but there is no clear association with this tumor syndrome at this time.

PMAs are astrocytic neoplasms composed of piloid cells in an abundant myxoid matrix (Figure 3-2C and D). PMAs lack the characteristic biphasic appearance of PAs. Rather, they have a distinct angiocentric pattern described as piloid cells aligning perpendicular to the vascular axis (Figure 3-2A).[21] In some areas, the architecture may resemble the perivascular pseudorosettes of ependymomas.[15] Rosenthal fibers, which are common in PAs, are almost universally absent in PMAs. EGBs are rare but have been described (Figure 3-2B).[21,25] The tumor cells are strongly and diffusely immunoreactive for GFAP.[25] Synaptophysin immunoreactivity is variable and cannot be reliably used to differentiate PMA from PA.[25–27] Mitotic activity is infrequent, usually 0 to 2 mitoses per 10 high-power fields, with a low MIB-1 labeling index (2% to 5%).[15] Similar to a PA, tumor necrosis and microvascular proliferation may be seen.[15,26]

Multiple reports of PMAs diagnosed as PAs on subsequent resection have given rise to the idea of a "maturation phenomenon," also referred to in the literature as "perceived maturation."[25]

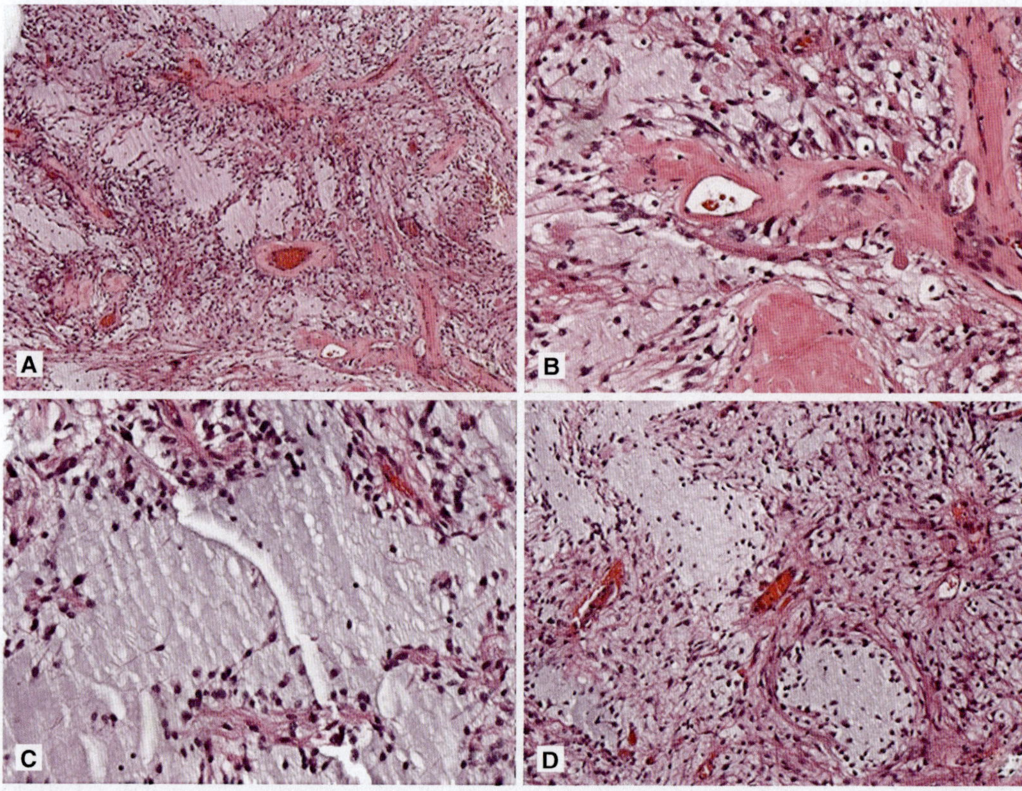

FIGURE 3-2: Medium-power H&E image of a PMA with angiocentric pattern (**A**). High-power H&E image of a PMA with densely hyalinized blood vessels and scattered EGBs (**B**). High-power H&E image of a PMA with monotonous bipolar cells in an abundant myxoid background (**C**). Medium-power H&E image of a PMA with an abundant myxoid background (**D**).

Most of these cases were diagnosed as PMA on initial resection based on the histologic features described above but, on recurrence, were found to have the classic morphology of a PA.[26,28] Furthermore, cases of intermediate tumors containing distinct regions of both PMA and PA have been described, suggesting that these tumors may exist along a spectrum.[20,25] Johnson et al.[25] report the histology of intermediate tumors ranging from prominently myxoid and monomorphous to extensively fibrillar with a dense growth pattern. In these cases, Rosenthal fibers could be seen in the more PA-like regions. The presence of the maturation phenomenon and the intermediate tumors suggests a common origin with PA[28]; however, an ependymal origin has also been suggested.[27]

Multiple studies have shown PMAs to have an increased incidence of CSF dissemination,[29] increased rate of recurrence, and shorter progression-free survival and overall survival than PAs.[21] In addition, PMAs have a higher incidence of leptomeningeal disease.[20,24] These findings support the WHO grade II designation.

Gross total resection, whenever possible, is the primary treatment modality for PMAs. Multiple studies suggest that the diagnosis of PMA should prompt closer follow-up, with evaluation for CSF dissemination.[19,30] Given the limited long-term follow-up data for PMAs, the behavior cannot be reliably predicted. As such, the presence of a PMA component should always be reported.[25]

PLEOMORPHIC XANTHOASTROCYTOMA

Pleomorphic xanthoastrocytoma (PXA) is a well-circumscribed, low-grade astrocytoma that occurs in children and young adults. It usually involves the leptomeninges and the cortex. PXAs frequently present with a seizure disorder, owing to the involvement of the cortex. It may be solid or cystic with a mural nodule. It predominantly arises supratentorially with a predilection for the temporal lobe. MRI frequently shows a cyst with an enhancing mural nodule, usually with some degree of leptomeningeal involvement.

PXAs are composed of pleomorphic giant cells with a dense deposition of intercellular reticulin (Figure 3-3A and C).[31] Xanthomatous change, or cytoplasmic lipid accumulation, may be inconspicuous and is not required for the diagnosis (Figure 3-3B). EGBs are frequently present (Figure 3-3D).[31] Anaplastic changes, including necrosis and increased mitotic activity, may be seen and should always be mentioned when present. These changes become more common with every tumor recurrence.[32,33] Glioblastoma has been reported to arise in PXA.

Gross total resection is the primary treatment in PXA.[32,33] Tumors that recur or show anaplastic features may warrant chemotherapy and/or radiation treatment.[33,34] The overall survival rate is 80% at 5 years and 70% at 10 years.[35,36] The tendency to recur and potential for malignant transformation are why PXA corresponds to WHO grade II.

Recent studies have shown *BRAF* V600E mutations to be present in more than half of PXAs[37,38] with a high sensitivity and specificity for PXA.[39] Immunohistochemistry for the *BRAF* V600E mutation has made evaluation for this mutation in PXAs rapid and readily available in many labs. Immunopositivity may be a useful tool in distinguishing PXA from giant cell glioblastoma.

SUBEPENDYMAL GIANT CELL ASTROCYTOMA AND SUBEPENDYMAL NODULE

Subependymal nodules (SENs) and subependymal giant cell astrocytomas (SEGAs) arise primarily in the setting of tuberous sclerosis complex (TSC), a genetic disorder caused by mutations in the *TSC1* or *TSC2* genes. SENs are small nodules (<1 cm) that are found on the surface of the ventricles (Figure 3-4A). SEGAs are larger than 1 cm and may grow to obstruct the foramen of Monro, causing hydrocephalus. SEGAs are the most common brain tumors in patients with TSC[40] and typically occur within the first two decades of life. Patients may present with signs of increased intracranial pressure or a change in seizure activity. MRI typically shows a

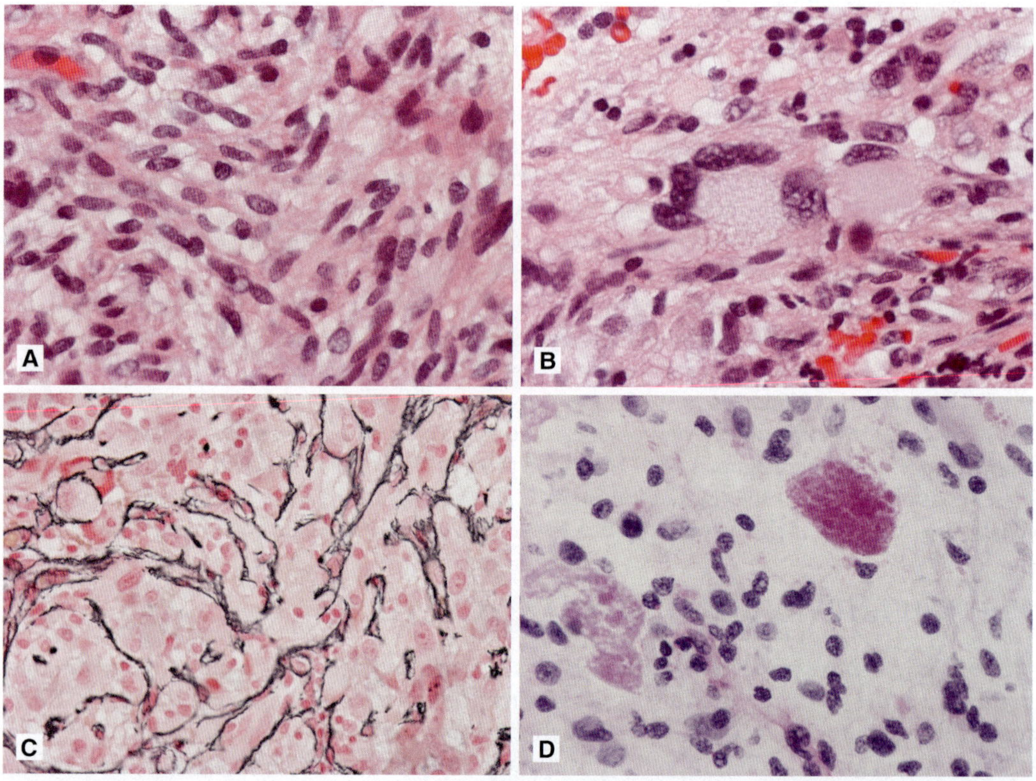

FIGURE 3-3: High-power H&E image of spindled morphology in a PXA (**A**). High-power H&E image of xanthomatous change in a PXA (**B**). High-power image of a reticulin stain showing dense reticulin deposition in a PXA (**C**). High-power image of a PAS stain showing PAS-positive EGBs in a PXA (**D**).

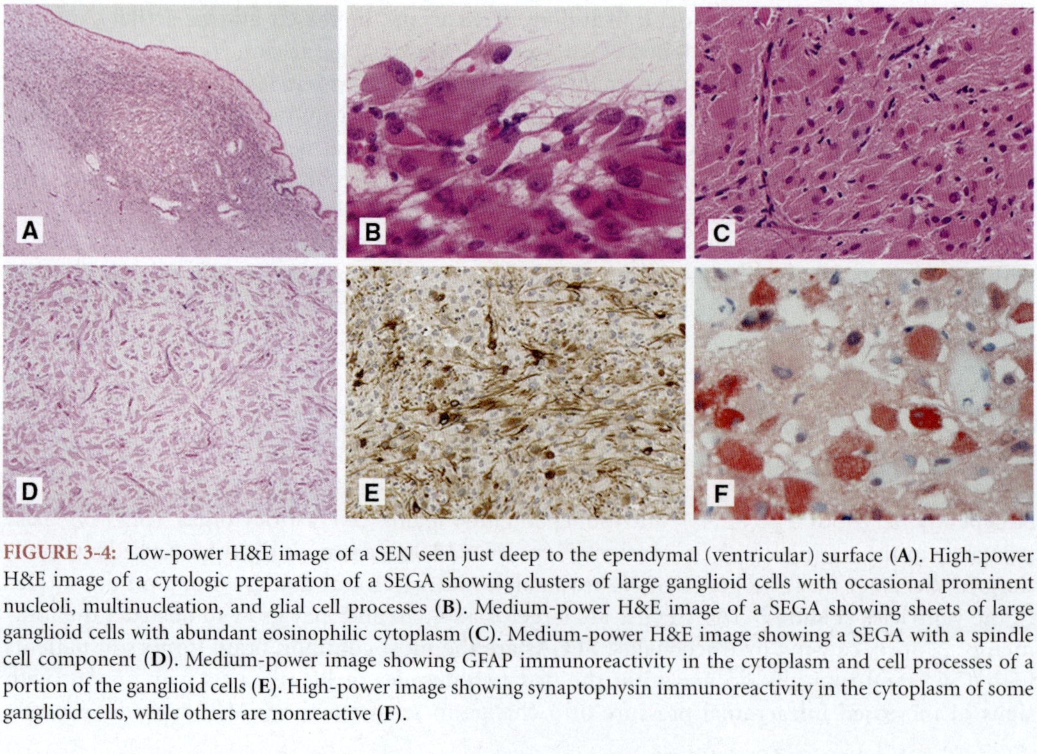

FIGURE 3-4: Low-power H&E image of a SEN seen just deep to the ependymal (ventricular) surface (**A**). High-power H&E image of a cytologic preparation of a SEGA showing clusters of large ganglioid cells with occasional prominent nucleoli, multinucleation, and glial cell processes (**B**). Medium-power H&E image of a SEGA showing sheets of large ganglioid cells with abundant eosinophilic cytoplasm (**C**). Medium-power H&E image showing a SEGA with a spindle cell component (**D**). Medium-power image showing GFAP immunoreactivity in the cytoplasm and cell processes of a portion of the ganglioid cells (**E**). High-power image showing synaptophysin immunoreactivity in the cytoplasm of some ganglioid cells, while others are nonreactive (**F**).

circumscribed mass near the foramen of Monro, frequently with avid contrast enhancement. Hydrocephalus may be present.

Histologically, SENs and SEGAs are indistinguishable. They are well-circumscribed lesions composed of large ganglioid cells with abundant eosinophilic cytoplasm resembling gemistocytic astrocytes (Figure 3-4C). A spindle cell component may be prominent (Figure 3-4D). On cytologic preparations, clusters of large ganglioid cells are present with glial cytoplasmic processes (Figure 3-4B). Multinucleation and nuclear pleomorphism are common. Microvascular proliferation and tumor necrosis are not typical of SEGAs and may warrant consideration of other diagnoses such as glioblastoma. Mitotic activity is uncommon.

The origin of these tumors is controversial. The immunostaining pattern is typically that of a glioneuronal tumor, with variable GFAP, neuron specific enolase (NSE), neurofilament, and synaptophysin positivity (Figures 3-4E and F).[41,42] Ultrastructural studies have shown features of neuronal differentiation, including dense core granules[41] and occasional synapses.[43] As such, the term subependymal giant cell tumor may be more appropriate than SEGA.

Gross total resection of symptomatic SEGAs is generally successful, as the lesions rarely regrow. In recent years, nonsurgical treatment options have become available, including mTOR inhibitor therapy and Gamma Knife therapy. mTOR inhibitor therapy has been shown to significantly reduce the size of SEGAs in most patients. However, upon cessation of the mTOR inhibitor therapy, the lesions tend to recur. The choice of which therapeutic option to implement is based upon many factors, including prior therapeutic interventions, surgical resectability, and patient comorbidities, to name a few.[44] SEGAs correspond to WHO grade I.

References

1. Central Brain Tumor Registry of the United States 1995. First annual report.
2. Ohgaki H, Kleihues P. Population-based studies on incidence, survival rates, and genetic alterations in astrocytic and oligodendroglial gliomas. *J Neuropathol Exp Neurol* 2005;65:479–489.
3. Rosemberg S, Fujiwara D. Epidemiology of pediatric tumors of the nervous system according to the WHO 2000 classification: a report of 1,195 cases from a single institution. *Childs Nerv Syst* 2005;21:940–944.
4. Listernick R, Louis DN, Packer RJ, et al. Optic pathway gliomas in children with neurofibromatosis type 1: consensus statement from the NF1 Optic Glioma Task Force. *Ann Neurol* 1997;41:143–149.
5. Miller NR. Primary tumours of the optic nerve and its sheath. *Eye* 2004;18:1026–1037.
6. Minehan KJ, Shaw EG, Scheithauer BW, et al. Spinal cord astrocytoma: pathological and treatment considerations. *J Neurosurg* 1995;83:590–595.
7. Fulham MJ, Melisi JW, Nishimiya J, et al. Neuroimaging of juvenile pilocytic astrocytomas: an enigma. *Radiology* 1993;189:221–225.
8. Lee YY, Van Tassel P, Bruner JM, et al. Juvenile pilocytic astrocytomas: CT and MR characteristics. *AJR Am J Roentgenol* 1989;152:1263–1270.
9. Burger PC, Breiter SN, Fisher PG. Pilocytic and fibrillary astrocytomas of the brain stemva—comparative clinical, radiological and pathological study. *J Neuropathol Exp Neurol* 1996;55:640.
10. Mamelak AN, Prados MD, Obana WG, et al. Treatment options and prognosis for multicentric juvenile pilocytic astrocytoma. *J Neurosurg* 1994;81:24–30.
11. Wallner KE, Gonzales MF, Edwards MS, et al. Treatment results of juvenile pilocytic astrocytoma. *J Neurosurg* 1988;69:171–176.
12. Listernick R, Charrow J, Greenwald M, et al. Natural history of optic pathway tumors in children with neurofibromatosis type 1: a longitudinal study. *J Pediatr* 1994;125:63–66.
13. Rosser T, Packer RJ. Intracranial neoplasms in children with neurofibromatosis 1. *J Child Neurol* 2002;17:630–637.
14. Cottingham SL, Boesel CP, Yates AJ. Pilocytic astrocytoma in infants: a distinctive histological pattern. (abstract) *J Neuropathol Exp Neurol* 1996;55:654.
15. Tihan T, Fisher PG, Kepner JL, et al. Pediatric astrocytomas with monomorphous pilomyxoid features and a less favorable outcome. *J Neuropathol Exp Neurol* 1999;58:1061–1068.

16. Nagaishi M, Yokoo H, Hirato J, et al. Clinico-pathological feature of pilomyxoid astrocytomas: three case reports. *Neuropathology* 2011;31:152–157.
17. Skovrlj B, Pain M, Bederson JB, et al. Pilomyxoid astrocytoma of the cerebellar vermis in an elderly patient. *Surg Neurol Int* 2014;5:29.
18. Paraskevopoulos D, Patsalas I, Karkavelas G, et al. Pilomyxoid astrocytoma of the cervical spinal cord in a child with rapid progression into glioblastoma: case report and literature review. *Childs Nerv Syst* 2011;27:313–321.
19. Garber ST, Bollo RJ, Riva-Cambrin JK. Pediatric spinal pilomyxoid astrocytoma. *J Neurosurg Pediatr* 2013;12:511–516.
20. Forbes JA, Mobley BC, O'Lynnger TM, et al. Pediatric cerebellar pilomyxoid-spectrum astrocytomas. *J Neurosurg Pediatr* 2011;8:90–96.
21. Komotar RJ, Burger PC, Carson BS, et al. Pilocytic and pilomyxoid hypothalamic/chiasmatic astrocytomas. *Neurosurgery* 2004;54:72–80.
22. Komotar RJ, Zacharia BE, Sughrue ME, et al. Magnetic resonance imaging characteristics of pilomyxoid astrocytoma. *Neurol Res* 2008;30:945–951.
23. Linscott LL, Osborn AG, Blaser S, et al. Pilomyxoid astrocytoma: expanding the imaging spectrum. *AJNR Am J Neuroradiol* 2008;29:1861–1866.
24. Lee IH, Kim JH, Suh YL, et al. Imaging characteristics of pilomyxoid astrocytomas in comparison with pilocytic astrocytomas. *Eur J Radiol* 2011;79:311–316.
25. Johnson MW, Eberhart CG, Perry A, et al. Spectrum of pilomyxoid astrocytomas: intermediate pilomyxoid tumors. *Am J Surg Pathol* 2010;34:1783–1791.
26. Amatya VJ, Akazawa R, Sumimoto Y, et al. Clinicopathological and immunohistochemical features of three pilomyxoid astrocytomas: comparative study with 11 pilocytic astrocytomas. *Pathol Int* 2009;59:80–85.
27. Fuller CE, Frankel B, Smith M, et al. Suprasellar monomorphous pilomyxoid neoplasm: an ultrastructural analysis. *Clin Neuropathol* 2001;20:256–262.
28. Ceppa EP, Bouffet E, Griebel R, et al. The pilomyxoid astrocytoma and its relationship to pilocytic astrocytoma: report of a case and a critical review of the entity. *J Neurooncol* 2007;81:191–196.
29. Komotar RJ, Mocco J, Carson BS, et al. Pilomyxoid astrocytoma: a review. *MedGenMed* 2004;6:42.
30. Tsugu H, Oshiro S, Yanai F, et al. Management of pilomyxoid astrocytomas: our experience. *Anticancer Res* 2009;29:919–926.
31. Kros JM, Vecht CJ, Stefanko SZ. The pleomorphic xanthoastrocytomas and its differential diagnosis: a study of five cases. *Hum Pathol* 1991;22:1128–1135.
32. Giannini C, Scheithauer BW, Burger PC, et al. Pleomorphic xanthoastrocytomas: what do we really know about it? *Cancer* 1999;85:2033–2045.
33. Pahapill PA, Ramsay DA, Del Maestro RF. Pleomorphic xanthoastrocytomas: case report and analysis of the literature concerning the efficacy of resection and the significance of necrosis. *Neurosurgery* 1996;38:822–828.
34. Koga T, Morita A, Maruyama K, et al. Long-term control of disseminated pleomorphic xanthoastrocytomas with anaplastic features by means of stereotactic irradiation. *Neuro Oncol* 2009;11:446–451.
35. Kepes JJ, Rubinstein LJ, Eng LF. Pleomorphic xanthoastrocytomas: a distinctive meningocerebral glioma of young subjects with relatively favorable prognosis. A study of 12 cases. *Cancer* 1979;44:1839–1852.
36. Rao AA, Laack NN, Giannini C, et al. Pleomorphic xanthoastrocytomas in children and adolescents. *Pediatr Blood Cancer* 2010;55:290–294.
37. Dias-Santagata D, Lam Q, Vernovsky K, et al. BRAF V600E mutations are common in pleomorphic xanthoastrocytoma: diagnostic and therapeutic implications. *PLoS ONE* 2011;6:1–9.
38. Koelsche C, Sahm F, Wohrer A, et al. BRAF-mutated pleomorphic xanthoastrocytoma is associated with temporal location, reticulin fiber deposition and CD34 expression. *Brain Pathol* 2014;24:221–229.
39. Ida CM, Vrana JA, Rodriguez FJ, et al. Immunohistochemistry is highly sensitive and specific for detection of BRAF V600E mutation in pleomorphic xanthoastrocytoma. *Acta Neuropathol Comm* 2013;1:1–7.
40. Shepherd CW, Scheithauer BW, Gomez MR, et al. Subependymal giant cell astrocytoma: a clinical, pathological, and flow cytometric study. *Neurosurgery* 1991;28:864–868.
41. Buccoliero AM, Franchi A, Castiglione F, et al. Subependymal giant cell astrocytoma (SEGA): is it an astrocytoma? Morphological, immunohistochemical and ultrastructural study. *Neuropathology* 2009;29:25–30.
42. You H, Kim YI, Im SY, et al. Immunohistochemical study of central neurocytoma, subependymoma, and subependymal giant cell astrocytoma. *J Neurooncol* 2005;74:1–8.
43. Jozwiak J, Jozwiak S, Skopinski P. Immunohistochemical and microscopic studies on giant cells in tuberous sclerosis. *Histol Histopathol* 2005;20:1321–1326.
44. Campen CJ, Porter BE. Subependymal giant cell astrocytoma (SEGA) treatment update. *Curr Treat Options Neurol* 2011;13:380–385.

Ependymomas

4

▶ Wamidh Adwar
▶ Aditya Raghunathan

Ependymal tumors are rare primary glial tumors of the central nervous system (CNS), affecting the pediatric population more commonly than adults.[1,2] These tumors are believed to originate from ependymal cells that line the ventricles of the CNS and the spinal canal.[3,4] At present, the 7th edition of the World Health Organization (WHO) Classification of Tumors of the Central Nervous System recognizes four main entities of ependymal tumors: subependymoma (WHO grade I), myxopapillary ependymoma (WHO grade I), (conventional) ependymoma (WHO grade II), and anaplastic ependymoma (WHO grade III).[5]

EPIDEMIOLOGY OF EPENDYMAL TUMORS

Overall, ependymomas represent about 2% of all primary CNS tumors.[6] In the 0- to 14-year age group, these represent about 5.7% of all primary CNS tumors and most commonly occur in the posterior fossa.[6] Among adults, these represent about 4% of all primary CNS tumors, with the spinal cord being the most common location.[4,6] Ependymal tumors occur more commonly among males than females.[6]

SUBEPENDYMOMA

Subependymomas are WHO grade I tumors[5] and are benign, noninvasive, and indolent.[7] In general, these tumors are less common than other types of ependymal tumors and are often incidentally identified.[8] Most frequently, subependymomas arise within the fourth ventricle (50% to 60%) and lateral ventricles (30% to 40%).[9] Less common locations include the third ventricle and within the cervical and cervicothoracic spinal cord.[7,8,10] Subependymoma is most commonly identified in middle-aged and elderly men.[7] When symptomatic, usually due to obstruction to the cerebrospinal fluid flow and increased intracranial pressure, the most common presentations are ataxia, vertigo, headache, nausea, and vomiting.[8]

Radiologic Features

Subependymomas appear as a lobulated, well-demarcated mass with little or no vascularity and minimal surrounding edema (Figure 4-1A).[11] By magnetic resonance imaging (MRI), these tumors are iso- to hypointense on T1-weighted images, are hyperintense on T2-weighted images, and show slight-to-moderate postcontrast enhancement.[7] Cystic degeneration, calcification, and hemorrhage may be identified among larger tumors.[12]

Histologic Features

At low magnification, subependymomas appear to have a multinodular growth pattern, with an abundant fibrillary background that contains clusters of monomorphic tumor cells (Figure 4-1B).[5,9,13] Calcification, microcyst formation, and hemorrhage may be seen, particularly among larger tumors, and are thought to represent degenerative changes. On higher magnification, the nuclei are uniform

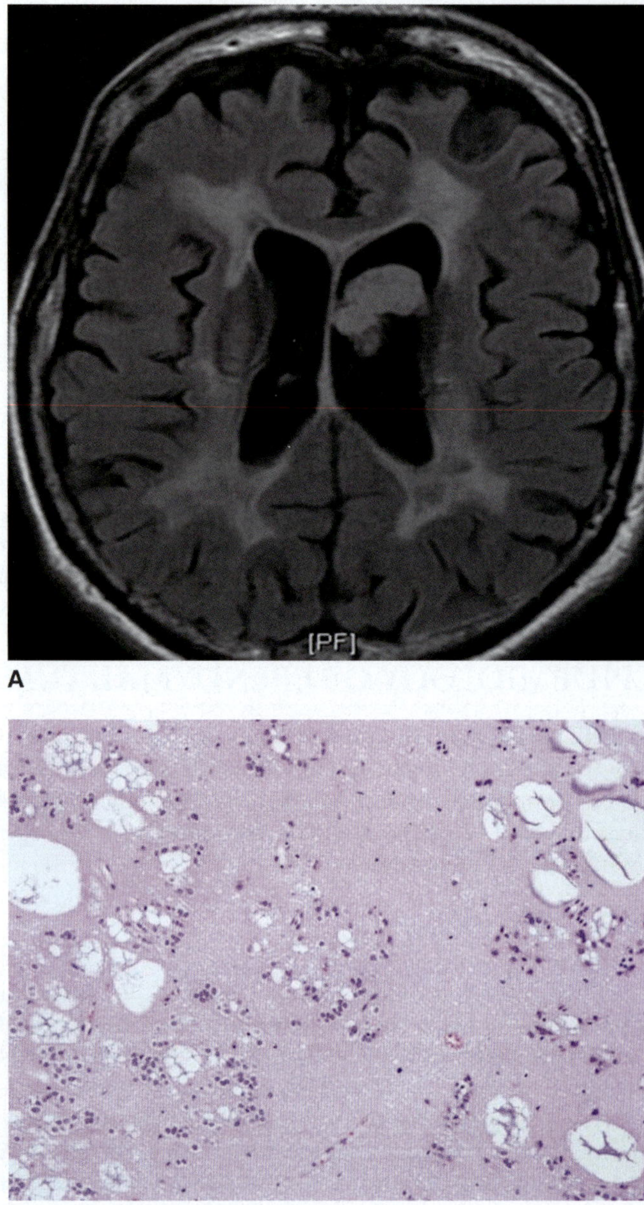

FIGURE 4-1: Subependymoma. Characteristically, the MRI shows a lobulated, well-demarcated mass within the lateral ventricle, without associated edema in the adjacent brain parenchyma (**A**). Histologically, groups of uniform cells with bland nuclei are seen in a predominant fibrillary background (**B**). Areas of microcystic degeneration may also be seen, as in this case.

and round to oval with punctuate, evenly distributed chromatin.[13] Mitotic activity is usually inconspicuous. Rare examples with nuclear pleomorphism, foci of tumor necrosis, and infiltrative borders have been reported.[5,7] However, these features are not indicative of worse prognosis.[13] By electron microscopy, subependymoma cells show cilia and microvillus formation and have abundant intermediate filaments—features that are typical of ependymal lineage.[5]

Prognosis

The prognosis of pure subependymoma is more favorable than cases with mixed ependymoma–subependymoma features. Prognosis is highly favorable in cases where complete surgical removal is feasible, more commonly tumors in the lateral ventricle than those that involve the floor of the fourth ventricle.[5,11]

MYXOPAPILLARY EPENDYMOMA

Myxopapillary ependymomas characteristically occur in the conus medullaris/filum terminale region of the spinal cord. A minority of cases have been described as involving the cervicothoracic spinal cord, while rare intracranial examples have been reported in the third ventricle,[14,15] fourth ventricle,[16] and cerebral hemispheres.[17] Rare cases of myxopapillary ependymoma have also been reported to involve the subcutaneous soft tissue at the sacrococcygeal region, perhaps originating from ectopic ependymal remnants.[18,19] These slowly growing tumors are categorized as WHO grade I.[5] Among ependymomas involving the spinal cord, over 25% are myxopapillary ependymomas, with a mean age at diagnosis of 36 years (6 to 82 years).[14] Clinically, patients predominantly present with low back pain, with or without sciatica. Sensorimotor disturbances in the lower limbs, loss of sphincter control, and impotence are also frequently reported.[14]

Radiologic Features

Myxopapillary ependymoma presents as a sausage-shaped, well-circumscribed mass in the cauda equina region (Figure 4-2A). Encasement of the cauda equina and erosion into adjacent bone structures may be seen in advanced cases.[13] By MRI, these tumors may show apparent cystic changes, postcontrast enhancement, and hemorrhage.[5,20]

Macroscopic Features

On macroscopic examination, these tumors are ovoid or sausage shaped and are usually encapsulated, with a smooth capsular surface. The cut surfaces may appear glistening, mucoid, or hemorrhagic.[14]

Histologic Features

Myxopapillary ependymoma is characterized by variably sized papillary formations, with frequently hyalinized fibrovascular cores that may also contain a pale blue, myxoid matrix (Figure 4-2B).[14,21] These are surrounded by flat, cuboidal, or columnar tumor cells arranged radially around the hyalinized fibrovascular cores, with centrally directed eosinophilic cytoplasmic processes and peripherally located nuclei (Figure 4-2C). The tumor cells have regular, round to oval nuclei, with fine, evenly distributed chromatin. Mucin may accumulate between and within the tumor cells, resulting in signet ring morphology. The mucin is highlighted with the periodic acid–Schiff (PAS), Alcian

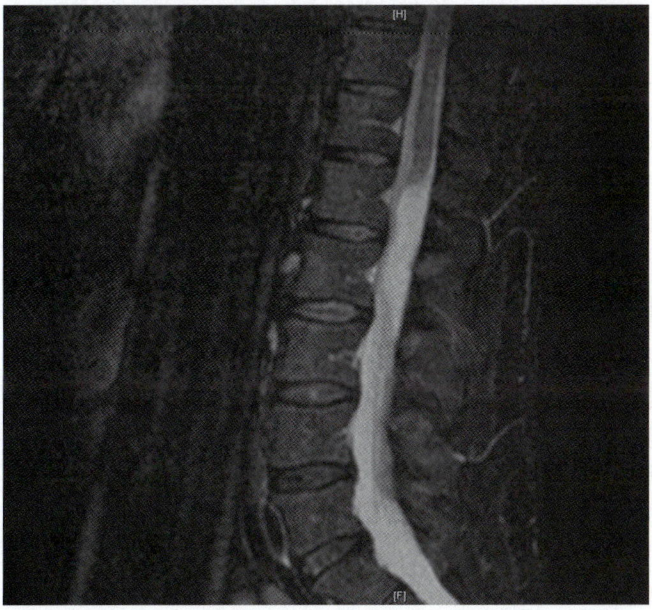

A

FIGURE 4-2: Myxopapillary ependymoma. MRI shows a well-circumscribed, "sausage-shaped" mass involving the cauda equina region (**A**).

FIGURE 4-2: (*Continued*) On low magnification, myxopapillary ependymoma demonstrates pale blue/myxoid matrix and papillary structures with hyalinized fibrovascular cores (**B**). Higher magnification showing elongated fibrillary processes forming the perivascular pseudorosettes, with myxoid matrix within the nucleus-free zone (**C**). Also note the uniform nuclei and the absence of mitotic activity and cytologic atypia.

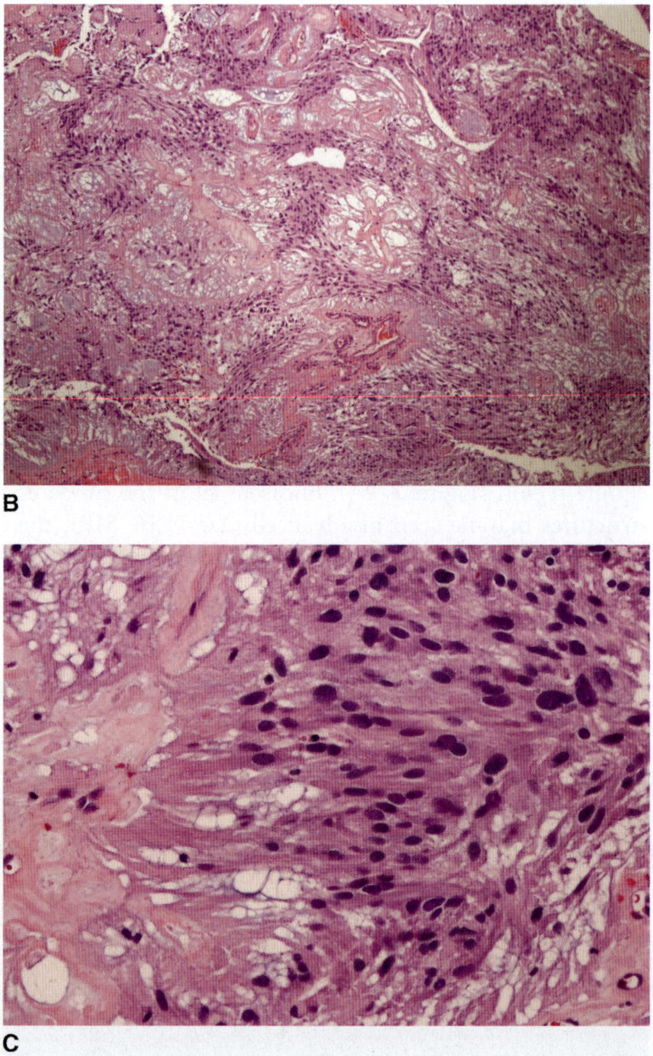

blue, and mucicarmine stains. On immunohistochemical staining, the tumor cells are positive for the glial fibrillary acid protein (GFAP) and the S100 protein. The absence of cytokeratin staining can help differentiate myxopapillary ependymoma from other neoplasia with myxoid stroma that may occur in this region, such as chordoma and papillary adenocarcinoma. The presence of GFAP immunostaining helps distinguish myxopapillary ependymoma from myxoid chondrosarcoma and paraganglioma. By electron microscopy, ependymal differentiation is evident by the identification of cytoplasmic microfilaments, intercellular microvilli, zonula adherens–type junctions, occasional microtubules, and extracellular basal laminae.[14]

Genetics

Myxopapillary ependymomas have been described to harbor loss of chromosomes 10q and 13.[22] However, in another study including six myxopapillary ependymomas, no evidence of allelic loss on chromosomes 10q and 22q were identified, and no mutations of *PTEN* or of the *NF2* tumor suppressors genes were identified.[23]

Prognosis

The overall survival (OS) rates among myxopapillary ependymomas are largely dependent on the completeness of tumor excision. In a study of 77 cases of myxopapillary ependymoma, the survival rates in patients who underwent complete excision (intact or piecemeal) were 19 to

19.5 years. In contrast, among those who underwent partial excision, the median OS rate was 14 years. Recurrences may be seen following resection of intact, encapsulated tumors and nonencapsulated tumors (10% vs. 19%, respectively). Rare cases of systemic metastasis have also been reported.[14]

EPENDYMOMA (CONVENTIONAL)

Ependymomas are slowly growing tumors, classified as WHO grade II. These are most common in the pediatric population and among young adults.[5,9] However, ependymomas can occur at any age. While these represent about 3% of primary CNS gliomas among adults, these are the third most common brain tumor in the pediatric population.[1] In adults, 50% to 60% of ependymomas are intraspinal, while among children, 80% of ependymomas are intracranial,[24] with the fourth ventricle being the most common site.[9] Though rare, cases of extra-axial ependymoma have been reported, including ependymoma of the lung, ovary, mediastinum, broad ligament, uterosacral ligament, and pelvic and perianal region.[25–30]

Radiologic Features

Ependymoma typically manifests as a relatively well-circumscribed intraventricular mass with variable, heterogenous postcontrast enhancement (Figure 4-3A). Within the posterior fossa, these tumors may fill the ventricle and grow through the foramina into the subarachnoid space of the ventral pons.[9,31] Spinal cord ependymomas tend to appear intra-axial, but are usually well demarcated (Figure 4-3B).[31] Areas of calcification may be identified, and these can occasionally be extensive.[9]

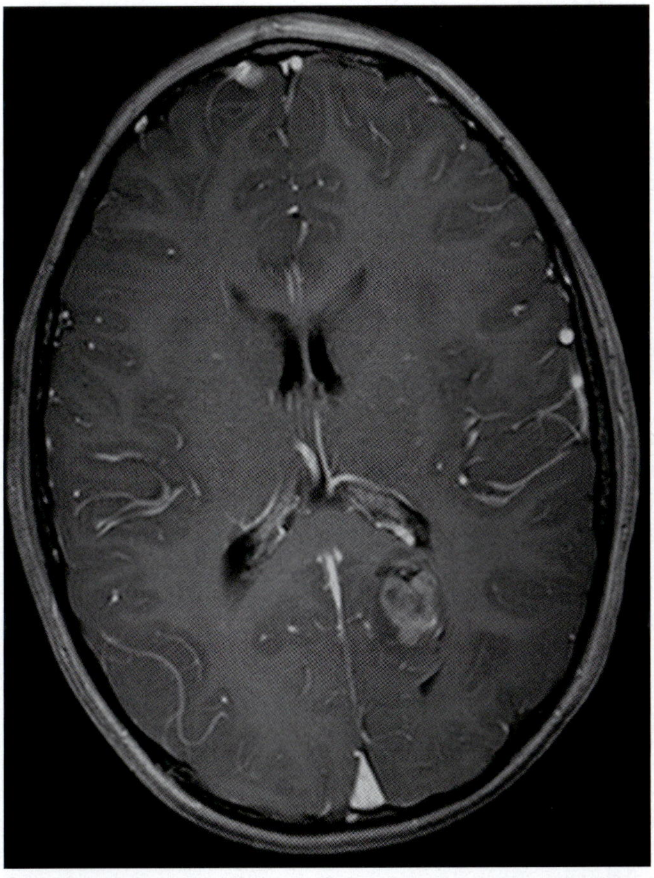

A

FIGURE 4-3: Ependymoma presenting as a circumscribed mass adjacent to occipital horn of the lateral ventricle. In this postcontrast MRI, the ependymoma shows enhancement (**A**).

FIGURE 4-3: (*Continued*) Spinal cord ependymoma, presenting as a well-circumscribed intramedullary mass (**B**).

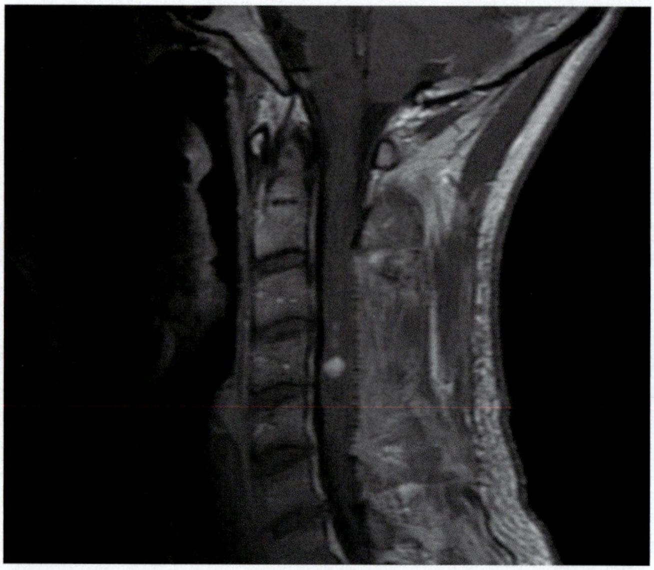

B

Macroscopic Features

Unlike infiltrating gliomas, ependymomas are well-demarcated, lobulated tumors, with a fleshy appearance to the cut surface.

Histologic Features

There are several described morphologic variants of ependymoma, including classical, cellular, tanycytic, papillary, giant cell, clear cell, signet ring cell, lipomatous, and melanotic variants.[1,9,13]

In classical ependymoma, the tumor cells grow in sheets and have elongated cytoplasm arranged radially around stromal blood vessels, forming a perivascular nucleus-free zone—a characteristic formation termed perivascular pseudorosettes (Figure 4-4A and B). This feature is the most useful diagnostic histologic feature for ependymomas.[1,9,31] In some cases, the tumor cells may be similarly arranged around an empty lumen, forming true ependymal rosettes (Figure 4-4C).

The constituent cells of ependymoma have uniform, round to oval nuclei with finely punctuate chromatin and distinct, small nucleoli. These cells have fibrillary cytoplasmic processes forming the background. Mitotic figures are rare, and there is usually no necrosis. Hemorrhage, calcifications, and formation of metaplastic bone or cartilage may be noted.[9]

By electron microscopy, ependymal differentiation is evident by the identification of cytoplasmic microfilaments, inter- and intracellular cilia and microvilli, zonula adherens–type junctions, microtubules, and extracellular basal laminae—features that are typical of ependymal lineage.[14] On immunohistochemical staining, all variants of ependymoma are positive for GFAP, underlining their glial origin. The GFAP stain might also help to highlight perivascular pseudorosette formation in cases where these structures are not readily identified. The epithelial membrane antigen (EMA) may show dot- or ring-like cytoplasmic staining and may also highlight the luminal aspects of true ependymal rosettes.

Ependymoma Variants

In *cellular ependymomas*, the cells are smaller and more crowded; hence, perivascular pseudorosettes may be less readily identified. However, there is no increase in mitotic activity.[1,9] Another rare subtype is the *tanycytic ependymoma*. These occur most commonly in the spinal cord, although intraventricular and supratentorial cases have been reported.[32,33] Histologically, these are characterized by fascicles of elongated cells with spindle-shaped nuclei and a densely fibrillary background formed by their cytoplasmic processes (Figure 4-4D). True ependymal rosettes and perivascular pseudorosettes are ill defined and may not be readily identified.[34] It has been postulated that the neoplastic cells are derived from tanycytes, which are elongated, bipolar ependymal cells of the floor of the third ventricle.[35] Tanycytic ependymoma needs to be distinguished from other tumors with "spindle cell" morphology, such as schwannoma, fibrous meningioma, and pilocytic astrocytoma. As their name might suggest, *papillary ependymomas* demonstrate

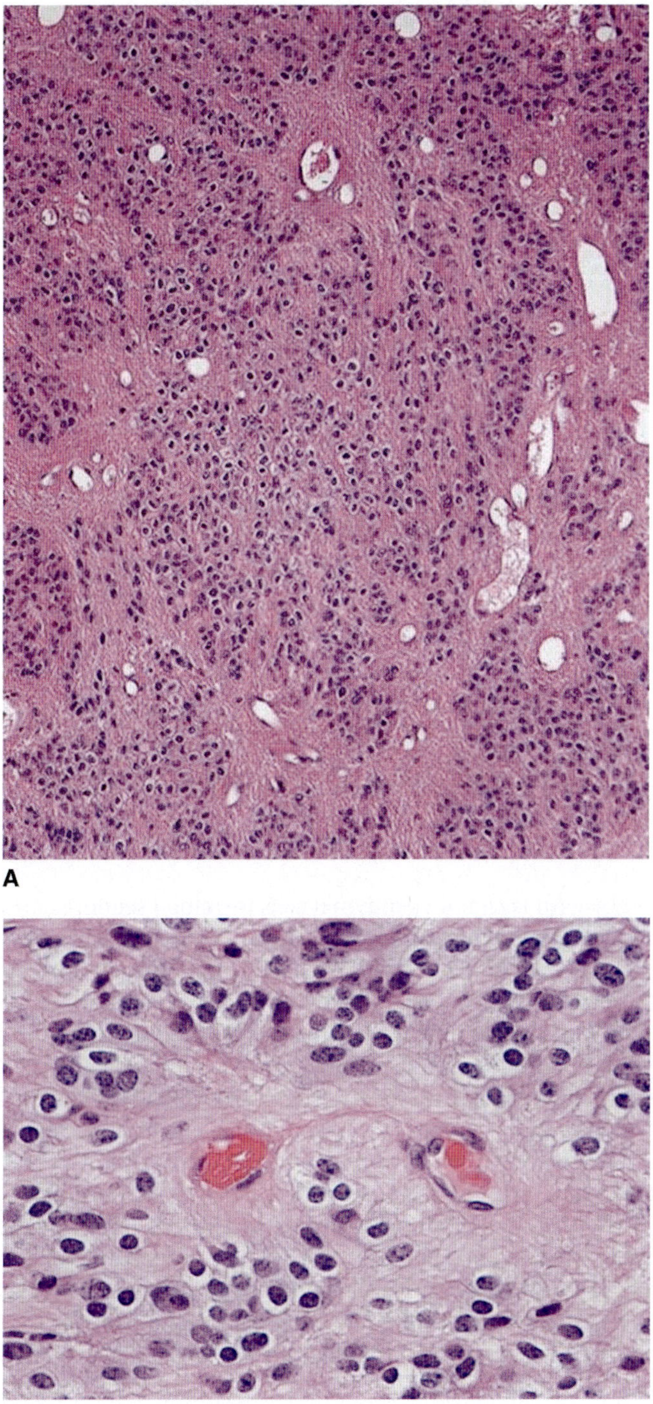

A

B

FIGURE 4-4: Ependymoma, WHO grade II, showing a moderately cellular neoplasm with perivascular nucleus-free zones (**A**). High magnification view of the perivascular pseudorosettes, where the ependymoma cell processes are oriented around blood vessels and nuclei are peripherally placed (**B**). Note the bland nuclear features of the ependymoma.

FIGURE 4-4: (*Continued*) True ependymal canals may also be identified (**C**). Tanycytic ependymoma, characterized by spindle-shaped tumor cells, densely fibrillary background, and ill-defined perivascular pseudorosettes (**D**).

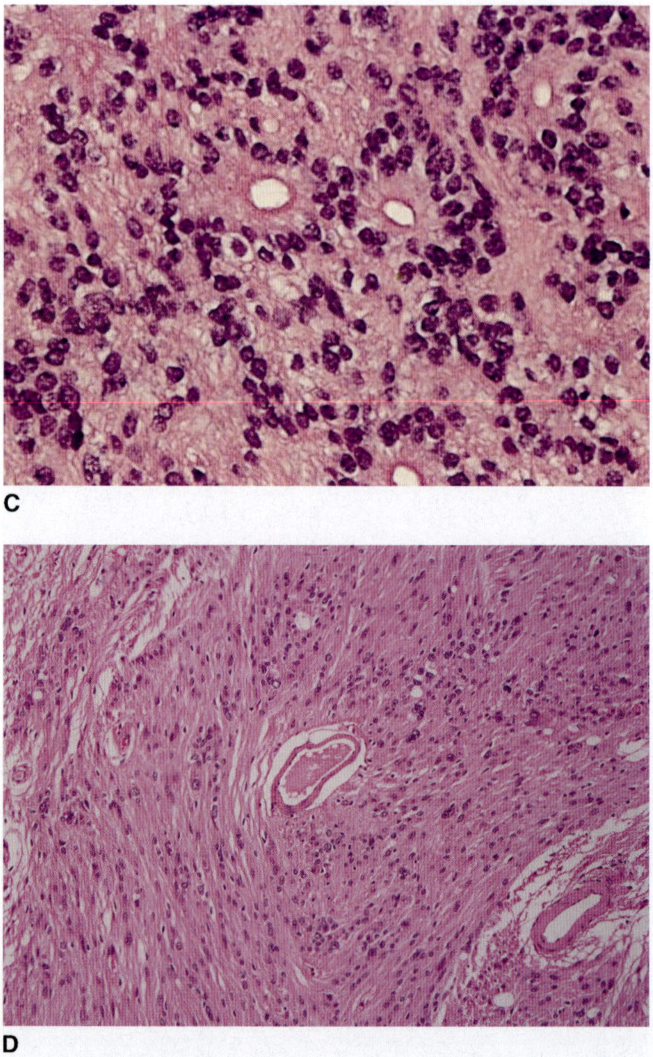

abundant papillary structures, formed by with layers of ependymal cells forming pseudorosettes around central vascular cores. These tumors should be differentiated from choroid plexus papilloma, metastatic carcinoma, and papillary carcinoma.[36] Diffuse GFAP immunoreactivity in a papillary ependymoma, and focal or absent GFAP immunoreactivity in choroid plexus papilloma or metastatic carcinoma, can help in this regard. An uncommon variant of ependymoma is *clear cell ependymoma*, a tumor with a predilection for the supratentorial compartment and a higher risk of recurrence. This variant is characterized by sheets of uniform cells with small-to-moderate amounts of clear to focally eosinophilic cytoplasm and round nuclei with identifiable nucleoli.[37,38] Perivascular pseudorosettes, ependymal rosette formation, highlighting perivascular pseudorosettes with the GFAP immunostain, and the characteristic dot-like EMA immunoreactivity can help in differentiating this variant from other tumors with clear cell morphology, such as oligodendroglioma, central neurocytoma, hemangioblastoma, and metastatic renal cell carcinoma.[9,37] *Giant cell ependymoma* is another rare variant of ependymoma, and in most of the reported cases, this tumor is located intracranially.[39] Histologically, these tumors are characterized by moderate-to-high cellularity, composed of two distinct populations of tumor cells. The first, from which this tumor derives its name, consists of giant cells with large, hyperchromatic, bizarre nuclei and abundant eosinophilic cytoplasm. The second, usually more abundant, population is composed of monomorphic cells with round to oval-shaped nuclei with inconspicuous nucleoli and eosinophilic cytoplasm forming the background.[39] In some areas, cytoplasmic clearing and eosinophilic intranuclear cytoplasmic pseudoinclusions may also be seen. Perivascular pseudorosette formation, true rosette formation, and GFAP and EMA immunoreactivity patterns can be of help in distinguishing this tumor from other tumor with giant cells, such as pleomorphic xanthoastrocytoma, giant cell glioblastoma, and subependymal giant cell astrocytoma.[9,39]

ANAPLASTIC EPENDYMOMA

Anaplastic ependymoma is a malignant ependymal tumor that shows accelerated growth and unfavorable prognosis and is classified as a WHO grade III tumor. It is found most commonly among children and involving the posterior fossa. The clinical presentation is similar to WHO grade II ependymomas. By radiology, areas of necrosis and postcontrast enhancement may be identified.[5]

Histologic Features

Anaplastic ependymomas show the hallmark histologic features of ependymomas, including perivascular pseudorosettes and ependymal canal formation. There have been different case series describing histologic features that characterize aggressive behavior of ependymomas, and most of the criteria might be subjective. Generally accepted criteria, described in the current WHO guidelines, include finding a predominance of areas with hypercellularity (Figure 4-5A), brisk mitotic activity (Figure 4-5B), cytologic anaplasia (increased nucleus:cytoplasmic ratios, nuclear

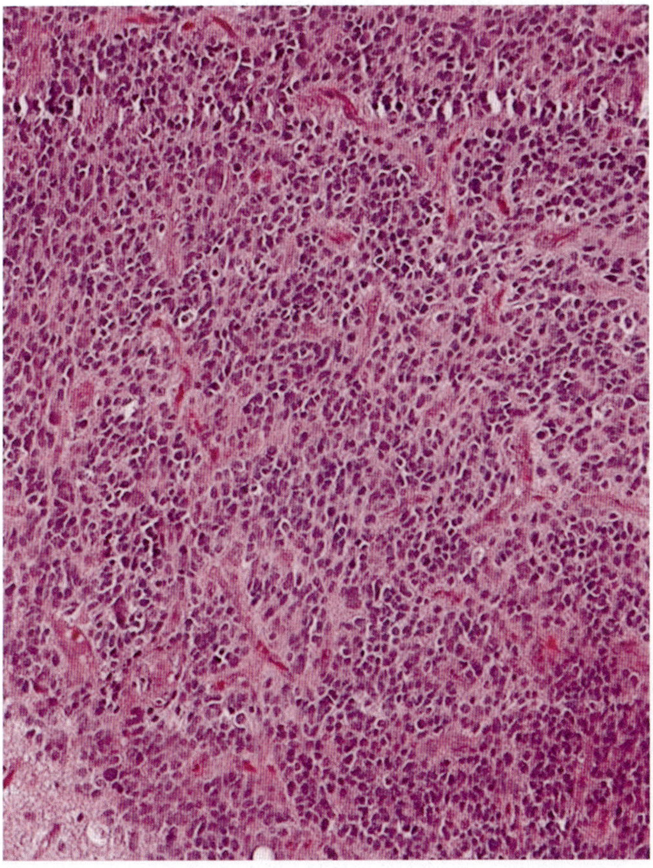

A

FIGURE 4-5: Anaplastic ependymoma, characterized by a predominance of areas of hypercellularity seen on low magnification (**A**).

FIGURE 4-5: (*Continued*) On higher magnification, mitotic figures are readily identified (**B**). The tumor nuclei show high nucleus: cytoplasmic ratios, pleomorphism, and dense, unevenly distributed chromatin. Microvascular proliferation, as seen in glioblastoma, may be identified within or outside areas of hypercellularity (**C**).

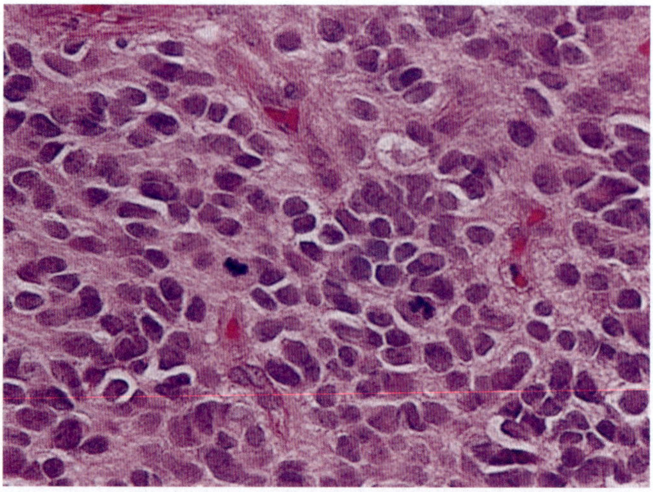

B

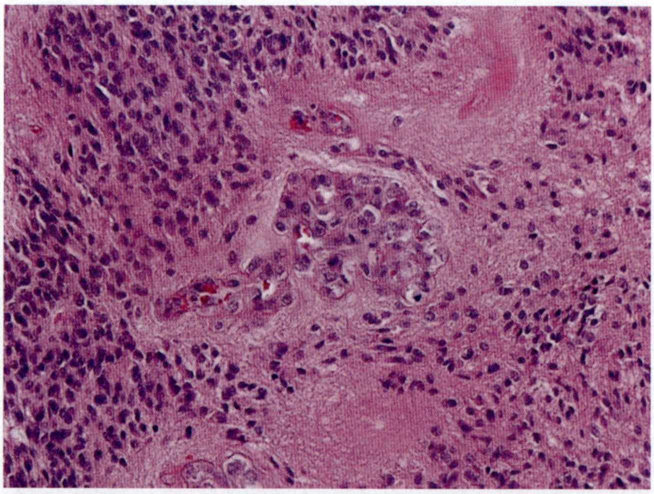

C

pleomorphism with hyperchromatic, coarse chromatin), tumor necrosis, and microvascular proliferation (Figure 4-5C) similar to that found in glioblastoma, within or outside the hypercellular regions.[5,40,41] Geographic tumor necrosis in the absence of other anaplastic features is not diagnostic of malignancy.[5] It bears emphasizing that the current WHO guidelines recommend grading ependymomas based on the predominance of areas with anaplastic features.

Prognostic Factors

There are multiple studies that describe different factors influencing the outcome of patients with ependymomas. The *age at presentation* has generally been accepted as a significant factor affecting outcome, with worse outcomes among children and improved outcomes with increasing age.[41–44] A cutoff of 3 years of age is generally accepted to be associated with worse OS and event-free survivals (EFS), with mean 5-year OS and EFS of 52% and 48%, respectively, for patients older than 3 years of age.[43] However, these findings are still under investigation.[45,46] *Tumor location* has also been identified by as an independent prognostic factor, regardless of the histology of the tumor.[47–49] Some studies have demonstrated supratentorial tumors in adults to have worse OS compared to infratentorial ependymomas.[41,42,49,50] The *extent of resection*, with or without concurrent radiation therapy, is another significant independent prognostic factor, with gross total resections being associated with better 5- and 10-year OS and EFS.[41,42,45,49]

Histologic grading (II vs. III) is also accepted as an independent prognostic factor, although different studies reached varying conclusions regarding the relative importance in conjunction with other clinical prognostic factors. In general, WHO grade II ependymomas are associated with better OS and EFS than anaplastic ependymomas (WHO grade III).[41,43,46,47] In a study exploring location-specific histologic predictors of outcome among 238 cases of ependymoma (excluding subependymoma and myxopapillary ependymoma), hypercellularity, increased mitotic activity (at a cutoff of 5 or more mitoses per 10 high-power fields), microvascular proliferation, and tumor necrosis were identified as significant histologic features associated with worse EFS among posterior fossa ependymomas.[51] However, among supratentorial ependymomas, not all of the same features were associated with worse outcomes. While microvascular proliferation and increased mitotic activity remained significant, hypercellularity and tumor necrosis were not found to be significantly associated with patient outcome. A novel finding was the presence of areas with well-formed ependymal canals being significantly associated with worse outcomes among supratentorial tumors, but not among posterior fossa and spinal cord tumors. Another study also identified the presence of infiltration into the adjacent brain parenchyma as being associated with worse outcomes among supratentorial ependymomas.[52] The presence of focal areas of anaplasia appeared to be associated with worse EFS than WHO grade II, but better outcome than when these areas were predominant. In other words, identifying areas of anaplasia might be indicative of worse patient outcome, irrespective of extent. Among spinal cord ependymomas, no histologic features associated with outcome were identified.[51]

Genetics

Cytogenetic changes in ependymoma have been well investigated. In one study of 86 ependymomas, tumors with balanced cytogenetic profiles were more common among children than in adults (41% compared to 9%, respectively) and were more commonly seen in intracranial ependymoma (32%) compared to spinal ependymoma (3%).[8] Other studies have reported similar proportions of cases with balanced cytogenetic profiles.[53,54] The loss of chromosome 22 was the most common cytogenetic abnormality, being described in about 25% to 26% of cases, more commonly seen in spinal ependymomas, and among WHO grade II ependymomas.[23,54] Gain of chromosomal arm 1q has also been described in 7% to 22% of ependymomas, more commonly found in children, in tumors arising in the posterior fossa, and in cases with anaplastic features.[22,53] The absence of 1q gain has been described to be associated with better OS than ependymomas that harbor chromosome 1q gains.[22] Other cytogenetic abnormalities described among ependymomas include loss of chromosomes 6q,[53] 10q, 12q, and 14q/14, the latter three being more commonly found among spinal cord ependymomas.[22]

Recently, two independent transcriptional profiling studies performed on posterior fossa ependymomas have identified two clinically and molecularly distinct subgroups.[4,55] Tumors belonging to the first subgroup tended to occur more commonly among younger patients, be more laterally located, and had balanced genomes. These ependymomas were found to harbor alterations of various genes related to response to wound healing, inflammation, migration, and cell adhesion and had a gene signature that was similar to the mesenchymal subgroup of glioblastoma. Ependymomas in the second subgroup primarily affected older children and adults, were more centrally located, and showed alterations in genes related to ciliogenesis and oxidative metabolism. Posterior fossa ependymomas in the first subgroup were found to have worse EFS and OS compared to the second. Among infants with posterior fossa ependymomas, a CpG island methylator phenotype has also been described as being associated with poor prognosis.[56] This CpG island methylation leads to silencing of transcription and, by trimethylation of the histone H3K27, decreased expression of differentiation genes.

Novel alterations are also being identified within supratentorial ependymomas. Oncogenic fusion between a principal effector of the canonical NF-kB signaling pathway, called RELA, and *C11orf95*, an as-yet uncharacterized gene, has been described in about two-thirds of supratentorial ependymomas.[57] In mice, the fusion protein activates nuclear NF-kB genes, leading to transformation of neural stem cells to ependymomas.

While these developments are all exciting, the challenge remains in identifying potential therapeutic targets and developing effective treatments against these in ependymomas.

References

1. Duff DJ, Miller DC. Ependymomas. *Pathol Case Rev* 2013;18:1–10.
2. Gilbert MR, Ruda R, Soffietti R. Ependymomas in adults. *Curr Neurol Neurosci Rep* 2010;10:240–247.
3. Rajaram V, Leuthardt E, Singh P, et al. 9p21 and 13q14 dosages in ependymomas: a clinicopathologic study of 101 cases. *Mod Pathol* 2004;17:9–14.
4. Wani K, Armstrong T, Vera-Bolanos E, et al. A prognostic gene expression signature in infratentorial ependymoma. *Acta Neuropathol* 2012;123:727–738.
5. McLendon RE, Schiffer D, Rosenblum MK, et al. Ependymal tumors. In: Louis DN, Ohgaki H, Wiestler OD, et al., eds. *World Health Organization Classification of Tumours of the Central Nervous System*. 4th ed. Lyon, France: International Agency for Research on Cancer; 2007;3:69–79.
6. Dolecek TA, Propp JM, Stroup NE, et al. CBTRUS statistical report: primary brain and central nervous system tumors diagnosed in the United States in 2005–2009. *Neuro Oncol* 2012;14:1–49.
7. Ragel BT, Osborn AG, Whang K, et al. Subependymomas: an analysis of clinical and imaging features. *Neurosurgery* 2006;58:881–890.
8. Prayson RA, Suh JH. Subependymomas: clinicopathologic study of 14 tumors, including comparative MIB-1 immunohistochemical analysis with other ependymal neoplasms. *Arch Pathol Lab Med* 1999;123:306–309.
9. Vogel H. Brain tumors. In: Weiss L, ed. *Nervous System*. 1st ed. New York: Cambridge University Press; 2009;3:122–139.
10. Schiffer D. *Brain Tumor Pathology: Current Diagnostic Hotspots and Pitfalls*. Dordrecht, The Netherlands: Springer; 2006:113–121.
11. Lombardi D, Scheithauer BW, Meyer FB, et al. Symptomatic subependymoma: a clinicopathological and flow cytometric study. *J Neurosurg* 1991;75:583–588.
12. Scheithauer BW. Symptomatic ependymoma: report of 21 cases with review of the literature. *J Neurosurg* 1978;49:689–696.
13. Rosai J. Central nervous system. In: Rosai J, ed. *Rosai and Ackerman's Surgical Pathology*. 10th ed. China: Elsevier Mosby; 2011:2355–2359.
14. Sonneland PR, Scheithauer BW, Onforid BM, et al. Myxopapillary ependymoma: a clinicopathologic and immunocytochemical study of 77 cases. *Cancer* 1985;56:883–893.
15. Sato H, Mizushima M, Ito J, et al. Myxopapillary ependymoma of the lateral ventricle: a study on the mechanism of its stromal myxoid change. *Acta Pathol Jpn* 1983;33:1017–1025.
16. Lim SC, Jang SJ. Case report. Myxopapillary ependymoma of the fourth ventricle. *Clin Neurol Neurosurg* 2006;108:211–214.
17. Warnick RE, et al. Intracranial myxopapillary ependymoma: case report. *J Neurooncol* 1993;15:251–256.
18. Helwig EB, Stern JB. Subcutaneous sacrococcygeal myxopapillary ependymoma: a clinicopathologic study of 32 cases. *Am J Clin Pathol* 1984;81:156–161.
19. Ilhan I, Berberoglu S, Kutluay L, et al. Subcutaneous sacrococcygeal myxopapillary ependymoma. *Med Pediatr Oncol* 1998;30:81–84.
20. Kahan H, Sklar EM, Post M, et al. MR Characteristics of histopathologic subtypes of spinal ependymoma. *AJNR Am J Neuroradiol* 1996;17:143–150.
21. Chan HS, Becker LE, Hoffman HJ, et al. Myxopapillary ependymoma of the filum terminale and cauda equina in childhood: report of seven cases and review of literature. *Neurosurgery* 1984;14:204–210.
22. Carter M, Nicholson J, Ross J, et al. Genetic abnormalities detected in ependymomas by comparative genomic hybridization. *Br J Cancer* 2002;86:929–939.
23. Ebert C, Von Haken M, Meyer-Puttlitz B, et al. Molecular genetic analysis of ependymal tumors NF2 mutations and chromosome 22q loss occur preferentially in intramedullary spinal ependymomas. *Am J Pathol* 1999;155:627–632.
24. Villano JL, Parker CK, Dolecek TA. Descriptive epidemiology of ependymal tumours in the United States. *Br J Cancer* 2013;108:2367–2371.
25. Bell DA, Woodruff JM, Scully RE. Ependymoma of the broad ligament: a report of two cases. *Am J Surg Pathol* 1984;3:203–209.
26. Duggan MA, et al. Ependymoma of the uterosacral ligament. *Cancer* 1989;64:2565–2571.

27. Guerrieri C, Jarlsfelt I. Ependymoma of the ovary: a case report with immunohistochemical, ultrastructural, and DNA cytometric findings, as well as histogenetic considerations. *Am J Surg Pathol* 1993;17:623–632.
28. Kleinman GM, Young RH, Scully RE. Primary neuroectodermal tumors of the ovary: a report of 25 cases. *Am J Surg Pathol* 1993;17:764–778.
29. Hofman V, Isnard V, Chevallier A, et al. Pelvic ependymoma arising from the small bowel. *Pathology* 2001;33:26–29.
30. Webber EM, Fraser RB, Resch L, et al. Perianal ependymoma presenting in the neonatal period. *Pediatr Pathol Lab Med* 1997;17:283–291.
31. Nelson JS, Mena H, Parisi JE, et al. CNS tumors. In: Nelson JS, Mena H, Parisi JE, et al., eds. *Principles and Practice of Neuropathology*. 2nd ed. New York: Oxford University Press; 2003:327–332.
32. Shuangshoti S, Rushing EJ, Mena H, et al. Supratentorial extraventricular ependymal neoplasms: a clinicopathologic study of 32 patients. *Cancer* 2005;103:2598–2605.
33. Ragel BT, Townsend JJ, Arthur AS, et al. Intraventricular tanycytic ependymoma: case report and review of the literature. *J Neurooncol* 2005;71:189–193.
34. Zhang S, Wang X, Zhang Z, et al. Tanycytic ependymoma arising from the right lateral ventricle: a case report and review of the literature. *Neuropathology* 2008;28:427–432.
35. Rodríguez EM, Blazquez JL, Pastor FE, et al. Hypothalamic tanycytes: a key component of brain–endocrine interaction. *Int Rev Cytol* 2005;247:89–164.
36. Park SH, Park HR, Chi JG. Papillary ependymoma: its differential diagnosis from choroid plexus papilloma. *J Korean Med Sci* 1996;11:415–421.
37. Fouladi M, Helton K, Dalton J, et al. Clear cell ependymoma: a clinicopathologic and radiographic analysis of 10 patients. *Cancer* 2003;15:2032–2244.
38. Min KW, Scheithauer BW. Clear cell ependymoma: a mimic of oligodendroglioma: clinicopathologic and ultrastructural considerations. *Am J Surg Pathol* 1997;21:820–826.
39. Adamek D, Dec M, Sobol G, et al. Giant cell ependymoma: a case report. *Clin Neurol Neurosurg* 2008;110:176–181.
40. Merchant TE, Jenkins JJ, Burger PC, et al. Influence of tumor grade on time to progression after irradiation for localized ependymoma in children. *Int J Radiat Oncol Biol Phys* 2002;53:52–57.
41. Korshunov A, Golanov A, Sycheva R, et al. The histologic grade is a main prognostic factor for patients with intracranial ependymomas treated in the microneurosurgical era: an analysis of 258 patients. *Cancer* 2004;100:1230–1237.
42. Mridha AR, Sharma MC, Sarkar C, et al. Anaplastic ependymoma with cartilaginous and osseous metaplasia: report of a rare case and review of literature. *J Neurooncol* 2007;82:75–80.
43. Tihan T, Zhou T, Holmes E, et al. The prognostic value of histological grading of posterior fossa ependymomas in children: a Children's Oncology Group study and a review of prognostic factors. *Mod Pathol* 2008;21:165–177.
44. McGuire C, Sainani KL, Fisher PG. Both location and age predict survival in ependymoma: a SEER study. *Pediatr Blood Cancer* 2009;52:65–69.
45. Kurt E, Zheng P, Hop W, et al. Identification of relevant prognostic histopathologic features in 69 intracranial ependymomas, excluding myxopapillary ependymomas and subependymomas. *Cancer* 2006;106:388–395.
46. Guyotat J, Metellus P, Giorgi R, et al. Infratentorial ependymomas: prognostic factors and outcome analysis in a multi-center retrospective series of 106 adult patients. *Acta Neurochir* 2009;151:947–960.
47. Guyotat J, Signorelli F, Desme S, et al. Intracranial ependymomas in adult patients: analyses of prognostic factors. *J Neurooncol* 2002;60:255–268.
48. Schild SE, Nisi K, Scheithauer BW, et al. The results of radiotherapy for ependymomas: the mayo clinic experience. *Int J Radiat Oncol Biol Phys* 1998;42:953–958.
49. Metellus P, Guyotat J, Chinot O, et al. Adult intracranial WHO grade II ependymomas: long-term outcome and prognostic factor analysis in a series of 114 patients. *Neuro Oncol* 2010;12:976–984.
50. Amirian ES, Armstrong T, Gilbert M, et al. Predictors of survival among older adults with ependymoma. *J Neurooncol* 2012;107:183–189.
51. Raghunathan A, Wani Khalida, Armstrong T, et al. Histological predictors of outcome in ependymoma are dependent on anatomic site within the central nervous system. *Brain Pathol* 2013;23:584–594.
52. Godfraind C, Kaczmarska JM, Kocak M, et al. Distinct disease-risk groups in pediatric supratentorial and posterior fossa ependymomas. *Acta Neuropathol* 2012;124:247–257.

53. Reardon DA, Entrekin RE, Sublett J, et al. Chromosome arm 6q loss is the most common recurrent autosomal alteration detected in primary pediatric ependymoma. *Genes Chromosomes Cancer* 1999;24:230–237.
54. Ward S, Harding B, Wilkins P, et al. Gain of 1q and loss of 22 re the most common changes detected by comparative genomic hybridization in pediatric ependymoma. *Genes Chromosomes Cancer* 2001; 32:59–66.
55. Witt H, Mack SC, Ryzhova M, et al. Delineation of two clinically and molecularly distinct subgroups of posterior fossa ependymoma. *Cancer Cell* 2011;20:143–157.
56. Mack SC, Witt H, Piro RM, et al. Epigenomic alterations define lethal CIMP-positive ependymomas of infancy. *Nature* 2014;506:445–453.
57. Parker M, Mohankumar KM, Punchihewa C, et al. C11orf95–RELA fusions drive oncogenic NF-kB signaling in ependymoma. *Nature* 2014;506:451–465.

Other Neuroepithelial Tumors (Chordoid Glioma, Astroblastoma, Angiocentric Glioma)

5

▶ Abir Mukherjee

CHORDOID GLIOMA

Chordoid glioma is a rare low-grade neoplasm first described as a distinctive clinicopathologic entity by Brat et al.[1] in 1998. An earlier suprasellar tumor described by Wanschiz[2] in 1995 had similar features. Less than 100 cases have been reported in the literature to date, almost all occurring in adults.

The tumor occurs almost exclusively in adults (mean age 46 years; range 35 to 60 years) with a female-to-male ratio of 2:1.[1] Pediatric examples are rare.[3] Almost all cases arise from anterior third ventricle, except rare cases reported in the lateral ventricle and thalamus.[4,5] Clinical features result from obstructive hydrocephalus (nausea and vomiting) and pressure on the optic chiasm (defects in visual acuity and field), hypothalamus (endocrine abnormalities), and medial temporal lobe (memory loss). MRI shows a well-demarcated oval mass in the suprasellar/anterior third ventricular region, with diffuse and uniform contrast enhancement. They are usually hyperintense on T2 and isointense on T1. Histogenesis of this tumor is uncertain, but ultrastructural studies suggest origin from specialized ependymal cells of organum vasculosum in the lamina terminalis.[6] Putative origin from tanycytes has also been suggested.[7]

Intraoperative cytologic smears are typically cellular with background mucinous/myxoid matrix. The neoplastic cells are "biphasic" with a predominant population of epithelioid cells with distinct cell border, forming monolayers. A minor population of "gliofibrillary" cells with coarse cytoplasmic processes is seen (Figure 5-1A). Both the cell types have a central round to oval bland nucleus with finely granular chromatin and inconspicuous nucleoli. Takei et al.[8] has reported frequent binucleation and "Touton"-type giant cells. Lymphocytes and plasma cells are frequently seen in the background. The histology is characterized by cords and clusters of epithelioid cells with moderate amount of eosinophilic cytoplasm and bland nucleus (Figure 5-1B). The mucinous stroma (positive for PAS and Alcian blue) in between the tumor cells show infiltration by lymphocytes and plasma cells (with and without Russell bodies). The tumor is noninfiltrative, with adjacent neural parenchyma showing astrogliosis and presence of rosenthal fibers. Atypical histopathologic features described in the literature include presence of "papillary structures"[9] and chondroid metaplasia.[3] The neoplastic cells are usually strongly immunoreactive to GFAP (Figure 5-1C), vimentin, and CD34. The neoplastic cells have been described variably immunoreactive to cytokeratins, EMA, S100 protein, D2-40, CD99, synaptophysin, and neurofilament protein. The percentages of Ki-67–positive cells are generally low (<5%). Ultrastructural studies have demonstrated presence of intermediate filaments, intracellular lumina, apical microvilli, hemidesmosomes, and focal basal lamina in the tumor cells.[7] Few studies done have suggested a different molecular genetic signature of these tumors from gliomas with no alterations detected in tumor suppressor genes *TP53* and *CDKN2A* nor amplifications in protooncogenes *EGFR, CDK4,* and *MDM2.*[10] Recent array CGH studies have shown loss at several loci including 9p21 and 11q13.[11] Follow-up data are limited by small number

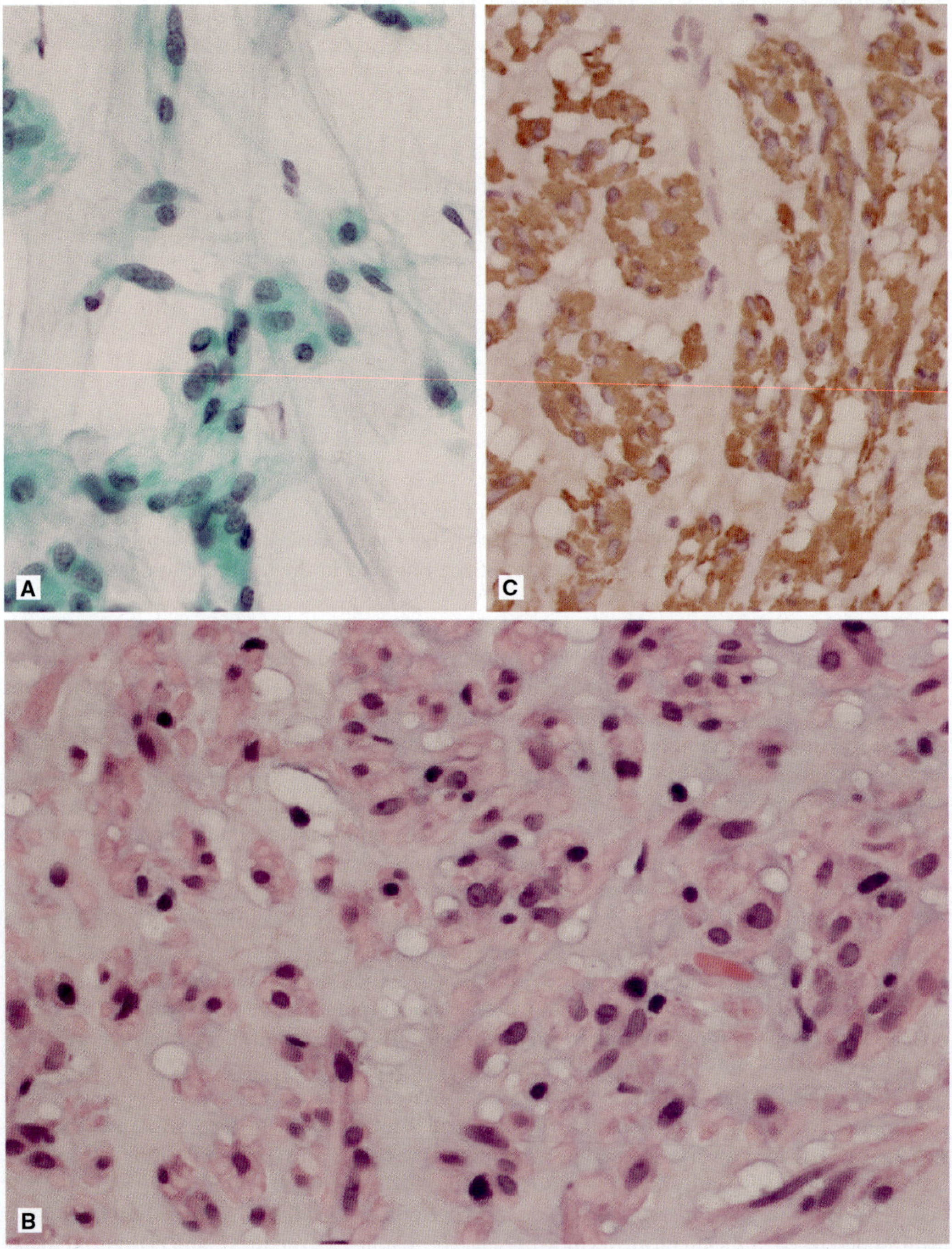

FIGURE 5-1: Chordoid glioma. Cytologic touch imprint showing epithelioid cells as well as few gliofibrillary cells with coarse processes (Papanicolaou stain) (**A**). Histologic section showing cords of epithelioid tumor cells in a myxoid stroma (H&E stain) (**B**). GFAP immunohistochemistry: Tumor cells strongly expressing GFAP (**C**).

of cases, but these tumors are considered as grade II by the WHO with potential for recurrences. Histologic differential diagnosis includes chordoid meningioma (dura based, strongly EMA positive, and GFAP negative) and chordoma (bone invasive, positive for brachyury, and GFAP negative). Multiple modalities have been used in combination for treatment including surgery (gross or subtotal resection), stereotactic radiosurgery, and conventional radiotherapy. Immediate postsurgical morbidity and mortality, especially after gross total resection, is high.[12]

ASTROBLASTOMA

Astroblastoma is a rare and controversial entity first mentioned in 1928 by Bailey and Cushing[13] and further described in 1930 by Bailey and Bucy.[14] The original term encompassed a heterogeneous group of tumors having "astroblastic rosettes." In 1989, Bonnin and Rubenstein[15] published the first large series of pure astroblastomas and discussed histopathologic diagnostic criteria. Little over 100 cases have been reported with scant follow-up data.[16]

The tumor typically occurs in young adults and in the pediatric age group (peak in 21 to 30 years) with female preponderance.[16] The location of this tumor is mostly supratentorial in the frontal lobe, but rare brainstem, cerebellar, and intraventricular examples have been described.[17] Most patients present with nonlocalizing features like nausea and vomiting, suggestive of increased intracranial pressure. Typically, astroblastomas are large, supratentorial, solid and cystic mass with relatively little vasogenic edema. The solid component has a "bubbly" appearance and is contrast enhancing. Punctate calcifications are often present.[18] Astroblastomas are neither of bonafide astrocytic lineages nor are they blastic. Ultrastructural studies in some cases suggest an ependymal lineage, perhaps from tanycytes.[19]

Astroblastoma is a circumscribed tumor with "astroblastic pseudorosettes," prominent perivascular hyalinization, and lack of fibrillarity. Astroblastic pseudo rosettes are formed by spindle or columnar cells extending stout short processes up to the blood vessels (Figure 5-2A). The cross-section of the rosettes has a "cartwheel"-like radiating appearance, and longitudinal sections are ribbon-like. Similar structures have been described in a variety of infiltrating tumors, causing considerable confusion. In addition to theses rosettes, astroblastomas show very limited infiltration into adjacent brain tissue and often have prominent perivascular hyalinization (Figure 5-2B). They can have focally papillary architecture. Some case reports describe rhabdoid and signet ring cells.[20] Microcalcifications are not unusual. A minor subset of these cases show areas of brisk mitotic activity (>5/10 HPF), pseudopalisading necrosis, and microvascular proliferation and are regarded as high grade.[21] Of note, due to paucity of follow-up data, the WHO has declined to grade this tumor, but conventionally they are graded in to high and low grade based on the features described above. The neoplastic cells are strongly immunoreactive to GFAP (Figure 5-2C), vimentin, and S100 protein and are negative for neuronal markers. They can be focally immunoreactive to EMA (paranuclear "dot-like" pattern) and cytokeratins, just like ependymoma. INI-1 immunoexpression is retained. Ki-67 labeling is variable (depending on grade). Ultrastructural studies show presence of intermediate filaments and intracellular lumens with microvillus processes and surface microvillus processes. Comparative genomic hybridization has shown gains of 20q and 19.[22] Recent studies have shown lack of *IDH1/2* and *p53* mutation.[19] The main differential diagnosis is ependymoma, and there is considerable overlap of immunomorphologic features. However, lack of fibrillarity and prominent perivascular hyalization are two distinct features of astroblastoma. Most cases have been treated with gross total resection, and limited follow-up data suggest even the high-grade tumors have favorable prognosis.[16]

ANGIOCENTRIC GLIOMA

Angiocentric glioma is a low-grade, epilepsy-associated tumor, first described in 2005 by two groups independently and codified by the WHO in 2007.[23,24] Since then, over 50 cases has been reported.

The tumor typically occurs in children and young adults (median age 17 years), with no gender predilection.[25] The tumor is cerebrocortical in location, involving, the frontal, temporoparietal, and occipital lobes in order of frequency. Rare locations include the midbrain.[26] All patients have history of intractable partial/complex epilepsy. MRI shows a T2 hyperintense, nonenhancing lesion with minimal mass effect. A stalk-like extension toward the ventricle is characteristic.[24] Ultrastructural studies show ependymal differentiation, and origin from radial glia has been proposed.[24]

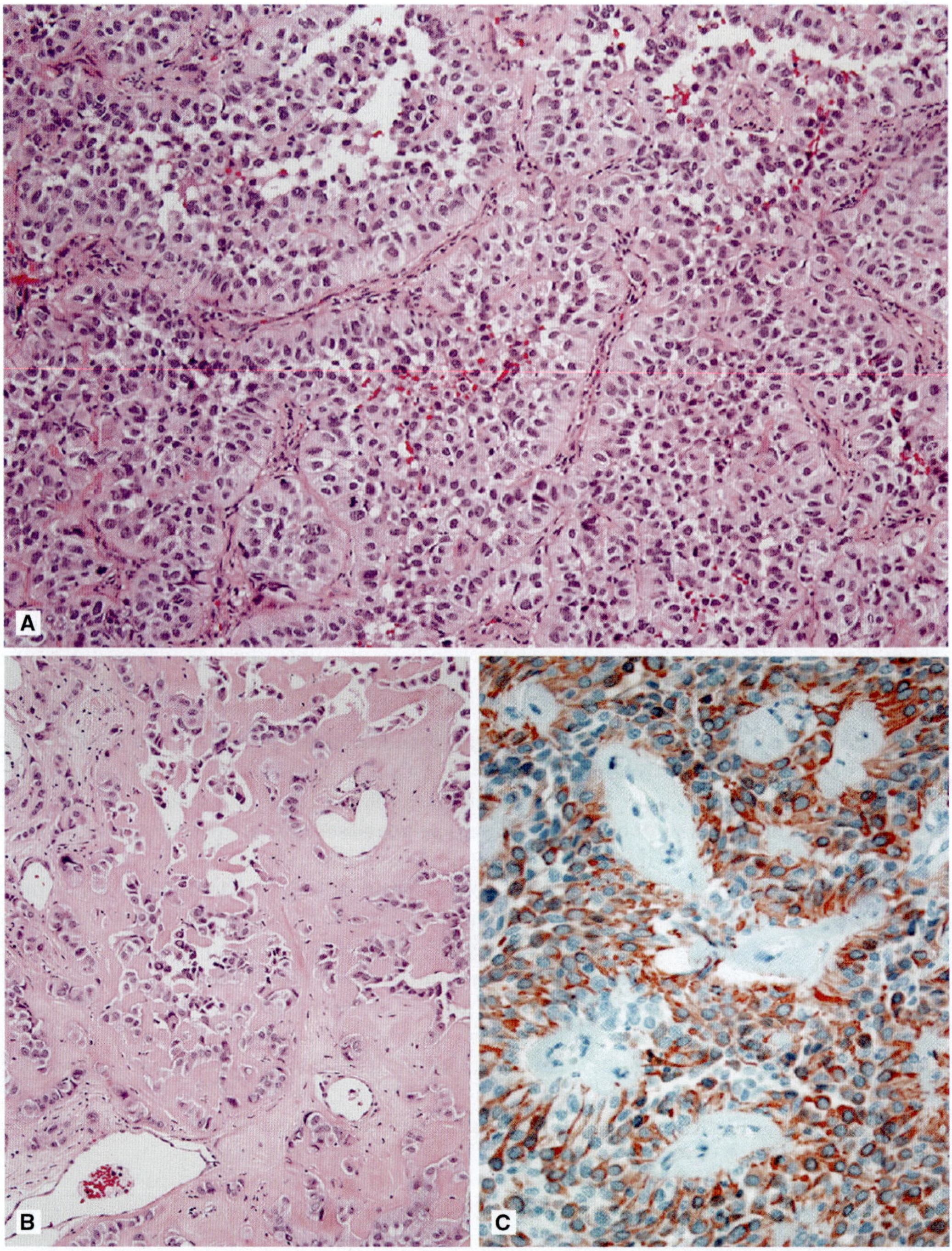

FIGURE 5-2: Astroblastoma. Tumor cells forming "astroblastic pseudorosettes" by extending stout short processes upto blood vessels (H&E stain) (**A**). Tumor cells with prominent perivascular hyalinization (H&E stain) (**B**). GFAP immunohistochemistry: Tumor cells with diffuse and strong positivity to GFAP (**C**). (Photos: Courtesy of Gregory Fuller, MD, PhD, MD Anderson Cancer Center, Texas.)

Cytologic preparations show monomorphic bland, bipolar cells with angiotropism (Figure 5-3A). Angiocentric glioma is an infiltrating tumor with variable cell density marked by condensation of the tumor cells around blood vessels of all calibers (Figure 5-3B). The neoplastic cells can be oriented parallel or radial to the blood vessels. In later case, they may resemble ependymal or astroblastic pseudorosettes. The neoplastic cells may also orient

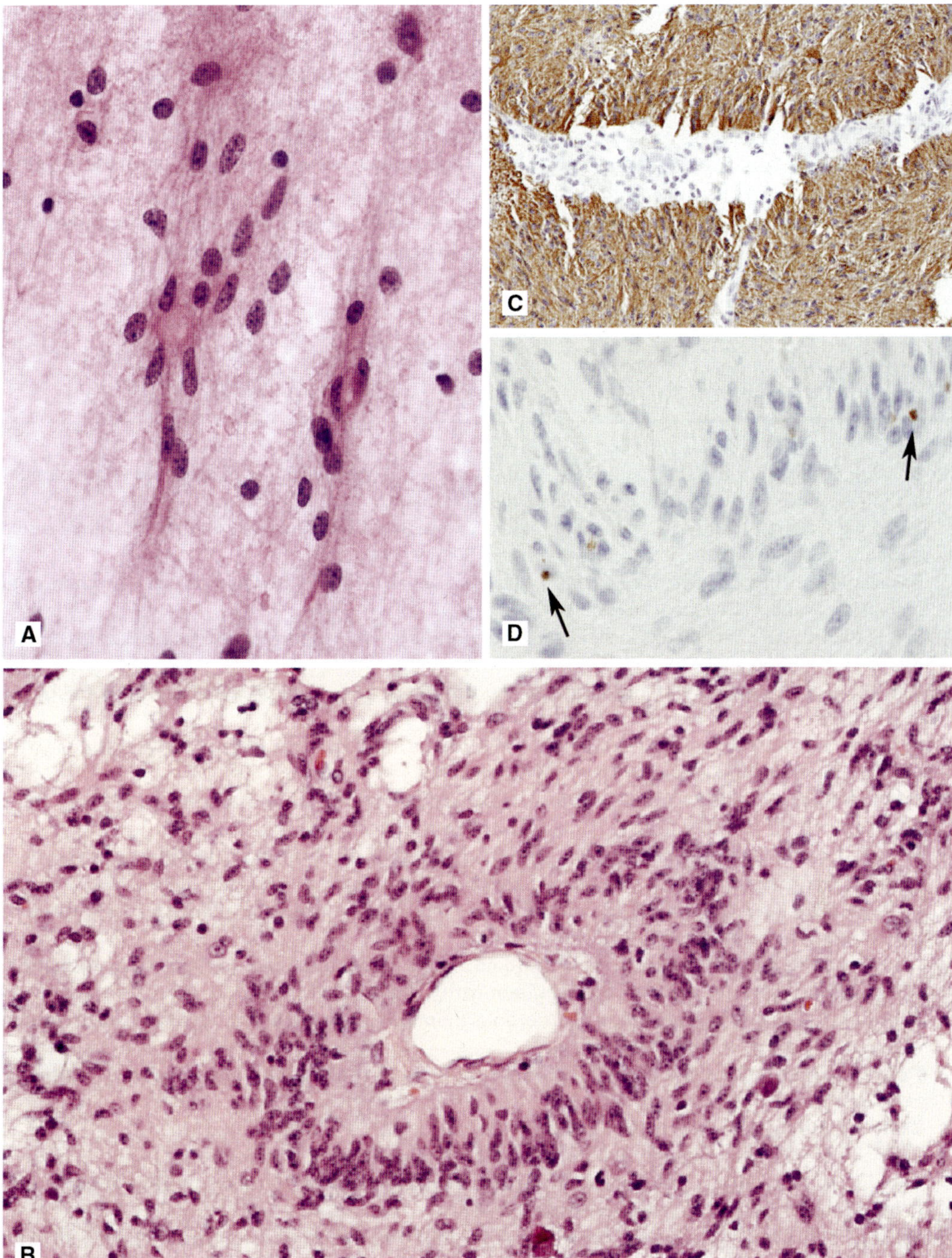

FIGURE 5-3: Angiocentric glioma. Cytologic preparation showing bland monomorphous bipolar neoplastic cells with vesicular chromatin (H&E stain) (**A**). Histologic section showing condensation of tumor cells around blood vessels, with most tumor cells oriented radially (H&E stain) (**B**). GFAP immunohistochemistry: Tumor cells show strong and diffuse expression of GFAP (**C**). EMA immunohistochemistry: Paranuclear "dot-like" immunoreactivity to EMA (*arrows*) (**D**).

perpendicular to the pial surface, creating a palisading appearance. Sometimes, the tumor cells can form compact areas resembling schwannoma. Some cells can show a paranuclear eosinophilic structure that correspond to "microlumens" highlighted by EMA immunostain. Some example show plumper epithelioid cells. Calcifications are uncommon. Rare examples can show high-grade anaplastic areas resembling glioblastoma.[27] The neoplastic cells are strongly immunoreactive to GFAP (Figure 5-3C) and vimentin. EMA shows paranuclear "dot-like," reactivity like ependymoma (Figure 5-3D). Neuronal markers, p53 and IDH-1, are negative. Rare examples can show high Ki-67 and PHH-3 labeling, but prognosis remains unchanged.[28] CGH has shown loss of 6q24-q25 in one tumor and gain of 11p11.2 in another (site of protein tyrosine phosphatase receptor J).[25] These tumors do not have *IDH-1* or *BRAFV* 600E mutations.[29,30] The WHO has codified this tumor as grade I. Differential diagnosis includes ependymoma and astroblastoma, which are circumscribed tumors. Pilocytic astrocytoma and pilomyxoid astrocytoma can also have bland bipolar cells but are circumscribed tumors without prominent angiotropism. Gross total resection is usually curative.

References

1. Brat DJ, Scheithauer BW, Staugaitis SM, et al. Third ventricular chordoid glioma: a distinct clinicopathologic entity. *J Neuropathol Exp Neurol* 1998;57:283–290.
2. Wanschiz J, Schmidbaur M, Maier H. Suprasellar meningioma with expression of glial fibrillary acidic protein: a peculiar variant. *Acta Neuropathol* 1995;90:539–544.
3. Castellano-Sanchez AA, Schemankewiitz E, Mazeski C, et al. Pediatric chordoid glioma with chondroid metaplasia. *Pediatr Dev Pathol* 2001;4:564–567.
4. Jain D, Sharma MC, Sarkar C. Chordoid glioma: report of two rare examples with unusual features. *Acta Neurochir* 2008;150:295–300.
5. Kim JM, Kim JH, Kim CY. Chordoid glioma: a case report of unusual location and neuroradiologic characteristics. *J Korean Neurosurg Soc* 2010;48:62–65.
6. Kawasaki K, Kohno M, Inenaga C. Chordoid glioma of the third ventricle: a report of two cases, one with ultrastructural findings. *Neuropathology* 2009;29:85–90.
7. Sato K, Kubota T, Ishida M. Immunohistochemical and ultrastructural study of chordoid glioma of the third ventricle: its tanycytic differentiation. *Acta Neuropathol* 2003;106:176–180.
8. Takei H, Bhattacharjee MB, Adesina AM. Chordoid glioma of the third ventricle: report of a case with cytologic features and utility during Intraoperative consultation. *Acta Cytol* 2006;50:691–696.
9. Ni H, Pio Y, Lu D, et al. Chordoid glioma of the third ventricle: four cases including one case with papillary features. *Neuropathology* 2013;33:134–139.
10. Reifenberger G, Weber T, Weber R, et al. Chordoid glioma of the third ventricle: immunohistochemical and molecular characterization of a novel tumor entity. *Brain Pathol* 1999;9:617–626.
11. Horbinski C, Dacic S, Mclendon R, et al. Chordoid glioma: a case report and molecular characterization of 5 cases. *Brain Pathol* 2009;19:439–448.
12. DeSouza R, Bodi I, Thomas N, et al. Chordoid glioma: ten years of a low grade tumor with high morbidity. *Skull Base* 2010;20:125–138.
13. Bailey P, Cushing H. *Tumors of the Glioma Group*. Philadelphia, PA: Lippincott; 1924.
14. Bailey P, Bucy PC. Astroblastomas of the brain. *Acta Psychiatr Neurol* 1930;5:439–461.
15. Bonnin JM, Rubinstein LJ. Astroblastomas: a pathological study of 23 tumors with a postoperative follow up in 13 patients. *Neurosurgery* 1989;25:6–13.
16. Saghrue ME, Choi J, Rutkowski MJ. Clinical features and postsurgical outcomes of patient with Astroblastomas. *J Clin Neurosci* 2011;18:750–754.
17. Denaro L, Gardiman M, Calderone M, et al. Intraventricular astroblastoma: case report. *J Neurosurg Pediatr* 2008;1:152–155.
18. Port J, Brat DJ, Burger PC, et al. Astroblastoma: radio-pathological correlation and distinction from ependymoma. *AJNR Am J Neuroradiol* 2002;23:243–247.
19. Fu Y, Taniguchi Y, Takeuchi Y, et al. Cerebral astroblastoma in an adult: an immunohistochemical, ultrastructural and genetic study. *Neuropathology* 2013;33:312–319.
20. Nasit JG, Trivedi P. Recurrent low–grade astroblastoma with signet ring like cells and high proliferation index. *Fetal Pediatr Pathol* 2013;32:284–292.
21. Thiessen B, Finlay J, Kulkarni R, et al. Astroblastoma: does histology predict biologic behavior? *J Neurooncol* 1998;40:59–65.

22. Brat DJ, Hirose Y, Cohen KJ, et al. Astroblastoma: clinicopathologic features and chromosomal abnormalities defined by comparative genomic hybridization. *Brain Pathol* 2000;10:342–352.
23. Wang M, Tihan T, Rojiani AM, et al. Monomorphous angiocentric glioma: a distinctive epileptogenic neoplasm with features of infiltrating astrocytoma and ependymoma. *J Neuropathol Exp Neurol* 2005;64:875–881.
24. Lellouch-Tubiana A, Boddaert N, Bourgeois M, et al. Angiocentric neuroepithelial tumor (ANET): a new epilepsy related clinicopathologic entity with distinct MRI. *Brain Pathol* 2005;15:281–286.
25. Preusser M, Hoischen A, Novak K, et al. Angiocentric glioma: report of clinico-pathologic and genetic findings in 8 cases. *Am J Surg Pathol* 2007;31:1709–1718.
26. Covington DD, Rosenblum MK, Brathwaite CD, et al. Angiocentric glioma like tumor of the midbrain. *Pediatr Neurosurg* 2009;45(6):429–433.
27. Lu JQ, Patel S, Wilson BA, et al. Malignant glioma with angiocentric features. *J Neurosurg Pediatr* 2013;11:350–355.
28. Li JY, Langford LA, Adesina A, et al. The high mitotic count detected by phosphor-histone H3 immunostain does not alter the benign behavior of angiocentric glioma. *Brain Tumor Pathol* 2012;29:68–72.
29. Raghunathan A, Olar A, Vogel H, et al. Isocitrate dehydrogenase 1 R132H mutation is not detected in angiocentric glioma. *Ann Diagn Pathol* 2012;16:255–259.
30. Buccoliero AM, Castiglione F, Deglinnocenti DR, et al. Angiocentric glioma: clinical, morphological, immunohistochemical and molecular features in three pediatric cases. *Clin Neuropathol* 2013;32:107–113.

6 Neuronal/Mixed Glioneuronal Tumors

Takashi Komori

OVERVIEW

Neuronal/mixed glioneuronal tumors are benign neuroepithelial tumors composed of mature neurons and glia.[1] Since pure neuronal tumors are usually accompanied by glial cells, and it is that are often difficult to determine whether they are a component of the tumor or reactive glia, neuronal tumors are classified in the same category. In the 1st edition of the World Health Organization (WHO) Classification of Tumors of the central nervous system (CNS), only six tumors, that is, gangliocytoma, ganglioglioma, ganglioneuroblastoma, anaplastic gangliocytoma and ganglioglioma, and neuroblastoma, were included within this category.[2] Ganglioneuroblastoma and neuroblastoma were reassigned to CNS primitive neuroectodermal tumors in the second WHO Classification.[3] With the development of electron microscopy and immunohistochemistry, new entities such as central neurocytoma have been identified in the past two decades. Furthermore, it became evident that even infiltrating gliomas occasionally exhibit neuronal differentiation. Nonetheless, such tumors have identical biologic behaviors and genetic signatures to those of their counterparts lacking neuronal differentiation, and thus, they are not included into this tumor category.

The current WHO Classification recognizes 12 tumor types.[1] Among those 12 tumors, paraganglioma of the film terminale is histologically identical to paraganglioma in the other anatomic sites, such as carotid body paraganglioma (chemodectoma), and thus, it is practically treated as a heterotopic tumor. It is rational to categorize these tumors into three subgroups based on their major constituents (Table 6-1).

The neuronal component can be divided into two categories: ganglion cells and small neurocytes. The cells of intermediate size between ganglion cells and small neurocytes are referred to as ganglioid cells, but they are essentially small ganglion cells. Ganglion cells share common features with large cortical neurons, whose features include single, prominent nucleoli and broad cytoplasm with Nissl substance, but are architecturally disorganized. They are abnormally clustered, have lost polarity, and are often swollen and vacuolated, with the nuclei being abnormally displaced. Neurocytes are mature small neurons; their nuclei are uniform in size and shape, have finely speckled chromatin, and are often surrounded by a perinuclear halo. Those features strikingly resemble to the appearance of oligodendroglioma. To confirm the neuronal nature of such cells, immunohistochemical analyses using neuronal markers are essential.

For the proper diagnosis of glioneuronal tumors, the most crucial step is the discrimination of neoplastic and/or hamartomatous neuronal cells from background entrapped neurons. When infiltrating glioma cells permeate into the cerebral parenchyma, the preexisting neurons in the background may show atypia, may lose polarity, and may look like ganglion or ganglioid cells. However, they maintain a laminar arrangement and uniformity in size. The presence of binucleation may help to identify abnormal neurons, but this is a rare feature and can also occur in maldevelopmental lesions, such as cortical dysplasia.

Immunohistochemistry is indispensable in identifying the neuronal and neoplastic nature of given abnormal cells. To distinguish entrapped neurons from truly neoplastic and/or

Table 6-1 Neuronal and Mixed Glioneuronal Tumors

	Major Constituents: Neuronal/Glial Components	Other Features	Genetics
Gangliocytoma and ganglioglioma	Ganglion cells/reactive or differentiated astrocytes, often pilocytic	Lymphocytic infiltrate, EGBs, CD34 (+) cells	*BRAF*^{V600E} mt in ganglioglioma
DIA and DIG	Ganglion cells (DIG)/elongated astrocytes	Superficial localization., fibroblasts in collagen-rich matrix, reticulin deposition	
Lhermitte-Duclos	Ganglion cells/absent	Enlargement of cerebellar folia, abnormal myelination in the molecular layer	*PTEN* mt
Central NC	Neurocytes/absent	Nucleus-free islands of neuropil	
Extraventricular NC	Neurocytes and occasional ganglion cells/variable differentiated astrocytes	Atypical features including brisk mitoses, vascular proliferation, and necrosis	1p/19q codeletion in limited cases
Cerebellar lipo-NC	Neurocytes/absent	Focal lipomatous differentiation	
PGNT	Neurocytic and ganglioid cells/astrocytic vascular papillae	Vascular hyalinization	*SLC44A1-PRKCA* fusion
RGNT	Neurocytic rosettes and differentiated astrocytes resembling pilocytic astrocytoma, often microcystic component dominant	Fourth ventricle and cerebellum	*FGFR1* mt in limited cases
DNT	Medium-sized, floating neurons/OLC ("specific glioneuronal element") in the simple form	Cerebral cortical localization, nodularity, variable differentiated astrocytes, diffuse or pilocytic, in the complex form	*BRAF*^{V600E} mt in the complex form

EGBs, eosinophilic granular bodies; mt, mutation; DIA, desmoplastic infantile astrocytoma; DIG, desmoplastic infantile ganglioglioma; NC, neurocytoma; PGNT, papillary glioneuronal tumor; RGNT, rosette-forming glioneuronal tumor; DNT, dysembryoplastic neuroepithelial tumor; OLC, oligodendroglia-like cells.

hamartomatous ones, chromogranin A cytoplasmic immunoreactivity is supportive,[4] although it is not sensitive. Chromogranin A staining is generally negative for the normal cortical neurons, but positive for some of normal neurons in the subcortical gray matter, such as the hypothalamus. The epiperikaryal immunoreactivity of synaptophysin, the major synaptic vesicle protein p38, is helpful to distinguish neoplastic neurons from background neurons in the cerebral cortex,[5] but it is not applicable in the subcortical gray matter and the posterior horn of the spinal cord where normal neurons show the epiperikaryal immunoreactivity. Cytoplasmic staining for synaptophysin is also common in ganglioglioma, but such staining, including that in Golgi areas, can be an artifact. Pretreatment with heat often causes a false-positive reaction for synaptophysin.

Neurofilament proteins (NFPs) are positive findings for ganglion cells, as well as normal neurons, but positivity for NFP heavily depends on the antibody applied. A commonly used antibody that reacts with the 70-kDa subunit of NFP does not always label the ganglion cells in gangliocytoma and ganglioglioma. The neuronal nuclear protein, NeuN, is generally positive in mature and normal neurons, but often negative in neoplastic neuronal cells. Microtubule-associated protein-2 (MAP-2) and class III beta tubulin can be nonspecific. Ganglion cells and ganglioid cells are generally positive for all of the neuronal markers mentioned, but neurocytes are generally negative for chromogranin A and NFP. The immunoreactivity for synaptophysin in neurocytes is not present in the cell bodies, which causes difficulty into distinguishing neoplastic immunoreactivity from that of the background neuropil.

On electron microscopy, ganglion cells are characterized by their euchromatic nuclei and broad cytoplasm, with well-developed Golgi apparatus and stacked rough endoplasmic reticulum.[6] Lamellar mitochondria and free ribosomes are also abundant. The intermediate filaments and microtubules are generally scattered, whereas dense core granules (DCGs), ranging from 100 to 230 nm in diameter, are rich in both cell bodies and neurites. DCGs are not present in normal cortical neurons, but they can be sometimes difficult to distinguish from lysosomes. Synaptic attachment on cell bodies and/or neurites is the most reliable finding of neuronal differentiation, but these are rare and often difficult to distinguish from those on the normal neurites. Astrocytic tumor cells are poor in intracytoplasmic organelles, but are rich in bundles of intermediate filaments. The cell bodies are covered by basal lamina where they face to the extracellular matrix. Neoplastic neurocytes, which are considered to imitate granular cells that are normally present in the internal granular layer of the cerebellum, generally form synapses on the cytoplasmic processes, but not on the cell bodies. This is why neurocytomas tend to lack membranous immunoreactivity for synaptophysin. Neurocytes also often lack DCGs and thus lack reactivity for chromogranin A. Neurofilaments are generally scant in the cytoplasm of the neurocytes, which is the explanation for their poor reaction to NFP.

Neuronal and mixed neuronal and glial tumors do not harbor the isocitrate dehydrogenase (*IDH*) mutations that are common in diffuse gliomas,[7,8] whereas some tumors do have mutations in *BRAF*,[9] mutation whose protein that is part of a signaling pathway known as the RAS/MAPK pathway.

Gangliocytoma and Ganglioglioma

Gangliocytoma and ganglioglioma are indolent neoplasms consisting of mature but dysplastic ganglion cells, either alone (gangliocytoma) or with a well-differentiated glial component.[1] Because the distinction of neoplastic glia from reactive glia is not always clear, an umbrella term "ganglion cell tumors" may be applied.[10]

Both conditions predominately affect children and young adults and are common in the cerebral hemispheres, with a strong preference for the temporal lobe (60% to 70%).[11] Chronic and intractable epilepsies are major symptoms.[12] On imaging studies, these conditions often have a cyst–mural nodule configuration, whose nodule is diffusely enhancing.[13,14] Peritumoral edema and mass effects are rare.

The histologic appearance of ganglioglioma varies case by case (Figure 6-1A and B), since both glial and neuronal components have variable histologic architectures, and the secondary features such as inflammation (Figure 6-1A), degenerative changes such as hyaline droplets/eosinophilic granular bodies (EGBs) (Figure 6-1C), and desmoplasia are also quite heterogeneous. Therefore, a key to the proper diagnosis of ganglioglioma is precise identification of ganglion cells, based on their microscopic findings mentioned above. The distribution of ganglion cells is often uneven and can be very focal, which may cause a diagnostic challenge. The differential

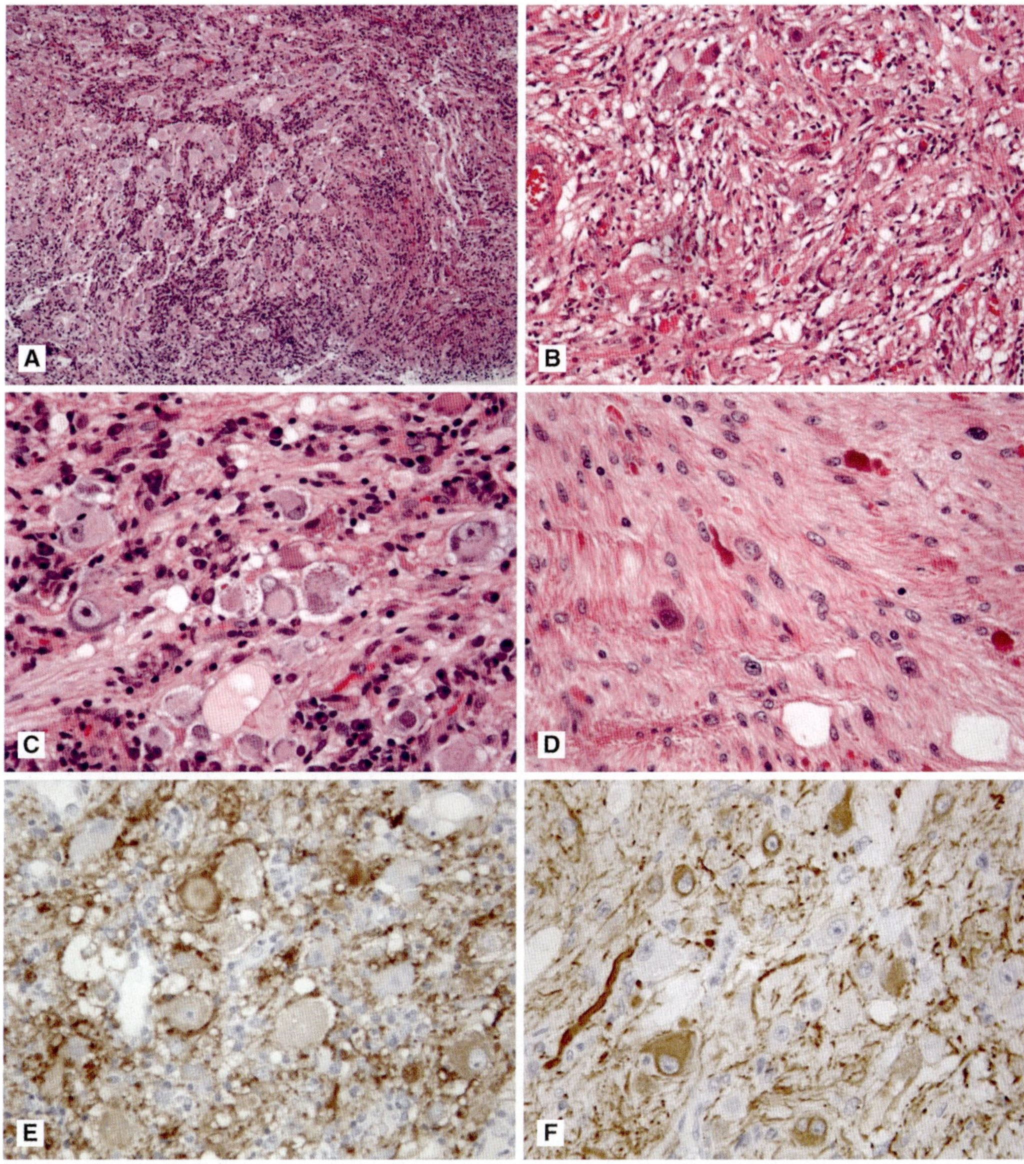

FIGURE 6-1: Ganglioglioma. Ganglioglioma showing a slightly lobular architecture and lymphocytic infiltrates (**A**). Fascicular or storiform fibrous stroma is common (**B**). The neurons are not obvious. Dysplastic ganglion cells exhibiting a prominent nucleolus, peripherally displaced heavy Nissl substance, and vacuolated cytoplasm in the fascicular background with abundant inflammatory cells (**C**). The astrocytic component often resembles pilocytic astrocytoma. Rosenthal fibers are present in such areas (**D**). Synaptophysin immunoreactivity is most prominent in the cell membrane (epiperikaryal immunoreactivity) although some neurons show cytoplasmic staining (**E**). Not all of the ganglion cells are positive for the antibody against 70-kD NFP, whereas the axons in the background are strongly positive (**F**).

diagnoses include pilocytic astrocytoma, pleomorphic xanthoastrocytoma (PXA), and diffuse astrocytoma. The absence of the *KIAA1549–BRAF* fusion and *IDH* mutation can distinguish either pilocytic astrocytoma or diffuse astrocytoma.[15] A neurocytic component is rare and is present in fewer than 5% of cases.[16] A glial component is generally astrocytic, low-grade fibrillary, stellate, or pilocytic in appearance (Figure 6-1D). Oligodendroglia-like cells (OLCs) are common but limited.[6,16] When an oligodendroglioma-like component is predominate, a molecular assessment is required to distinguish such examples from oligodendrogliomas with a ganglioglioma-like component.[17] Accompanying microscopic features such as lymphocyte cuffing and granular bodies

(Figure 6-1C) can be subtle, but are consistent and diagnostically useful features. Ganglioglioma may show some distinctive architectural features, including a lobular pattern (Figure 6-1A), a loose fascicular pattern (Figure 6-1B), and/or a microcyst-rich pattern.[10] Desmoplasia is also common in ganglioglioma, particularly in cases that involve the subarachnoid space. The involvement of the subarachnoid space is a common feature of glioneuronal tumors and does not indicate aggressive biology.

The immunohistochemical findings of the neuronal and glial components are essentially identical to those of the normal counterparts (Figure 6-1E and F), as mentioned previously. Again, discrimination of falsely positive reactions and normal reactions of entrapped neurons is the key for obtaining a proper diagnosis. Immunohistochemistry for CD34, one of the progenitor cell markers, highlights aberrant expression in star-shaped cells. CD34-positive cells are often identified in the periphery of the lesions.[11] Although CD34 expression is relatively specific for ganglioglioma and is rare and limited in other glioneuronal tumors, its significance is unclear. Mitotic activities, microvascular proliferation, and necrosis in the glial component are absent or limited. The Ki-67 labeling index ranges from 1.1% to 2.7%.[6,18,19]

Long-term tumor control can be achieved by total surgical resection alone in more than 80% of the patients,[20] and malignant transformation is considered to be extremely rare, although the true recurrence rate and prognosis of ganglioglioma are difficult to determine given the slow-growing nature of the tumor. Some data have suggested that conventional criteria used for grading of astrocytomas do not correlate well to the outcome of patients with ganglioglioma and the criteria for atypical or anaplastic ganglioglioma, which occasionally shows anaplastic features not only in the glial component but also in the neuronal component, have yet to be established.[21,22] One paper demonstrated that the histopathologic features associated with a shorter recurrence-free survival included an absence of oligodendroglial morphology, a higher glial cell density, microvascular proliferation, and the presence of a high lymphoplasmacytic inflammatory infiltrate.[23] This paper also suggested that *BRAFV600E* mutations are a negative prognostic factor in pediatric ganglioglioma.[23]

A subset of gangliogliomas (21%) possesses the *BRAFV600E* mutation, whereas no gangliocytomas possess this mutation.[9] PXA, low-grade localized astrocytoma that often shows neuronal differentiation and overlapping clinical as well as histologic features, harbors the *BRAFV600E* mutations in about 60% of cases.[9] This molecular link between ganglioglioma and PXA suggests the possibility of a shared molecular pathogenesis.

A recently described, rare variant of ganglion cell tumors is "multinodular and vacuolating neuronal tumors of the cerebrum."[24] This is a nonneurocytic, purely neuronal tumor affecting the adult cerebral hemispheres. Microscopically, the tumor cells were largely distributed into discrete and coalescent nodules exhibiting varying degrees of matrix vacuolization, principally within the deep cortical ribbon and superficial subcortical white matter. The populating elements ranged from morphologically ambiguous to recognizably neuronal, with only two cases manifesting overt ganglion cell cytology. Follow-up data indicated that this unusual neuronal lesion behaves in a benign manner and is amenable to surgical control.

Desmoplastic Infantile Astrocytoma and Ganglioglioma

Desmoplastic infantile astrocytoma (DIA) and desmoplastic infantile ganglioglioma (DIG) are large cystic tumors involving the superficial cerebral cortex and leptomeninges.[1] DIA and DIG are separately described entities,[25–27] but since the clinical, biologic, and histologic features are highly overlapping, except for the presence and absence of neurons, they have been categorized together. DIA is solely composed of astrocytes, whereas DIG is composed of both astrocytes and neurons.

The majority of the DIA and DIG patients present within the first year of life.[25] There is a male–female ratio of about 1.5:1. An increasing head circumference, tense fontanels, and lethargy are common clinical manifestations. DIA/DIG arises in the supratentorial region, preferentially involving the frontoparietal lobes. They are commonly superficial, multiloculated, and massive, often attaching to the dura with contrast enhancement. The signal intensities of the

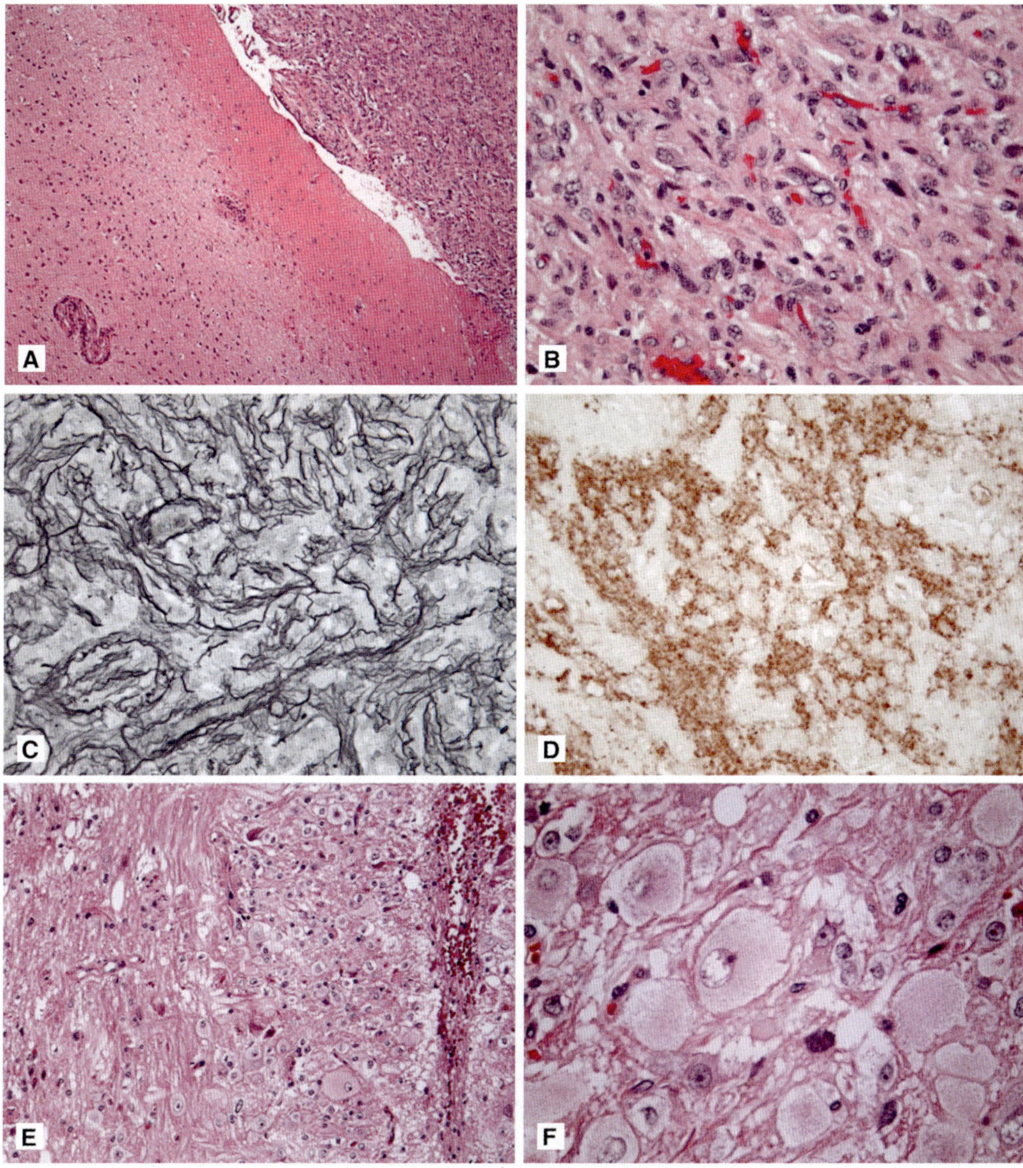

FIGURE 6-2: Desmoplastic infantile ganglioglioma (DIG) Lhermitte-Duclos disease (LDD). DIG occupying the leptomeningeal space (*right upper corner*). Note that tumor cells extend along Virchow-Robin space (*left lower corner*) (**A**). Spindle-shaped astrocytes and fibroblasts arrange in fascicular pattern. Neuronal differentiation is not readily appreciable. Marked deposition of reticulin fibers surrounding the nests of tumor cells is evident in silver impregnation staining (**B**). Synaptophysin immunohistochemistry highlights the surface positivity in the small neurons (**C**). Replacement of the Purkinje cell and the granular cell layers by dysplastic large ganglion as well as ganglioid cells in the cerebellum of LDD. Note the abnormal myelinated axons running in parallel to the pia surface (*left half*) (**D**). The dysplastic ganglion and ganglioid cells in LDD resemble Purkinje cells and granular cells, respectively (**E**). Clusters of dysplastic ganglion cells showing swollen cytoplasm. They have morphologic similarity to gangliocytomas (**F**).

solid components are heterogeneous in T2-weighted and FLAIR images.[28] The mass effect may be strong, but edema is generally mild. Erosion of the inner table of the skull, which suggests the lesions are long-standing, is common.

The bulk of the tumor cells are located in the leptomeningeal spaces (Figure 6-2A), where spindle-shaped astrocytes and fibroblasts are arranged in a fascicular or storiform pattern (Figure 6-2B). Silver impregnation shows marked deposition of reticulin fibers surrounding the tumor cells (Figure 6-2C). Those features give a mesenchymal appearance. The neuronal cells are often inconspicuous, ranging from small polygonal cells to atypical ganglionic cells, and require immunohistochemical studies to confirm their neuronal nature (Figure 6-2D). In the underlying cortex where tumor cells extend along the Virchow-Robin space, DIA/DIG shows a rather diffuse appearance. In such areas, small astrocytic, oligodendroglia-like, or immature-looking neuroepithelial cells with hypercellularity are often present. Mitotic activity and necrosis are uncommon. Neoplastic astrocytes are positive for GFAP and S100 protein, whereas fibroblasts are negative for such glial antigens, but are positive for vimentin. The neuronal component is consistently positive for synaptophysin and class III beta tubulin, but there is variable expression of other neuronal markers. OLCs are Olig2 positive. The Ki-67 index is quite low, but may be high in the immature-looking components. The prognosis is generally favorable with resection alone,[29] but unrespectable cases can be fatal.[30] The presence of immature-looking neuroepithelial cells and anaplastic features do not appear to correlate with a worse prognosis.

Mesenchymal neoplasms affecting the superficial cerebrum including fibroblastic meningioma and fibrohistiocytic tumors would be primary differential diagnoses. Nonetheless, they do not contain the neuroepithelial constituents that are identified by immunohistochemistry for GFAP and other neuroepithelial markers. Distinction between DIA and "gliofibroma" that is a poorly characterized and controversial entity may be problematic.[31,32] Reported gliofibromas do not have the typical localization and clinical findings of DIA/DIG. Although DIA/DIG shares some clinical and pathologic features with ganglioglioma and PXA, the *BRAFV600E* mutation is rare.[33] A recent genome-wide DNA copy number analysis failed to clearly separate the DIA and DIG according to their molecular profiles and suggested that these two represent a histologic spectrum of the same tumor rather than two separate entities.[34]

Dysplastic Gangliocytoma of the Cerebellum (Lhermitte-Duclos Disease)

The dysplastic gangliocytoma of the cerebellum is a benign cerebellar mass composed of dysplastic ganglion cells. It is commonly called Lhermitte-Duclos disease (LDD) and is a component of Cowden syndrome. LDD corresponds to WHO grade I.[1]

Most LDD patients are identified in middle age. The symptoms are related to cerebellar dysfunction and obstructive hydrocephalus.[35] LDD can be an initial clinical presentation of Cowden disease.[36] The cerebellar lesions are curable by resection alone, but it may regrow after resection. MRI typically demonstrates a unilateral nonenhancing zone of hemispheric expansion where parallel linear stripes are present.[37] Such striation is considered to represent thickening of the cerebellar folia and is almost pathognomonic to LDD.

Histologically, the striation corresponds to a nonneoplastic enlargement of the cerebellar folia, which is characterized by replacement of the internal granular cell layer by mature, but medium-to-large stratified dysplastic Purkinje cells (Figure 6-2E). Preservation of the cerebellar cortical architecture indicates a hamartomatous or maldevelopmental nature. The extent of replacement gradually increases from the edge to the center, where the outer layer is also filled with abnormal, variable-sized neurons (Figure 6-2F). Another conspicuous feature is abnormal myelinated axons that run in parallel to the pial surface (Figure 6-2E), whose appearance yields an inverted cerebellar cortex-like feature. Microcalcification and white matter vacuolation are often present. Abnormal neurons are positive for various neuronal markers, including synaptophysin and NFP. GFAP labels abundant reactive astrocytes and gliosis. Mitotic activities are very rare, and the Ki-67 labeling index is low.

About 80% of the patients with Cowden disease possess *PTEN/NMAC1* mutations, and the remaining harbor *PTEN* promoter mutations.[36] Of note, pediatric patients with dysplastic gangliocytoma of the cerebellum often do not possess those mutations.[36] At the same time, not all the patients with Cowden disease suffered from dysplastic gangliocytoma. The precise mechanisms underlying the mutations into dysplastic gangliocytoma and their impact on the natural history of the disease require further investigations.

Neurocytomas: Central Neurocytomas, Extraventricular Neurocytomas, and Cerebellar Liponeurocytomas

Neurocytomas are low-grade neoplasms mainly composed of uniform small round cells with neuronal differentiation.[1,38] They may occur in any site of the CNS. Central neurocytoma, the most common, preferentially occurs in the lateral and third ventricles. It is considered to originate from the medial aspect of the ventricles, such as the foramen of Monro, the septum pellucidum, and the corpus callosum. Central neurocytoma is solely comprised of neoplastic neurocytes, although reactive astrocytes and small vessels are always intermingled within the tumor. Tumors with similar histology occasionally occur outside of the ventricles, which include the cerebral hemisphere, brainstem, cerebellum, and spinal cord. Such examples are termed extraventricular neurocytomas.[39] Cerebellar liponeurocytoma, originally reported as lipomatous medulloblastoma, is a rare but unique well-differentiated neurocytoma that occurs in the cerebellum of the adults.[40,41] It exhibits neurocytic differentiation as well as focal cytoplasmic lipidization that resembles fat metaplasia. Neurocytomas correspond to WHO grade II.

Central neurocytoma mainly occurs in young adults.[42] The clinical symptoms are nonspecific and are essentially related to increased intracranial pressure, resulting in headaches. Those symptoms of extraventricular neurocytomas depend on the location of each tumor affected. Cerebellar liponeurocytoma often causes cerebellar symptoms. On imaging studies, central neurocytoma is heterogeneously hypointense on T1- and hyperintense on T2-weighted MRI, with good demarcation. It has a multiple bubble-like or lobulated appearance. Heavy calcification is common. These tumors almost always show irregular weak-to-moderate contrast enhancement. The images of extraventricular neurocytomas resemble those of ganglioglioma, although the inner signals are more heterogeneous. They can be cystic or nodular. The radiologic features of cerebellar liponeurocytoma are heterogeneous and nonspecific. The signal intensity and contrast enhancement depend on the given lipomatous tissue in each tumor.

Neurocytomas are small cell neoplasms that are arranged in a sheet-like architecture in a solid area (Figure 6-3A). The tumor tissue is often interrupted focally or regionally by fine fibrillary, neuropil-like matrices around the small vessels (Figure 6-3B and C). These are called "neuropil-like islands" that corresponds to large neurocytic rosettes. Linear or ribbon-like patterns are common. Halos, round uniform nuclei, and a fine capillary network yield an oligodendroglioma-like appearance, and immunohistochemical confirmation of neuronal differentiation is required for a proper diagnosis (Figure 6-3D and E), although intraventricular oligodendroglioma is extremely rare.

Neurocytomas arising from typical locations, such as the medial aspect of the third lateral ventricles, are almost always comprised of only neurocytes, whereas those arising in lateral areas of the ventricles, including the deep white matter around the anterior horns of the lateral ventricles, may have heterogeneous constituents, such as ganglion cells and glial components (Figure 6-3F). Extraventricular neurocytomas are comprised of not only neurocytes but also ganglion cells and astrocytes in variable proportions. Atypical features are also not uncommon (Figure 6-3G). Those features lead to a heterogeneous appearance in each tumor. The histologic features of cerebellar liponeurocytoma are essentially identical to those of central neurocytoma, except for the presence of lipid-laden cells that resemble adipocytes, resembling fat metaplasia (Figure 6-3H).

On immunohistochemistry, synaptophysin is positive in the tumor matrix or "neuropil-like islands" (Figure 6-3C). Although the former is difficult to distinguish from the background staining of the gray matter, the intraventricular localization of central neurocytoma can make the diagnosis easier. Neuron specific enolase (NSE), class III beta tubulin, and MAP-2 are also positive, but their specificity for neuronal differentiation is not satisfactory. Olig2, a basic helix–loop–helix transcriptional factor that is indispensable for the generation of motor neurons and oligodendrocytes, is negative (Figure 6-3D). NeuN, a marker of advanced neuronal

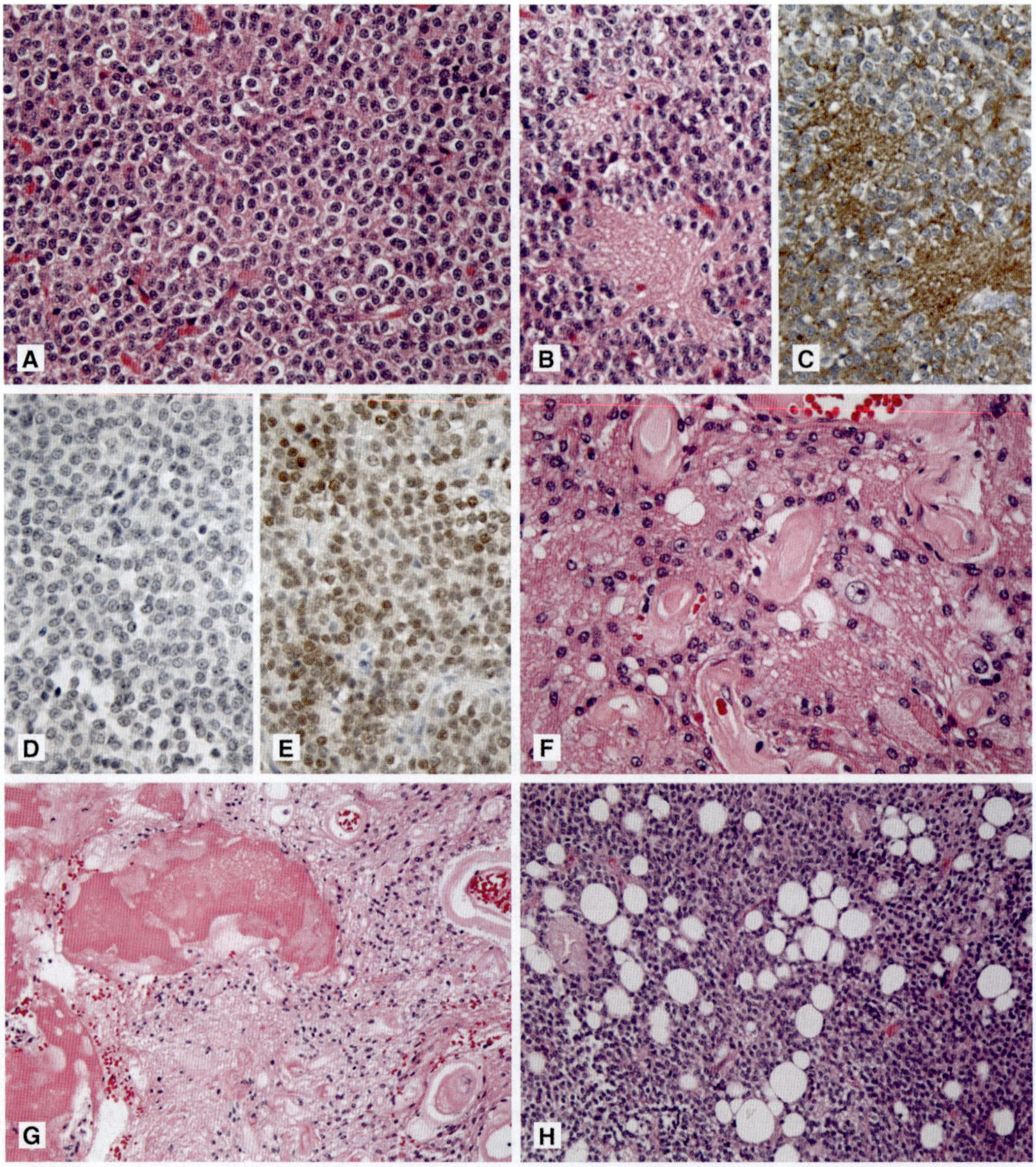

FIGURE 6-3: Neurocytomas. A sheet-like proliferation of uniform small round cells is the typical feature. A chicken-wire vasculature often seen in oligodendrogliomas is present (**A**). Anuclear neuropil-like zones ("neuropil-like islands") corresponding to large neurocytic rosettes (**B**). The "neuropil-like islands" as well as the matrix are positive for synaptophysin, the latter being indistinguishable from that of the preexisting background. No epiperikaryal immunoreactivity is present in those neurocytes (**C**). Olig2 is generally negative (**D**) whereas NeuN is often diffusely positive (**E**). Extraventricular neurocytoma showing ganglionic differentiation. Hyalinized vessels, coarse fibrillary background, and nuclear irregularity give a heterogeneous appearance (**F**). Coagulation necrosis as well as an astrocytic component is not uncommon in extraventricular neurocytoma (**G**). Liponeurocytoma showing lipidization of neoplastic cells (**H**).

differentiation, is moderately positive (Figure 6-3E). GFAP is only positive for reactive astrocytes around the vessels. Overall, neurocytomas exhibit only mild nuclear atypia, and mitoses are rare. The Ki-67 indices are low. Extraventricular tumors tend to have higher cellularity, atypia, and Ki-67 labeling indices. Neurocytomas with hypercellularity along with frank atypia and mitotic activity with/without microvascular proliferation and necrosis are designated "atypical neurocytomas" (Figure 6-3G).

Central neurocytoma is curable by resection alone, but may recur. True malignant transformation has not been recognized. Atypical neurocytomas pose a worse prognosis as a group, but the prognosis does not correlate well with the pathologic features. Extraventricular neurocytomas behave more aggressively than their intraventricular counterparts, and some subjects may succumb to the tumor.[43]

IDH and *TP53* mutations are absent. Rare examples of extraventricular neurocytoma show 1p/19q codeletion.[44] The relationship with oligodendroglioma in terms of the pathogenesis remained unknown.

Papillary Glioneuronal Tumor

A papillary glioneuronal tumor (PGNT) is a rare, benign glioneuronal tumor composed of two distinctive components; one is unique gliovascular papillae and the other an intervening neuronal component.[1,45] PGNT corresponds to WHO grade I.

The vast majority of PGNT occurs in the cerebral hemisphere, preferentially the temporal lobe, and often situates in the deep white matter adjacent to the ventricles. The patients are mainly young to middle-aged adults. In spite of the generally large size of the tumors, neurologic deficits are rare. Headaches and a single episode of seizures are the most common symptoms. The radiologic features of PGNT are similar to those of ganglioglioma. On imaging studies, the tumors present as a discrete solid mass or a cystic mass with a mural nodule with contrast enhancement.[45] Peritumoral edema and mass effects are minimal.

PGNT is associated with compact pseudopapillae composed of hyalinized vessels covered by a single layer of spindle or cuboidal astrocytes (Figure 6-4A and B) that are positive for astrocytic markers such as GFAP, S100 protein, and nestin (Figure 6-4C). The radiating cytoplasmic processes or anuclear zones positive for GFAP seen in ependymomas and astroblastoma are absent. Neuronal cells, mainly of neurocytic or ganglioid cells, fill the interstices between the pseudopapillae or form solid sheets (Figure 6-4B). The background can be fibrillary or loosely textured. The neuronal cells are diffusely positive for synaptophysin (Figure 6-4D) and class III beta tubulin. Minigemistocytes and Olig2-positive cells have also been recognized.[46] The vast majority show no or little mitotic activity and lack atypia, microvascular proliferation, or necrosis. There have been a few reports of recurrence and examples with anaplasia and high proliferation (Ki-67 index >10%).[47]

Recently, a novel translocation, t(9;17)(q31;q24), as the sole karyotypic anomaly, was identified in PGNT.[48] A reverse transcription–polymerase chain reaction (RT-PCR) analysis using a forward primer from *SLC44A1* and a reverse primer from *PRKCA* confirmed the presence of an *SLC44A1-PRKCA* fusion product, suggesting that this novel fusion, *SLC44A1-PRKCA*, is the defining and oncogenic molecular feature of PGNT.

Rosette-Forming Glioneuronal Tumor

Rosette-forming glioneuronal tumor (RGNT) is a benign glioneuronal tumor that is mainly located in the fourth ventricle and cerebral aqueduct. RGNT is composed of neuronal and astrocytic components, the former being neuronal rosettes composed of neurocytes and the latter being an astrocytoma resembling pilocytic astrocytoma.[1,49,50] RGNT corresponds to WHO grade I.

RGNT occurs in adolescents to young adults. Females are reportedly affected slightly more often than males. The major symptoms are cerebellar dysfunctions and those related to obstructive hydrocephalus. The radiologic features are rather unique, not only in terms of the location but also in appearance. On MRI, the tumor represents a well-circumscribed, fourth ventricular mass with vague central cysts or multiloculation with thick walls and often shows heterogeneous contrast enhancement. In a sagittal section, linear contrast enhancement in the center may be seen. Multiple solid nodules in the cerebellum have also been reported.[49] Other rare locations include the optic chiasm, pineal region, cerebral hemisphere, and spinal cord.[51]

The neuronal components in RGNT are neurocytic and/or perivascular rosettes (Figure 6-5A). The neurocytic rosettes contain a fine fibrillary matrix in the center that is surrounded by

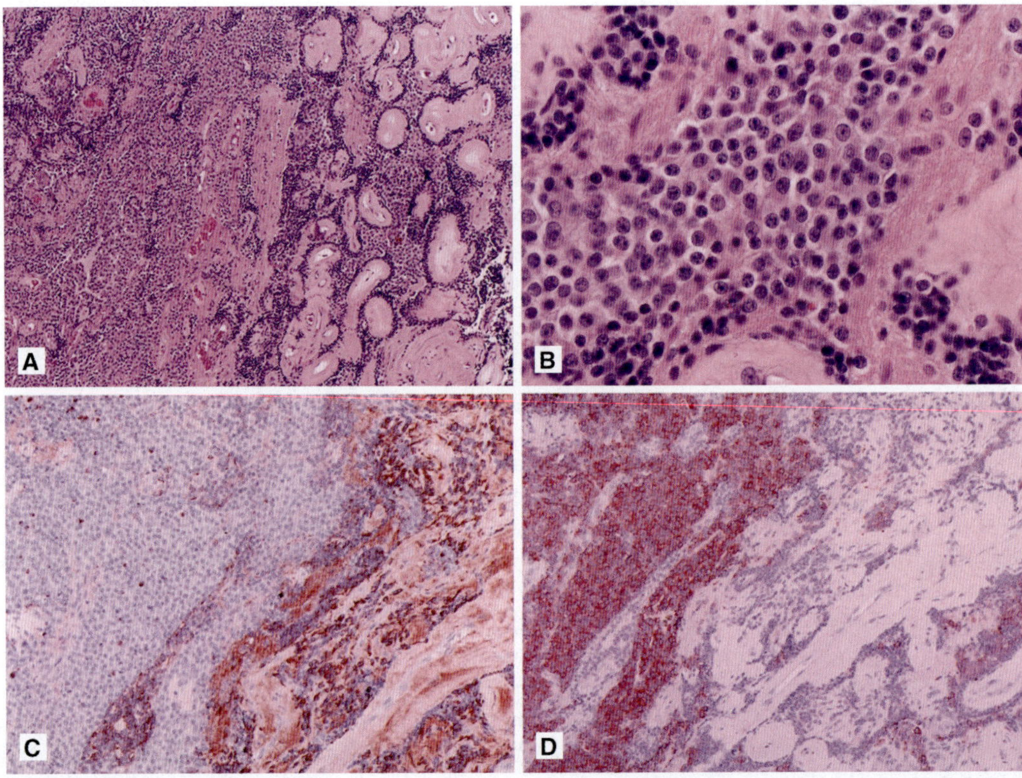

FIGURE 6-4: Papillary glioneuronal tumor (PGNT). PGNT harbors two distinctive components: the neuronal component in the left half and the gliovascular papillae in the right half. The gliovascular papillae. The neuronal component is a sheet-like proliferation of neurocytes intervening between the gliovascular papillae. The latter composes of hyalinized vessels covered by a single layer of astrocytes (**A**). A sheet of neurocytes showing uniform round nuclei with speckled chromatin (**B**). The astrocytes (*left upper corner*) show denser chromatin. Astrocytes covering hyalinized vessels are positive for glial fibrillary acidic proteins (**C**). A sheet of neurocytes are diffusely positive for synaptophysin (**D**).

neurocytes.[52] The perivascular rosettes are pseudopapillary structures of small vessels lined by neurocytes radiating fine cytoplasmic processes toward the vessels. The astrocytic component possesses a biphasic pattern—a compact area composed of piloid cells (Figure 6-5B) and a microcytic area with OLCs (Figure 6-5C). Although this is identical to the architecture of pilocytic astrocytoma, the compact area is generally small or often lacking. Rosenthal fibers, granular bodies, and microcalcification may be present, but generally are not conspicuous. Since the astrocytic component, particularly the microcytic area, is dominant compared to the neuronal component in the vast majority of cases, there may be diagnostic difficulty caused by sampling errors. If the neuronal component is absent in the specimen, a final diagnosis cannot be made. The differential diagnosis includes pilocytic astrocytoma and oligodendroglioma, although the latter is extremely rare in the cerebellum. The fine matrix present in the center of the neurocytic and/or perivascular rosettes is weakly or faintly positive for synaptophysin (Figure 6-5D), class III beta tubulin, and NSE. Such weak reactions for neuronal markers parallel the scantiness of synaptic vesicles within the rosettes on electron microscopy. The neurocytes in the rosettes are negative or weakly positive for NeuN (Figure 6-5E) but are consistently positive for Olig2 (Figure 6-5F), which are a characteristic features of RGNT and may reflect a biphasic differentiation of neurocytes. Gross total resection cannot always be accomplished due to the presence of brainstem infiltration. Although the overall survival is generally favorable, some cases cause neuronal deficits. RGNT may not be a fully indolent tumor.[53,54]

RGNT lacks the *KIAA1549-BRAF* gene fusion or *BRAFV600E* mutation,[55] both of which represent the most common genetic alterations in pilocytic astrocytoma. Recently, fibroblast

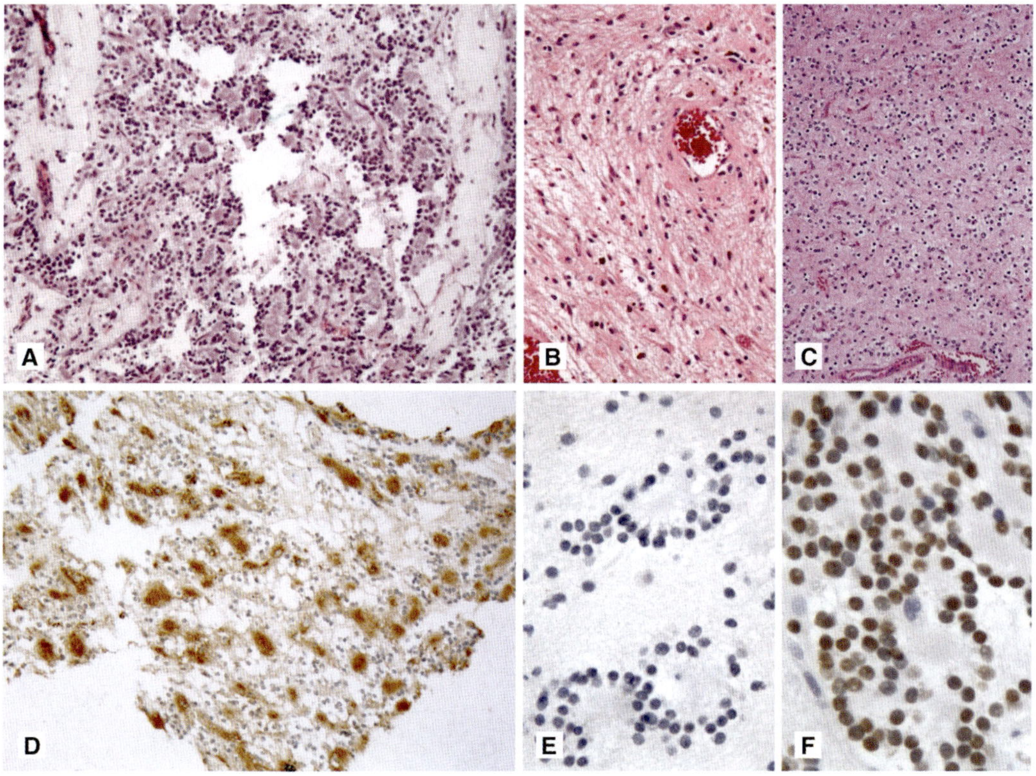

FIGURE 6-5: Rosette-forming glioneuronal tumor (RGNT). Neurocytic and/or perivascular rosettes, with fine fibrillary matrix in the center formed by neurocytes, are distinctive components of RGNT (**A**). Pilocytic appearance of the astrocytic component (**B**). Microcystic areas with oligodendroglia-like cells often predominate (**C**). Fine fibrillary matrix is positive for synaptophysin, but it can be faint (**D**). NeuN is often negative in neurocytes (**E**). Olig2 is consistently positive for nuclei of neurocytic rosettes, which is a distinctive feature of RGNT (**F**).

growth factor receptor 1 (*FGFR1*) mutations have been described in three out of eight patients with RGNT.[56] *FGFR1* mutations are considered to be the most frequent mechanism underlying mitogen-activated protein kinase activation and are an alternative to *KIAA1549-BRAF* fusion and *BRAFV600E* mutations in pilocytic astrocytoma. Notably, one of the three *FGFR1*-mutated RGNT patients had undergone a resection of a diencephalic pilocytic astrocytoma with pilomyxoid features 5 years before the discovery of the fourth ventricle tumor. The mutational analysis uncovered the presence of the same *FGFR1* mutation in the diencephalic tumor. These results indicate that, in addition to histologic similarities, at least a subgroup of RGNT may show close molecular relationships with pilocytic astrocytoma.

Dysembryoplastic Neuroepithelial Tumor

Dysembryoplastic neuroepithelial tumor (DNT) is a benign or hamartomatous tumor of the cerebral hemisphere that is characterized by a multinodular architecture made up of the specific glioneuronal element (SGNE).[1,57] The SGNE is composed of OLCs and floating neurons. The tumors that are comprised of nodules made of SGNE alone are called the simple form, whereas those with nodules of other glial cells in addition to SGNE nodules are called the complex form.[58]

Although the original report described that the patients were all under 20 years old and had intractable epilepsy, which were often complex partial seizures, the progress in imaging investigations has made it possible to identify older patients and those with ones having a single episode of epilepsy. Neurologic deficits are absent in affected cases. Some data suggest that DNT is the second most common cause of intractable epilepsy. The imaging features are characteristic and

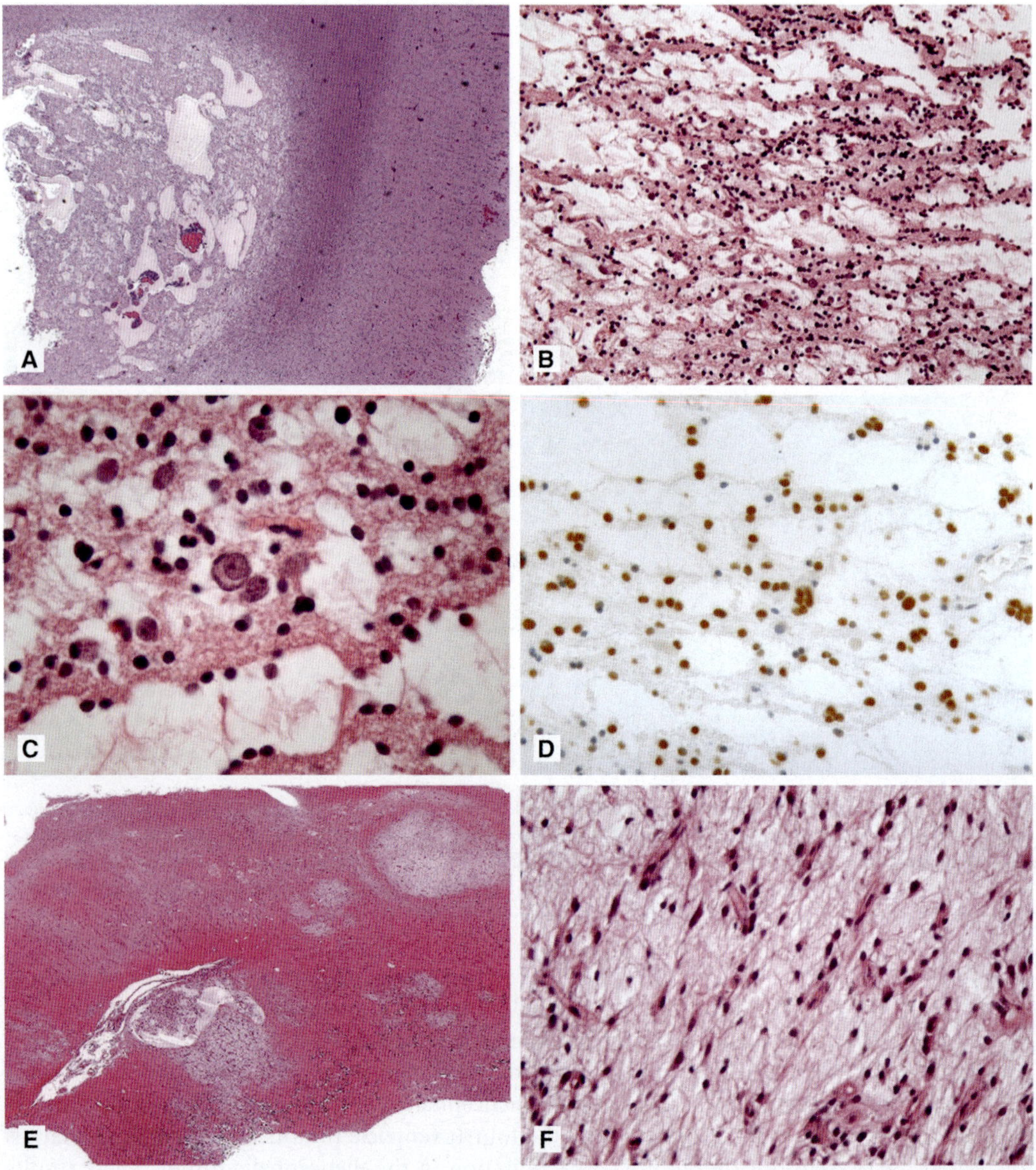

FIGURE 6-6: Dysembryoplastic neuroepithelial tumor (DNT). Well-defined nodular or patchy architecture is an essential feature of DNT. This nodule is solely composed of the specific glioneuronal element (SGNE) corresponding a simple form of DNT (**A**). A characteristic striped pattern of SGNE. Oligodendroglia-like cells (OLC) line along trabeculae of thin neuropil in the myxoid matrix (**B**). "Floating neurons" do not show atypia or swelling (**C**). OLC are diffusely positive for Olig2. Some cells with OLC-like configuration are negative. They are small neurons positive for NeuN (**D**). Complex form of DNT comprising of heterogeneous nodules (**E**). Some nodules look like diffuse astrocytoma (**F**).

parallel the gross pathologic appearance. The thickened cerebral cortex shows slightly lobular or nodular areas that are low on T1-weighted images. Generally, neither contrast enhancement nor surrounding edema is present.

Histologically, well-demarcated nodules or patches of SGNE are present in the cerebral cortex or the subcortical white matter (Figure 6-6A). Occasionally, the entire cortex is replaced by SGNE. Those cortices are thickened and disorganized, with the loss of distinction between the gray and the white matter. Nevertheless, the overall configuration of the cerebral cortex remains, suggesting that DNT is hamartomatous in nature. SGNE exhibits an alveolar or microcytic pattern made of the neuropil matrix in a mucinous or myxoid background having loose capillaries. OLCs lining along the trabecular neuropil matrix or vessels yield a characteristic striped pattern (Figure 6-6B–D), which is seen in the sections cut perpendicular to the cortical surface. "Floating neurons" that lack cellular atypia, or swelling of the cytoplasm, which are common features in ganglioglioma, are present in a mucinous background (Figure 6-6C). Since "floating neurons" occasionally show continuous lamination with the adjacent cortex, some investigators have considered them to be entrapped neurons.[59] In the complex form (Figure 6-6E), some of the nodules are comprised of glial cells, mainly astrocytes (Figure 6-6F), which are occasionally pilocytic in appearance. The nodules of ganglion cells are also found. When the nodularity is unclear, distinction between the complex form and other types of gliomas, including pilocytic astrocytoma, ganglioglioma, and oligodendroglioma, is often difficult. The microscopic feature of SGNT is essentially indistinguishable from that of low-grade oligodendroglioma. Since 1p/19q codeletion, a hallmark for classic oligodendroglioma, is absent in infants and children, the presence of nodularity is essential for the precise pathologic diagnosis of DNT of the patients in those ages. OLCs are diffusely positive for Olig2 and S100 protein (Figure 6-6D), but negative for NeuN. Occasional NeuN-positive small cells may be entrapped small neurons in the background rather than a tumor component.[59] The "floating neurons" are positive for NFP, synaptophysin, and NeuN. The immunohistochemical profile of the glial cells in the complex form depends on the characteristics of the glial cells. The overall survival is extremely favorable. Rare malignant transformation has been reported in the complex form, but it is unclear in such cases whether the initial lesions are truly DNT.

Some cases of DNT, the complex form in particular, harbor the *BRAFV600E* mutation.[60] Whether DNT with such mutations is a variant of DNT or ganglioglioma remains to be determined.

ACKNOWLEDGMENT

This chapter is dedicated to the memory of my mentor, late Dr. Bernd W. Scheithauer.

References

1. Louis DN, Ohgaki H, Wiestler OD, et al. *WHO Classification of Tumours of the Central Nervous System*. Lyon, France: IARC; 2007.
2. Zülch KJ. *Histological Typing of Tumours of the Central Nervous System*. Geneva, Switzerland: World Health Organization; 1979.
3. Kleihues P, Burger PC, Scheithauer BW. *Histological Typing of Tumours of the Central Nervous System*. 2nd ed. Berlin, Germany: Springer-Verlag; 1993.
4. Lloyd RV, Jin L. In situ hybridization analysis of chromogranin A and B mRNAs in neuroendocrine tumors with digoxigenin-labeled oligonucleotide probe cocktails. *Diagn Mol Pathol* 1995;4(2):143–151.
5. Miller DC, Koslow M, Budzilovich GN, et al. Synaptophysin: a sensitive and specific marker for ganglion cells in central nervous system neoplasms. *Hum Pathol* 1990;21(1):93–98.
6. Hirose T, Scheithauer B, Lopes M, et al. Ganglioglioma. An ultrastructural and immunohistochemical study. *Cancer* 1997;79(5):989–1003.
7. Yan H, Parsons DW, Jin G, et al. IDH1 and IDH2 mutations in gliomas. *N Engl J Med* 2009;360(8): 765–773.
8. Mukasa A, Takayanagi S, Saito K, et al. Significance of IDH mutations varies with tumor histology, grade, and genetics in Japanese glioma patients. *Cancer Sci* 2012;103(3):587–592.
9. Schindler G, Capper D, Meyer J, et al. Analysis of BRAF V600E mutation in 1,320 nervous system tumors reveals high mutation frequencies in pleomorphic xanthoastrocytoma, ganglioglioma and extra-cerebellar pilocytic astrocytoma. *Acta Neuropathol* 2011;121(3):397–405.
10. Burger PC, Scheithauer BW. *Tumors of the Central Nervous System*. Washington, DC: Armed Forces Institute of Pathology; 2007.
11. Blumcke I, Wiestler OD. Gangliogliomas: an intriguing tumor entity associated with focal epilepsies. *J Neuropathol Exp Neurol* 2002;61(7):575–584.

12. Wolf HK, Campos MG, Zentner J, et al. Surgical pathology of temporal lobe epilepsy. Experience with 216 cases. *J Neuropathol Exp Neurol* 1993;52(5):499–506.
13. Barkovich AJ, Raybaud C. *Pediatric Neuroimaging*. Philadelphia, PA: LWW; 2011.
14. Yousem DM, Grossman RI. *Neuroradiology*. 3rd ed. New York: Elsevier; 2010.
15. Horbinski C, Kofler J, Yeaney G, et al. Isocitrate dehydrogenase 1 analysis differentiates gangliogliomas from infiltrative gliomas. *Brain Pathol* 2011;21(5):564–574.
16. Miller DC, Lang FF, Epstein FJ. Central nervous system gangliogliomas. Part 1: pathology. *J Neurosurg* 1993;79(6):859–866.
17. Perry A, Burton SS, Fuller GN, et al. Oligodendroglial neoplasms with ganglioglioma-like maturation: a diagnostic pitfall. *Acta Neuropathol* 2010;120(2):237–252.
18. Wolf HK, Muller MB, Spanle M, et al. Ganglioglioma: a detailed histopathological and immunohistochemical analysis of 61 cases. *Acta Neuropathol (Berlin)* 1994;88(2):166–173.
19. Prayson RA, Khajavi K, Comair YG. Cortical architectural abnormalities and MIB1 immunoreactivity in gangliogliomas: a study of 60 patients with intracranial tumors. *J Neuropathol Exp Neurol* 1995; 54(4):513–520.
20. Langford LA. Central nervous system neoplasms: indications for electron microscopy. *Ultrastruct Pathol* 1996;20(1):35–46.
21. Lang FF, Epstein FJ, Ransohoff J, et al. Central nervous system gangliogliomas. Part 2: clinical outcome. *J Neurosurg* 1993;79(6):867–873.
22. Luyken C, Blumcke I, Fimmers R, et al. Supratentorial gangliogliomas: histopathologic grading and tumor recurrence in 184 patients with a median follow-up of 8 years. *Cancer* 2004;101(1):146–155.
23. Dahiya S, Haydon DH, Alvarado D, et al. BRAF(V600E) mutation is a negative prognosticator in pediatric ganglioglioma. *Acta Neuropathol* 2013;125(6):901–910.
24. Huse JT, Edgar M, Halliday J, et al. Multinodular and vacuolating neuronal tumors of the cerebrum: 10 cases of a distinctive seizure-associated lesion. *Brain Pathol* 2013;23(5):515–524.
25. VandenBerg SR. Desmoplastic infantile ganglioglioma and desmoplastic cerebral astrocytoma of infancy. *Brain Pathol* 1993;3(3):275–281.
26. Taratuto AL, Monges J, Lylyk P, et al. Superficial cerebral astrocytoma attached to dura. Report of six cases in infants. *Cancer* 1984;54(11):2505–2512.
27. VandenBerg SR, May EE, Rubinstein LJ, et al. Desmoplastic supratentorial neuroepithelial tumors of infancy with divergent differentiation potential ("desmoplastic infantile gangliogliomas"). Report on 11 cases of a distinctive embryonal tumor with favorable prognosis. *J Neurosurg* 1987;66(1):58–71.
28. Trehan G, Bruge H, Vinchon M, et al. MR imaging in the diagnosis of desmoplastic infantile tumor: retrospective study of six cases. *AJNR Am J Neuroradiol* 2004;25(6):1028–1033.
29. Taratuto AL, Sevlever G, Schultz M, et al. Desmoplastic cerebral astrocytoma of infancy (DCAI). Survival data of the original series and report of two additional cases, DNA, kinetic and molecular genetic studies. *Brain Pathol* 1994;4:423.
30. Komori T, Scheithauer BW, Parisi JE, et al. Mixed conventional and desmoplastic infantile ganglioglioma: an autopsied case with 6-year follow-up. *Mod Pathol* 2001;14(7):720–726.
31. Prayson RA. Gliofibroma: a distinct entity or a subtype of desmoplastic astrocytoma? *Hum Pathol* 1996;27(6):610–613.
32. Cerda-Nicolas M, Kepes JJ. Gliofibromas (including malignant forms), and gliosarcomas: a comparative study and review of the literature. *Acta Neuropathol* 1993;85(4):349–361.
33. Koelsche C, Sahm F, Paulus W, et al. BRAF V600E expression and distribution in desmoplastic infantile astrocytoma/ganglioglioma. *Neuropathol Appl Neurobiol* 2014;40(3):337–344.
34. Gessi M, Zur Muhlen A, Hammes J, et al. Genome-wide DNA copy number analysis of desmoplastic infantile astrocytomas and desmoplastic infantile gangliogliomas. *J Neuropathol Exp Neurol* 2013; 72(9):807–815.
35. Eberhart CG, Wiestler OD, Eng C. *Cowden Disease and Dysplastic Gangliocytoma of the Cerebellum/Lhermitte-Duclos Disease*. 4th ed. Lyon, France: IARC; 2007.
36. Zhou XP, Marsh DJ, Morrison CD, et al. Germline inactivation of PTEN and dysregulation of the phosphoinositol-3-kinase/Akt pathway cause human Lhermitte-Duclos disease in adults. *Am J Hum Genet* 2003;73(5):1191–1198.
37. Klisch J, Juengling F, Spreer J, et al. Lhermitte-Duclos disease: assessment with MR imaging, positron emission tomography, single-photon emission CT, and MR spectroscopy. *AJNR Am J Neuroradiol* 2001; 22(5):824–830.

38. Hassoun J, Gambarelli D, Grisoli F, et al. Central neurocytoma. An electron-microscopic study of two cases. *Acta Neuropathol* 1982;56(2):151–156.
39. Giangaspero F, Cenacchi G, Losi L, et al. Extraventricular neoplasms with neurocytoma features. A clinicopathological study of 11 cases. *Am J Surg Pathol* 1997;21(2):206–212.
40. Giangaspero F, Cenacchi G, Roncaroli F, et al. Medullocytoma (lipidized medulloblastoma). A cerebellar neoplasm of adults with favorable prognosis. *Am J Surg Pathol* 1996;20(6):656–664.
41. Ellison DW, Zygmunt SC, Weller RO. Neurocytoma/lipoma (neurolipocytoma) of the cerebellum. *Neuropathol Appl Neurobiol* 1993;19(1):95–98.
42. Figarella-Branger D, Pellissier JF, Daumas Duport C, et al. Central neurocytomas. Critical evaluation of a small-cell neuronal tumor. *Am J Surg Pathol* 1992;16(2):97–109.
43. Brat DJ, Scheithauer BW, Eberhart CG, et al. Extraventricular neurocytomas: pathologic features and clinical outcome. *Am J Surg Pathol* 2001;25(10):1252–1260.
44. Rodriguez FJ, Mota RA, Scheithauer BW, et al. Interphase cytogenetics for 1p19q and t(1;19)(q10;p10) may distinguish prognostically relevant subgroups in extraventricular neurocytoma. *Brain Pathol* 2009;19(4):623–629.
45. Komori T, Scheithauer BW, Anthony DC, et al. Papillary glioneuronal tumor: a new variant of mixed neuronal-glial neoplasm. *Am J Surg Pathol* 1998;22(10):1171–1183.
46. Tanaka Y, Yokoo H, Komori T, et al. A distinct pattern of Olig2-positive cellular distribution in papillary glioneuronal tumors: a manifestation of the oligodendroglial phenotype? *Acta Neuropathol* 2005; 110(1):39–47.
47. Ishizawa T, Komori T, Shibahara J, et al. Papillary glioneuronal tumor with minigemistocytic components and increased proliferative activity. *Hum Pathol* 2006;37(5):627–630.
48. Bridge JA, Liu XQ, Sumegi J, et al. Identification of a novel, recurrent SLC44A1-PRKCA fusion in papillary glioneuronal tumor. *Brain Pathol* 2013;23(2):121–128.
49. Komori T, Scheithauer BW, Hirose T. A rosette-forming glioneuronal tumor of the fourth ventricle: infratentorial form of dysembryoplastic neuroepithelial tumor? *Am J Surg Pathol* 2002;26(5):582–591.
50. Kuchelmeister K, Bergmann M, von Wild K, et al. Desmoplastic ganglioglioma: report of two non-infantile cases. *Acta Neuropathol* 1993;85(2):199–204.
51. Hsu C, Kwan G, Lau Q, et al. Rosette-forming glioneuronal tumour: imaging features, histopathological correlation and a comprehensive review of literature. *Br J Neurosurg* 2012;26(5):668–673.
52. Kinno M, Ishizawa K, Shimada S, et al. Cytology is a useful tool for the diagnosis of rosette-forming glioneuronal tumour of the fourth ventricle: a report of two cases. *Cytopathology* 2010;21(3):194–197.
53. Chiba K, Aihara Y, Eguchi S, et al. Rosette-forming glioneuronal tumor of the fourth ventricle with neurocytoma component. *Childs Nerv Syst* 2014;30(2):351–356.
54. Schlamann A, von Bueren AO, Hagel C, et al. An individual patient data meta-analysis on characteristics and outcome of patients with papillary glioneuronal tumor, rosette glioneuronal tumor with neuropil-like islands and rosette forming glioneuronal tumor of the fourth ventricle. *PLoS One* 2014;9(7):e101211.
55. Gessi M, Lambert SR, Lauriola L, et al. Absence of KIAA1549-BRAF fusion in rosette-forming glioneuronal tumors of the fourth ventricle (RGNT). *J Neurooncol* 2012;110(1):21–25.
56. Gessi M, Moneim YA, Hammes J, et al. FGFR1 mutations in Rosette-forming glioneuronal tumors of the fourth ventricle. *J Neuropathol Exp Neurol* 2014;73(6):580–584.
57. Daumas-Duport C, Scheithauer BW, Chodkiewicz JP, et al. Dysembryoplastic neuroepithelial tumor: a surgically curable tumor of young patients with intractable partial seizures. Report of thirty-nine cases. *Neurosurgery* 1988;23(5):545–556.
58. Daumas-Duport C. Dysembryoplastic neuroepithelial tumours. *Brain Pathol* 1993;3(3):283–295.
59. Komori T, Arai N. Dysembryoplastic neuroepithelial tumor, a pure glial tumor? Immunohistochemical and morphometric studies. *Neuropathology* 2013;33(4):459–468.
60. Baar HS. Osseous hamartosis of dura mater resulting in epilepsy and hemiatrophy of the brain. *J Maine Med Assoc* 1962;53:2–7.

7 Embryonal Tumors

▶ Hidehiro Takei
▶ Adekunle M. Adesina

INTRODUCTION

Embryonal tumors of the central nervous system (CNS) are primitive, clinically aggressive tumors associated with significant morbidity and mortality and occur most commonly in children. They represent the most common group of malignant brain tumors especially in the 0- to 4-year age group.[1] Although they share the common histologic features of malignant "(small) blue cell tumors," these tumors comprise a biologically heterogeneous group of neoplasms with divergent patterns of differentiation. A common propensity exists for leptomeningeal invasion and subsequent cerebrospinal fluid (CSF) dissemination throughout the neuraxis. On the other hand, extraneural metastasis is very rarely reported. The histogenesis of CNS embryonal tumors has been a matter of debate. According to the current WHO classification, this group of tumors includes three main histologic entities—medulloblastoma (MB), atypical teratoid/rhabdoid tumor (AT/RT), and CNS primitive neuroectodermal tumors (PNETs)—all of which correspond to grade IV.[2] Of these entities, MB is the most commonly encountered tumor. Despite recent considerable advances in the understanding of the molecular biology of these tumors and in their treatment over the past few decades, CNS embryonal tumors in childhood remain the greatest challenge in pediatric neuro-oncology.

This chapter addresses primarily the clinical features and histopathologic findings of each histologic entity. The detailed molecular characteristics are described in the Molecular Pathology chapter.

MEDULLOBLASTOMA

MB is defined by the WHO as a malignant invasive embryonal tumor of the cerebellum, corresponding to grade IV, and is the most common malignant brain tumor in children.[2] MB accounts for 15% to 20% of all pediatric brain tumors[3] and occurs mostly during the first decade of life with a peak age of 7 years and with a slight male predominance. Approximately 10% to 15% of MBs are diagnosed in infancy.[3] This tumor can occur in adults with the highest incidence in 20 to 34 years, although it is very rare and accounts for less than 1% of adult intracranial tumors.[4] The vast majority of childhood MBs arise as midline tumors in the cerebellar vermis, often with extension into the fourth ventricle, whereas involvement of cerebellar hemispheres increases with age and is frequently seen in adult MBs. CSF dissemination reportedly occurs in as many as 30% of MB patients at the time of diagnosis, which is detected by imaging and/or CSF cytologic examination.[5]

Clinically, the most common early symptoms in patients with MB are nonspecific and nonlocalizing findings related to increased intracranial pressure due to obstruction of the fourth ventricle, which include headache, vomiting, and lethargy. Truncal ataxia manifesting as an unsteady gait is usually present early in the disease. With increasing tumor size, appendicular ataxia and signs and symptoms of brain stem deficits can occur.

There are a few rare, familial cancer predisposition syndromes that are associated with increased risk for developing MB, which include Gorlin syndrome (germline *PTCH1* mutation), Turcot syndrome (germline *APC* mutation), and Li-Fraumeni syndrome (germline *TP53* mutation). (Refer to Chapter 12 for details.)

Radiologically, MBs show heterogeneous hypointense or isointense signal on MR T1-weighted image (WI), often with heterogeneous enhancement. MR T2-WI shows a heterogeneous mass due to calcification, necrosis, and cystic degeneration. Restricted diffusion is seen on diffusion-weighted imaging (DWI).

Maximal safe resection is the mainstay of therapy followed by adjuvant chemotherapy and/or radiation therapy. Overall 5- and 10-year relative survival rates of patients with MB are reported to be 71.1% and 62.8%, respectively, during the period of 1995–2010 in the United States.[1] Currently, pediatric MB is classified clinically into high risk and average (standard) risk based on the patient's age, metastases, and extent of surgical resection.[6] The average-risk group includes children ≥3 years with postoperative residual tumor ≤1.5 cm^2 and no metastatic disease, whereas all others are considered high risk. Current therapeutic strategies for newly diagnosed childhood MB are mostly based on this clinical classification.[7] According to the National Cancer Institute scheme, children with MB histologically showing diffuse anaplasia are assigned to the high-risk group and treated as such.[8] Although this clinical stratification is a valuable prognostic indicator currently used in clinical practice, it does not adequately account for the prognostic variability that exists among patients ascribed to either of these risk groups.[9] It is also unable to identify or predict average-risk patients who will develop resistant disease or the number of high-risk patients who might be overtreated with current protocols.[10] (Please refer to Chapter 19 for detailed descriptions.)

Molecular studies clearly demonstrate that MB is not a single disease but comprises a collection of demographically, clinically, and molecularly distinct subgroups. More recently, a consensus conference in Boston in 2010 supported classification of the following four main subgroups of MBs based on molecular profiling: WNT subgroup, Sonic hedgehog (SHH) subgroup, group 3, and group 4.[11] This novel molecular classification may become increasingly important not only for more reliable prognostication but also for the design and implementation of molecular targeted therapies. The detailed molecular characteristics of MB are described in the Molecular Pathology chapter.

Adult MBs are different from childhood MBs by showing higher frequencies of lateral cerebellar location, desmoplastic histology, and SHH tumors and an exceptional rarity of group 3 tumors.[12] The 5- and 10-year relative survival rates of adult patients with MB are 64.9% and 52.1%, respectively, according to the population-based study analyzing 454 adult patients in the United States.[4] This study identifies age of diagnosis before 20 years, gross total resection, and radiation therapy as favorable prognostic factors.[4]

Histologically, classic MB is composed of diffuse sheets of densely packed, predominantly undifferentiated tumor cells. The tumor cells are characterized by small- to medium-sized, round to oval, or carrot-shaped, hyperchromatic nuclei and scant cytoplasm. Marked nuclear pleomorphism is usually not seen. Mitotic figures and apoptotic bodies are often readily observed. Necrosis may be present. Microvascular proliferation is uncommon. Although MBs are considered to be derived from embryonal precursor cells with a capacity for divergent differentiation, neuronal differentiation is most consistently seen. This is usually incipient in that it is restricted to the expression of neuronal immunohistochemical markers (described below), with rare cases showing overt ganglionic or mature neuronal cells. Homer Wright ("neuroblastic") rosettes, characterized by tumor cells surrounding a central region containing neuropil, are seen in less than a half of MBs (Figure 7-1A). These structures may be subtle or absent although they are unique histologic hallmarks of classic MB. Perivascular pseudorosettes and spongioblastic features, characterized by arrangement of tumor cells with their long axes in parallel rows, may be present. Glial (astrocytic) differentiation is restricted to small foci of some MBs without evidence of progressive differentiation to mature astrocytes.

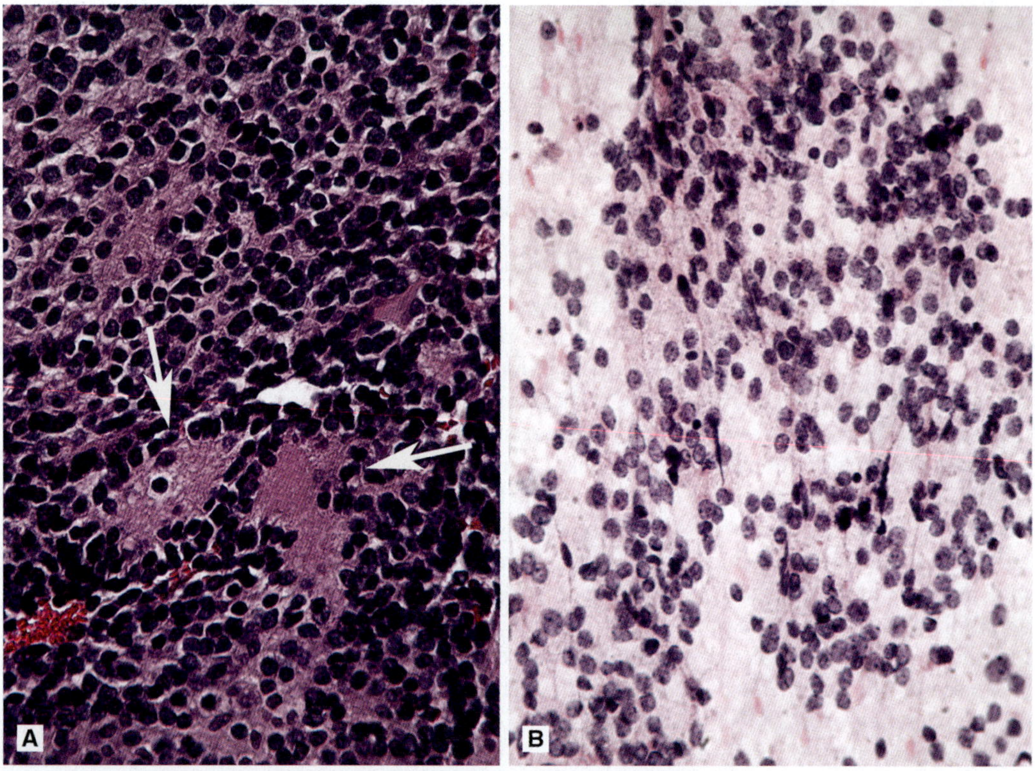

FIGURE 7-1: Classic medulloblastoma. Histologic section showing a diffuse sheet of small, round to oval tumor cells with hyperchromatic nuclei and scant cytoplasm (**A**). Homer Wright rosettes are present (*arrows*). Cytologic touch imprint showing a monolayered discohesive sheet of relatively uniform tumor cells with round to oval, occasionally elongated nuclei and fine hyperchromatic chromatin with some chromatin clumping (**B**).

Cytologic touch/squash preparations demonstrate monolayered discohesive sheets of relatively uniform tumor cells with round to oval, occasionally, elongated or carrot-shaped nuclei and a fine hyperchromatic chromatin pattern with some chromatin clumping (Figure 7-1B). The nuclei tended to mold to the shape of the adjacent tumor cells (molding). These features readily permit discrimination from cells of normal cerebellar internal granular layer. It is reported that these cytologic features are seen in both classic MB and desmoplastic/nodular MB described below, which are cytologically indistinguishable from each other.[12] Our study analyzing 43 cytologic smears, which include touch-and-squash preparations, reports that touch preparation is the preferred method compared to squash preparation given the significantly fewer artifacts and sufficient cellularity.[12]

Immunohistochemically, neuronal markers such as synaptophysin (Figure 7-2A) is of great importance for the confirmation of the histologic diagnosis of MB and is positive at least focally in the majority of MBs. Other neuronal markers such as neuron-specific enolase, class III tubulin, and microtubule-associated protein (MAP)-2 may be positive. Homer Wright rosettes and perivascular pseudorosettes are frequently labeled. In contrast, neurofilament protein (NFP) is rarely immunoreactive. Glial fibrillary acidic protein (GFAP) commonly highlights entrapped reactive astrocytes; however, a small proportion of MBs show small foci of tumor cells with GFAP immunoreactivity (Figure 7-2B). A Ki-67 (MIB-1) labeling index is generally high in MBs (Figure 7-2C), while it is very low in the pale islands. INI-1 protein expression is retained in the nuclei of all MBs, which is important to exclude AT/RT.

For assignment of MB molecular subgroups, immunohistochemical expression of beta-catenin (nuclear stain) and Dickkopf-related protein 1 (DKK1) for the identification of WNT MBs and of secreted frizzled-related protein 1 (SFRP1), GLI1, and GRB2-associated–binding protein 1 (GAB1) for SHH MBs is promising and is under extensive investigation.[9,11]

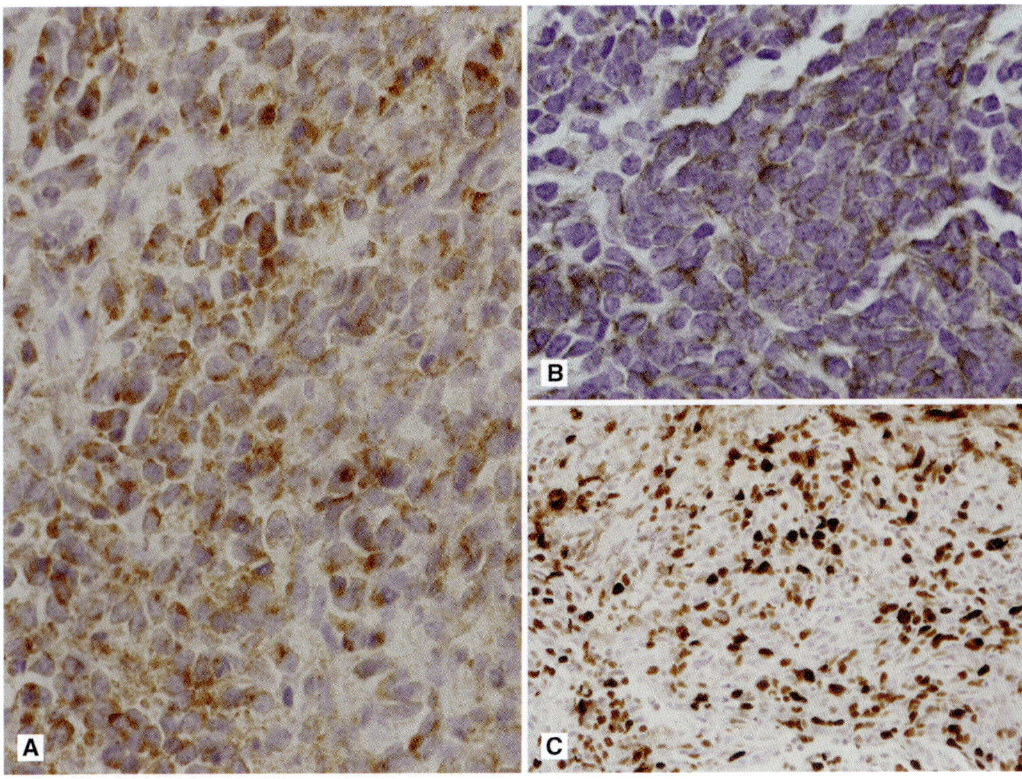

FIGURE 7-2: Classic medulloblastoma: Immunohistochemistry. Synaptophysin is positive in tumor cells (**A**). GFAP is focally positive in tumor cells (**B**). Ki-67 (MIB-1) labeling index is 40–50% (**C**).

Although the majority of MBs exhibit classic histology described above, the following four variants of MB are recognized in the current WHO classification.[2] In addition, MB with myogenic differentiation (previously termed medullomyoblastoma) (Figure 7-3) and MB with melanotic differentiation (previously termed melanocytic MB) are rarely seen as unique histologic patterns of differentiation of MBs, although not considered as separate variants. All these histologic variants/patterns of differentiation are classified as WHO grade IV.

i. *Desmoplastic/nodular MB* (Figure 7-4): This variant usually arises in the cerebellar hemisphere and is the most common variant in adult MBs. It has distinct molecular characteristics and is typified histologically by reticulin-free nodular zones (pale islands) that are surrounded by densely packed, hyperchromatic cells with brisk mitotic activity, producing a dense intercellular reticulin fiber network. These characteristic "pale islands" are composed of uniform tumor cells with reduced nuclear cytoplasmic ratio and reduced proliferation accompanied by a fibrillary matrix, which represent neuronal maturation. Immunohistochemically, these structures are predominantly highlighted with neuronal markers (e.g., synaptophysin). Desmoplasia is commonly seen to some degree in association with leptomeningeal invasion, but desmoplasia alone without nodules is not sufficient for a diagnosis of this variant.
ii. *Medulloblastoma with extensive nodularity* (Figure 7-5): This variant usually occurs almost exclusively in infants. It is associated with better prognosis in spite of the young age. On MRI, an extensive nodular grape-like appearance with contrast enhancement is observed. It is characterized histologically by an expanded lobular architecture of the classic reticulin-free zones that are enlarged with abundant fibrillary neuropil, with little or no desmoplastic internodular tissue.
iii. *Anaplastic MB* (Figure 7-6): This variant is biologically aggressive and is composed of markedly atypical large tumor cells with enlarged, markedly pleomorphic nuclei showing angulation, molding, and brisk mitotic activity with atypical forms, often present diffusely in the tumor. Distinctive

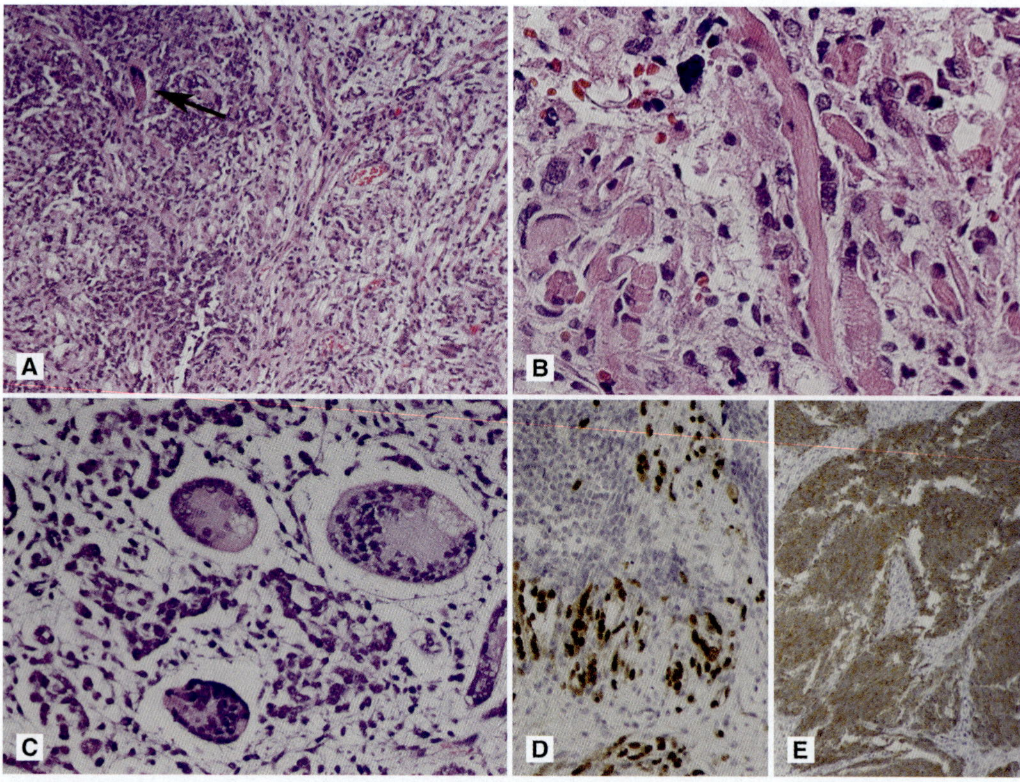

FIGURE 7-3: Medulloblastoma with myogenic differentiation. Sheets of small blue tumor cells (PNET component) in the *left half* (**A**). A multinucleated large myogenic cell is identified (*arrow*). Spindled tumor cells (i.e., myogenic tumor component) are predominantly seen in the *right half*. Abundant myogenic tumor cells, some with cytoplasmic striation, are seen (**B**). Multinucleated giant myogenic tumor cells are noted (**C**). Myogenin immunostain exhibiting nuclear positivity in the myogenic component (**D**). Synaptophysin immunostain revealing positivity in the PNET component (**E**).

cannibalism or "cell wrapping," characterized by the nucleus of one tumor cell "wrapped" around the degenerated nucleus of another one, and numerous apoptotic bodies are frequently seen.

iv. *Large cell MB* (Figure 7-7): This variant is composed of monotonous large polygonal tumor cells with vesicular nuclei and prominent nucleoli, with loss of cellular cohesion. These features bear superficial resemblance to those of malignant lymphoma (large cell type). High mitotic rate and extensive apoptosis is commonly seen. This variant frequently contains areas of anaplastic MB in varying proportions and is also known to be associated with worse prognosis.

Cytologic touch/squash preparations are very informative for a diagnosis of MB and can be used to differentiate aggressive tumor subtypes (anaplastic and large cell variants) from other subtypes. Our study showed that "cell wrapping," pleomorphism, macronucleoli, apoptosis, mitoses, and cytoplasmic vacuoles were more significantly observed in anaplastic and large cell variants than in other variants.[12]

The most important differential diagnosis in children includes ependymoma/anaplastic ependymoma arising from the fourth ventricle, which can present similar radiologic features to MB, and AT/RT. Anaplastic ependymoma, especially highly cellular one, needs to be distinguished from classic MB by lack of neuronal markers, strong GFAP positivity within the perivascular pseudorosettes, and occasional epithelial membrane antigen (EMA) dot-like immunoreactivity in tumor cells. Careful search for typical ependymal structures (i.e., ependymal rosettes) is also important. AT/RT should be excluded especially in very young children (<3 years old) and in small biopsy specimens, which may not be representative of the morphologic heterogeneity typical of AT/RT. AT/RTs occur in the cerebellum (although not typically midline) and may contain focal or prominent malignant

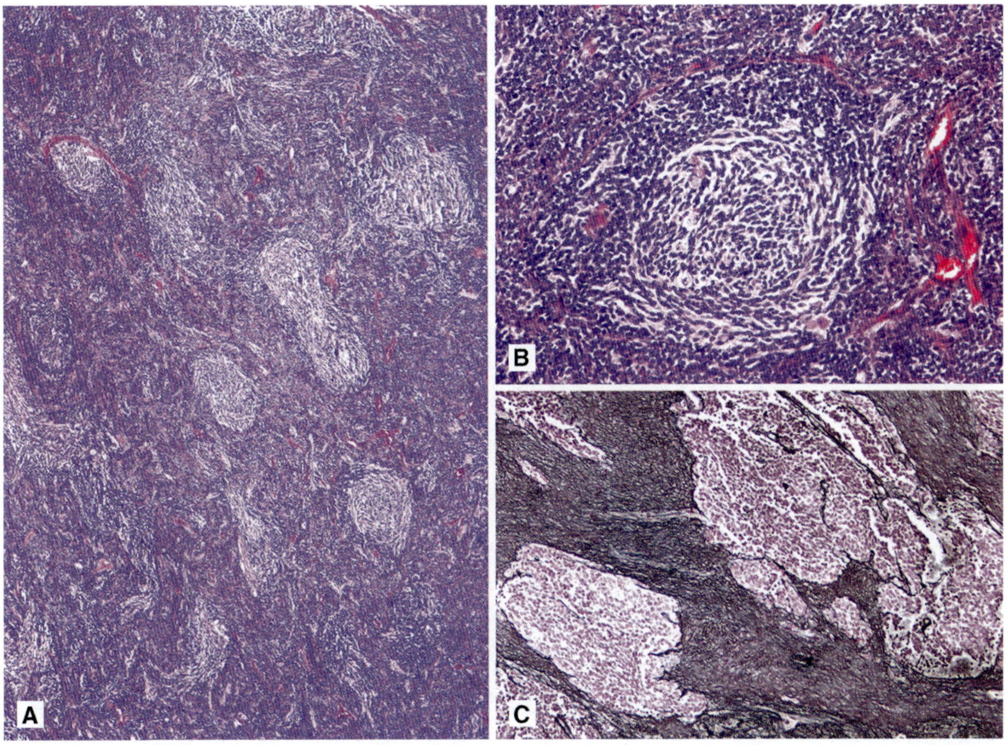

FIGURE 7-4: Desmoplastic/nodular medulloblastoma. Low-power view showing multiple characteristic "pale islands" (**A**). Intermediate-power view of a "pale island" showing a nodule of uniform tumor cells with a fibrillary matrix (**B**). Reticulin stain highlighting reticulin-free nodular zones (pale islands) surrounded by a dense reticulin fiber network (**C**).

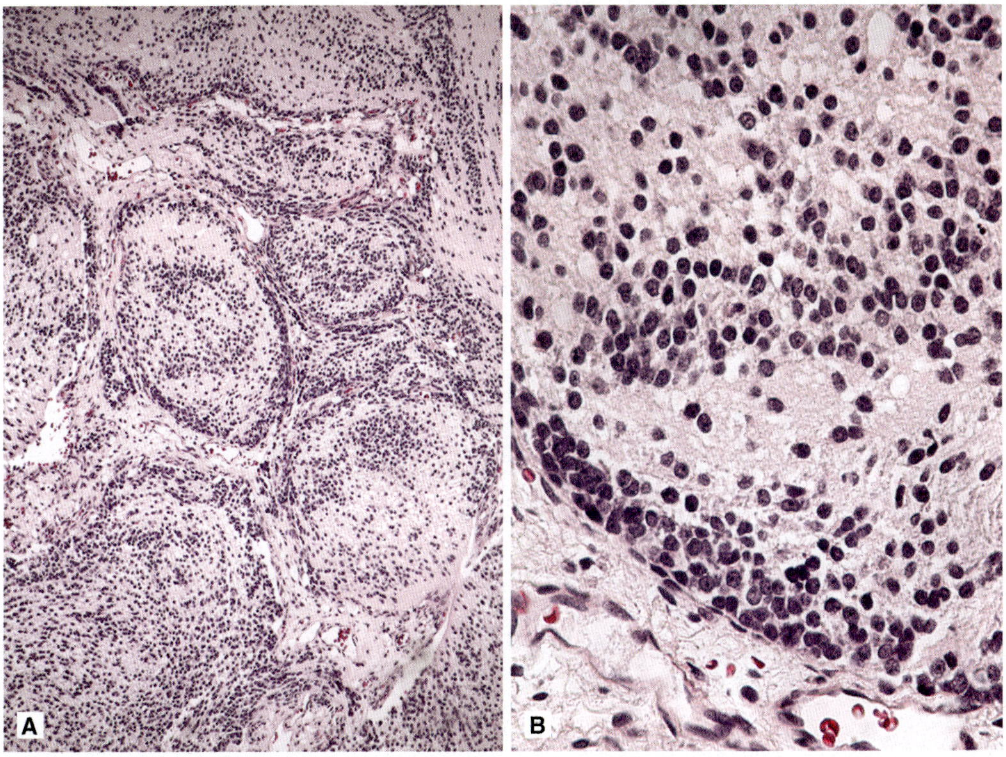

FIGURE 7-5: Medulloblastoma with extensive nodularity. Low-power view showing an expanded lobular architecture (**A**). Intermediate-power view showing lobules of monomorphic small tumor cells without desmoplastic internodular tissue (**B**).

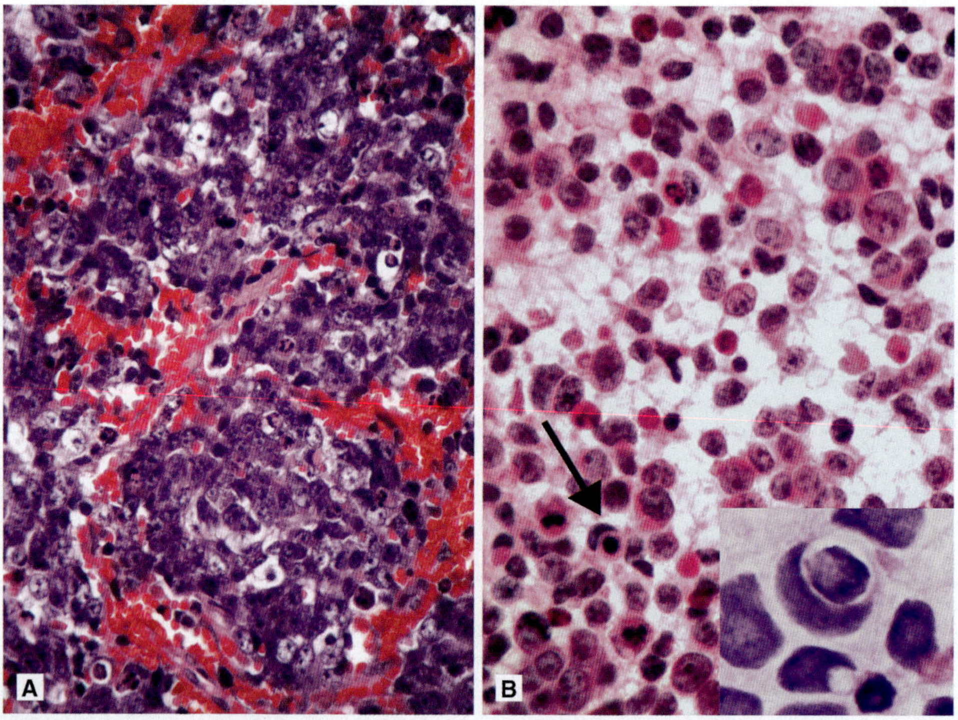

FIGURE 7-6: Anaplastic medulloblastoma. Histologic section showing cellular sheets of markedly atypical large tumor cells with brisk mitotic activity and many apoptotic bodies (**A**). Cytologic touch imprint showing a discohesive markedly atypical tumor cells with frequent apoptotic bodies and "cell wrapping" (*arrow* and **inset**) in a hemorrhagic background (**B**).

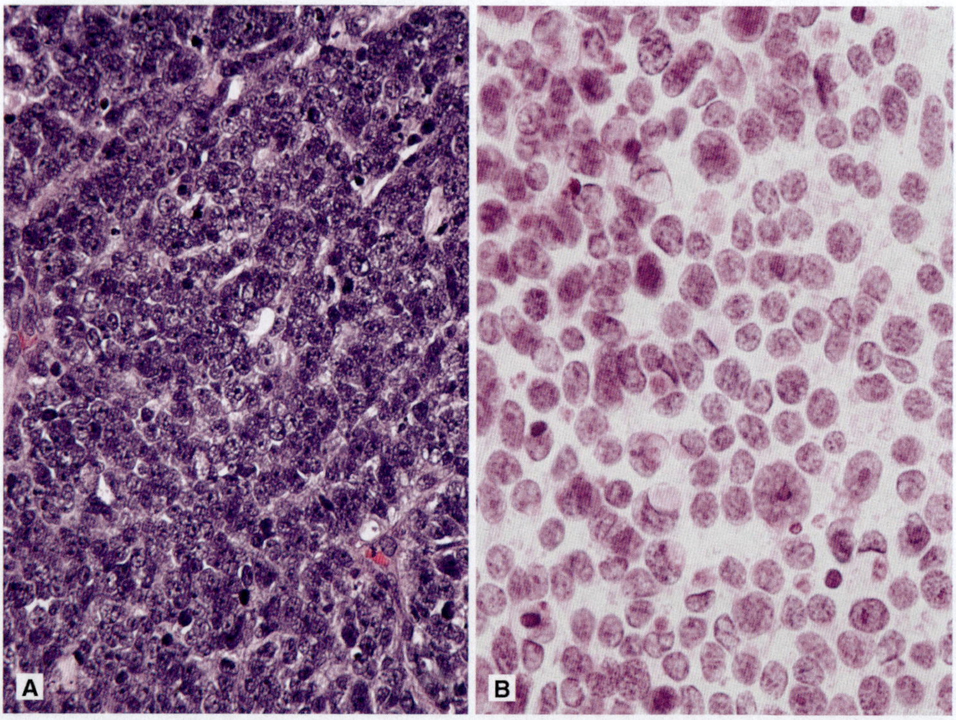

FIGURE 7-7: Large cell medulloblastoma. Histologic section showing very cellular sheets of large monomorphic polygonal tumor cells with vesicular nuclei and prominent nucleoli (**A**). Cytologic touch imprint showing discohesive tumor cells with vesicular chromatin and prominent nucleoli, bearing some resemblance to malignant lymphoma (diffuse large cell type) (**B**). Lymphoglandular bodies are not conspicuous in the background.

"(small) blue cell" (or PNET-like) components as seen in MBs in addition to the typical rhabdoid elements. In some examples of AT/RT, rhabdoid cells may be scarce. Immunohistochemistry is very helpful in the differential diagnosis. AT/RT characteristically demonstrates multilineage immunoreactivity for mesenchymal, epithelial, and neuroectodermal markers, whereas MBs have the capacity for neuronal, astrocytic, muscular, and melanocytic differentiation. The loss of INI-1 immunoreactivity is a characteristic feature of AT/RT, but not in MBs.

In adults, metastatic small cell carcinoma of the lung can be included in the differential diagnosis of MB especially in patients around 50 years of age. The histologic features are almost identical between these two tumors, with the exception of (vague) nodularity, which if present, favors a diagnosis of MB since it is extremely rare in small cell carcinomas. Pancytokeratin (panCK), CK-7, and thyroid transcription factor (TTF)-1 are immunoreactive in metastatic small cell carcinomas of the lung, but not in MBs. Clinical and radiologic information is usually most useful.

ATYPICAL TERATOID/RHABDOID TUMOR

AT/RT is a rare, highly malignant CNS tumor (WHO grade IV) of unknown histogenesis, with rhabdoid cells and divergent differentiation. AT/RT was the first pediatric brain tumor to have a candidate tumor suppressor gene identified. Virtually, all cases of AT/RT are characteristically associated with inactivation of the *INI1/hSNF5/SMARCB1* gene at 22q11.2, which is now the defining molecular feature of this tumor. A small fraction of cases occur in rhabdoid tumor predisposition syndrome (with germline mutation of the *INI1* gene). (Please refer to "Molecular Pathology, Non-glial Tumors" and "Hereditary Syndrome" chapters for detailed descriptions.)

AT/RT typically occurs in children aged 3 years and younger, and the posterior fossa (cerebellum and cerebellopontine angle) is a preferred site although it can originate anywhere throughout the neuraxis. Supratentorial AT/RTs can arise in the cerebral hemispheres, pineal gland, and sellar/suprasellar region, and are seen in higher age groups compared to infratentorial tumors. AT/RT can occur rarely in adults, and most reported cases are located in the cerebral hemispheres.[13]

Clinical symptoms are nonspecific, depending on the patient's age as well as the location and size of the tumor. In posterior fossa tumors, clinical and neuroimaging features are indistinguishable from those of MBs.[14] AT/RT is a large, heterogeneously contrast-enhancing tumor on MRI with restricted diffusion on DWI. Leptomeningeal dissemination (LD) can be detected by MRI. Although LD is frequently found in AT/RT at diagnosis or during/after treatment, there is no standard staging system to describe the extent or spread of tumor.

The current treatment options include surgery for debulking as well as for pathologic diagnosis, chemotherapy, radiation therapy, and high-dose chemotherapy with stem cell transplant.[15] Surgery followed by chemotherapy is commonly preferred. Radiation is an effective component of therapy but is avoided in patients younger than 3 years due to its long-term neurocognitive sequelae.[16] Despite intensive treatment, the prognosis is dismal with estimated overall survival of 10 months, which is significantly worse than that of other embryonal tumors.[16]

Histologically, AT/RTs are very cellular tumors that show marked regional heterogeneity, characteristically with primitive neuroepithelial, rhabdoid, epithelial, and mesenchymal components (Figures 7-8 and 7-9). Evidence of divergent differentiation is often limited to areas that appear sarcomatoid in quality on routine staining, or merely a polyphenotypic immunohistochemical pattern.[17] There is often a fibrovascular stroma separating lobules and sheets of tumor cells. The cellular morphology varies from those of primitive neuroepithelial type cells with hyperchromatic nuclei resembling those of MBs, to large cells with eosinophilic, pale or clear cytoplasm, and large round nuclei with more open chromatin and prominent nucleoli, including typical rhabdoid cells. Of note is that these typical rhabdoid cells may be sparse to absent, imparting histologic features virtually indistinguishable from those of CNS PNET or MB. Most lesions are focally necrotic.

Cytologically, AT/RT shows hypercellular smears composed of small to medium neuroblastic-type tumor cells with hyperchromatic fine chromatin and high N/C ratio (i.e., PNET component), as well as "plasmacytoid" tumor cells with eccentrically located nuclei and elongated

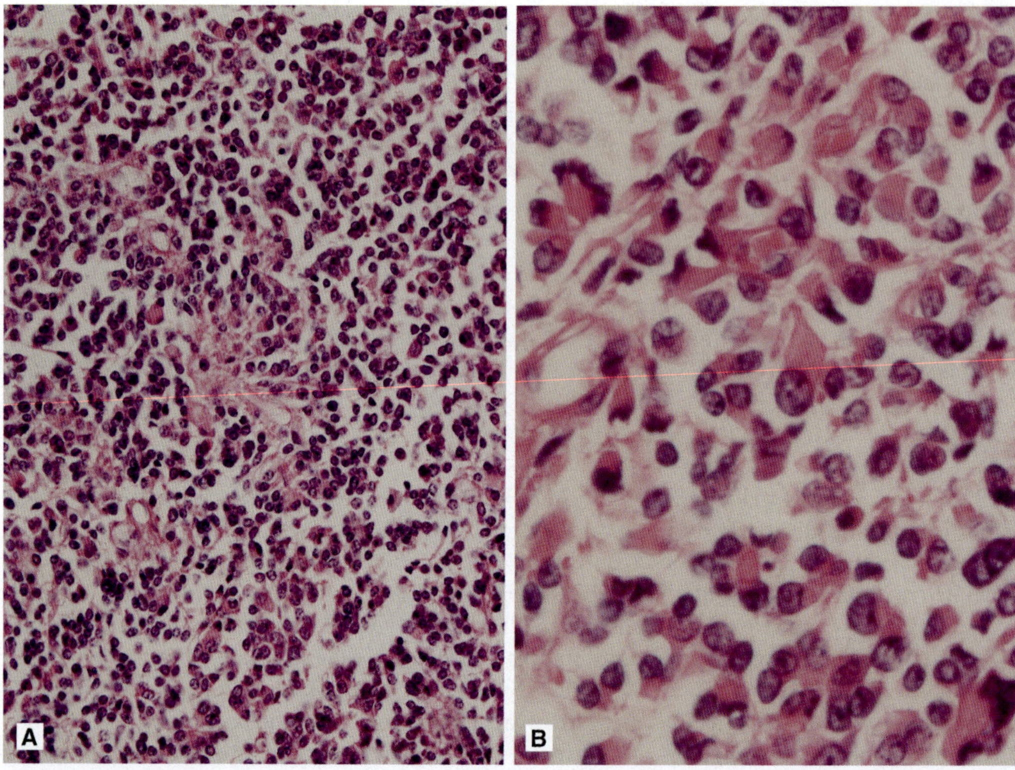

FIGURE 7-8: Atypical teratoid rhabdoid tumor. Low-power view showing cellular sheets of PNET component (**A**). High-power view showing many rhabdoid tumor cells of varying shapes and sizes (**B**).

cytoplasm. "Cell wrapping," apoptosis, mitosis, and necrosis are frequently seen. Neuropil background or lymphoglandular bodies are not a feature. Characteristic rhabdoid tumor cells, characterized by large, eccentrically placed nuclei, prominent nucleoli, and abundant brightly eosinophilic cytoplasm, are seen (Figure 7-9B and C). These cytomorphologic features are unique and lead to an accurate diagnosis in the right clinicoradiologic context.[18]

Immunohistochemically, AT/RT demonstrates immunoreactivity for a range of mesenchymal, epithelial, and neuroectodermal markers (Figures 7-10 and 7-11). Expression of EMA, CK, smooth muscle actin, and GFAP is frequently observed.[19] S100 protein, synaptophysin, chromogranin, NFP, desmin may be variably and focally expressed in AT/RT.[19] Vimentin is consistently expressed, whereas germ cell markers are consistently negative. Antibody to INI1 (with absent nuclear immunoreactivity in tumor cells in AT/RT) has been shown to correlate with *INI1* gene mutation in AT/RT. Loss of INI-1 expression has now become a standard feature for the confirmation of histologic diagnosis of AT/RT. Normally, positive cells in the background such as endothelium, fibroblasts, and inflammatory cells, are valuable internal controls. This immunohistochemical marker is of particular importance in the identification of rhabdoid cell–poor cases of AT/RT or in the diagnosis of examples with indeterminate histologic features and in small biopsies that might not be representative of the morphologic heterogeneity typical of AT/RTs.

Given the histologic variability of AT/RTs, there is significant histologic overlap with the appearances of other embryonal tumors of CNS. Currently, the recommendation is that all embryonal CNS tumors should be systematically screened for INI-1 expression, with the exception of conventional desmoplastic/nodular MBs.[20] However, recently, cases of AT/RT with nodularity mimicking beta-catenin–positive nodular MB have been recorded and support the notion that INI-1 immunostain should be performed in all CNS embryonal tumors including nodular MBs, especially in very young patients.[21]

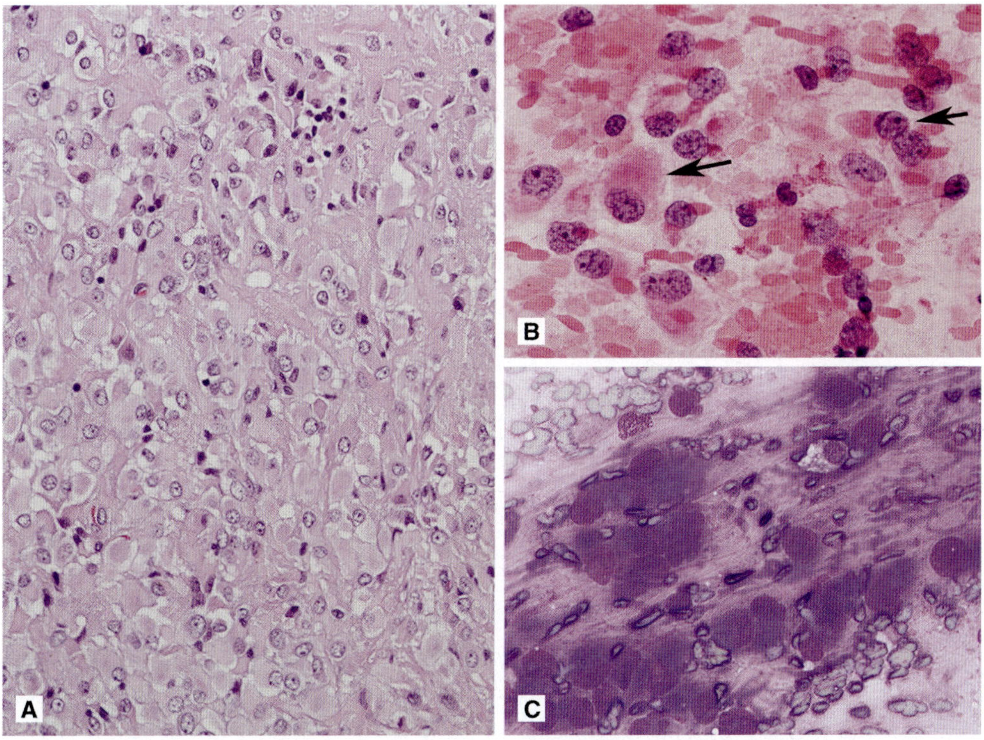

FIGURE 7-9: Atypical teratoid rhabdoid tumor. Histologic section showing a densely packed sheet that is composed almost exclusively of rhabdoid tumor cells with abundant eosinophilic cytoplasm (**A**). Cytologic touch imprint showing discohesive rhabdoid tumor cells with abundant cytoplasm (*arrows*) in a hemorrhagic background (**B**). Cytologic touch imprint (Diff-Quik stain) showing many rhabdoid tumor cells with a gray nodular area in the cytoplasm (**C**).

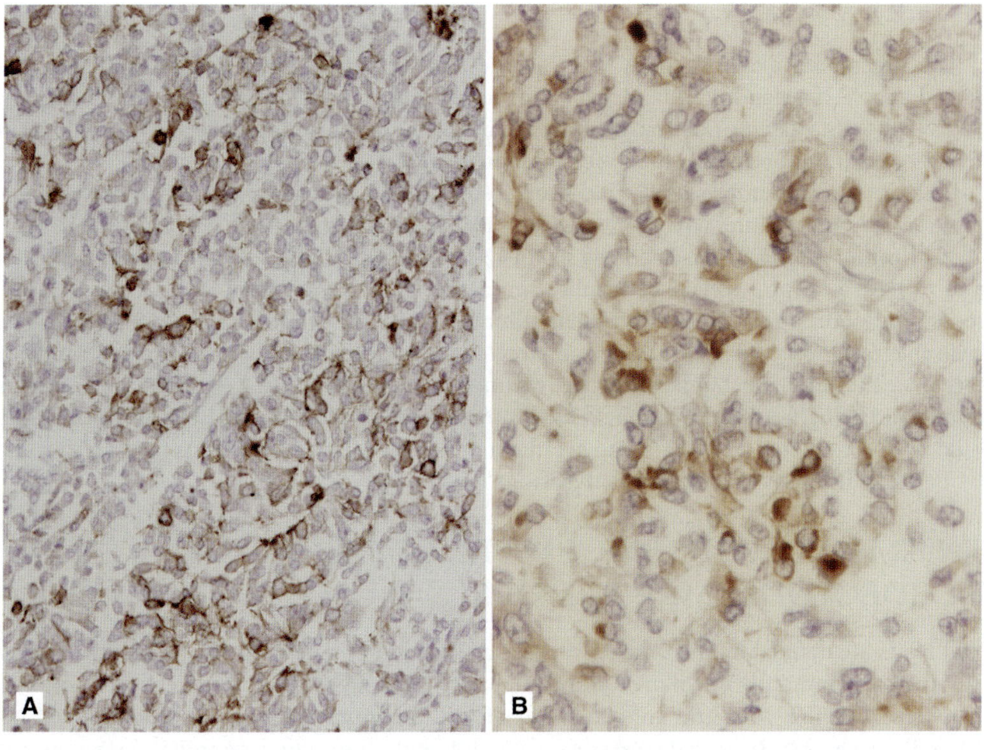

FIGURE 7-10: Atypical teratoid rhabdoid tumor (same case as shown in Figure 7-8). Immunohistochemistry. EMA is focally positive in tumor cells (**A**). GFAP is focally expressed in tumor cells (**B**).

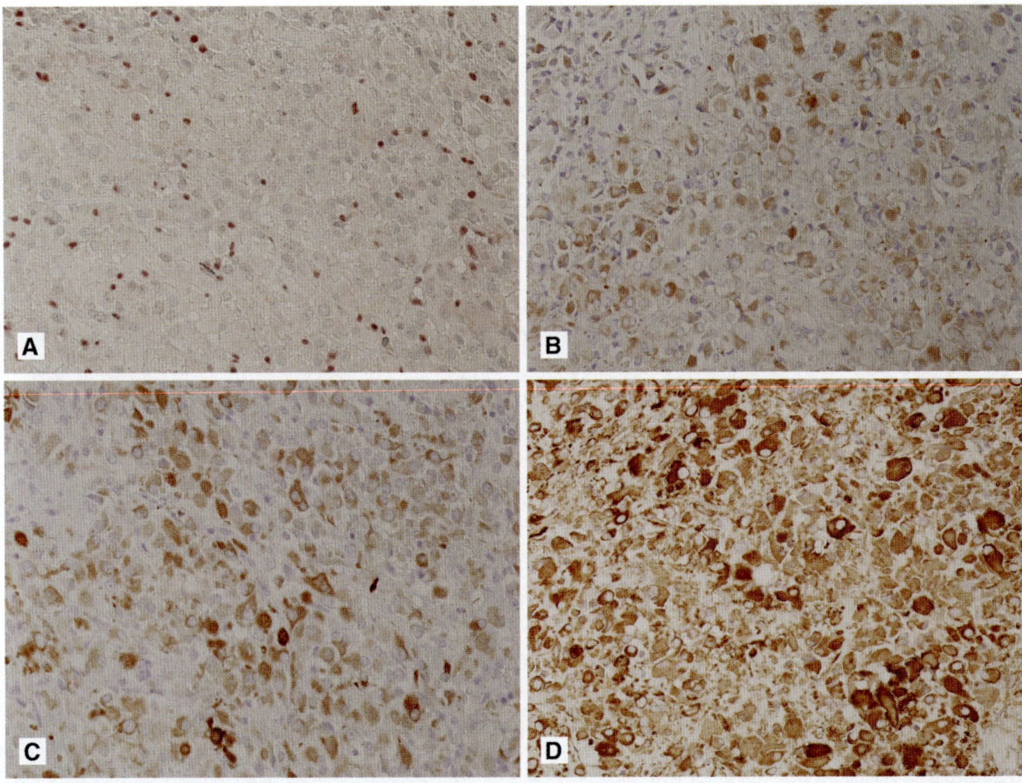

FIGURE 7-11: Atypical teratoid rhabdoid tumor (same case as shown in Figure 7-10). Immunohistochemistry. INI-1 is not expressed in tumor cells. Inflammatory cells and endothelial cells are positive (i.e., internal control) (**A**). Neurofilament protein is positive in subsets of tumor cells (**B**). Pancytokeratin is positive in subsets of tumor cells (**C**). Vimentin is diffusely and strongly positive in tumor cells (**D**).

The differential diagnosis of AT/RT includes MB especially the large cell/anaplastic variants and anaplastic ependymoma for posterior fossa tumors, and choroid plexus carcinoma and CNS PNETs for supratentorial tumors. Immunohistochemical profile (especially INI1) described above is of great importance in the differential diagnosis.

Lack of INI1 immunoreactivity has been seen in non-CNS tumors such as renal medullary carcinoma and epithelioid sarcoma (especially proximal type). In the CNS, cribriform neuroepithelial tumor (CRINET) is reported as an INI1-deficient PNET.[22] One case was reportedly found to have a homozygous 4-bp duplication in the *INI-1* gene (exon 4).[22] CRINET is a very rare, unique nonrhabdoid intraventricular tumor in young children characteristically carrying a favorable prognosis.[21,22] This tumor is characterized histologically by cribriform strands and trabeculae, immunohistochemically by well-defined EMA-positive surfaces, absence of GFAP and inwardly rectifying potassium channel (Kir7.1) reactivity, and loss of INI1 expression. CRINET should be differentiated from AT/RT to avoid potential overtreatment given its favorable prognosis with probable better response to conventional chemotherapy regimens.

CENTRAL NERVOUS SYSTEM PRIMITIVE NEUROECTODERMAL TUMORS

CNS PNETs are defined by the current WHO classification as a heterogeneous group of tumors occurring predominantly in children and adolescents that may arise in the cerebral hemispheres, brain stem, or spinal cord and are composed of undifferentiated or poorly differentiated neuroepithelial cells, which may display divergent differentiation along neuronal, astrocytic, and ependymal lines.[2] CNS PNETs are basically noncerebellar and nonpineal PNETs, encompassing previously termed, supratentorial PNET, and histologically similar PNETs occurring in the brain stem and spinal cord. These tumors are much less common than MBs. The signs and symptoms depend on the site of origin of the tumor and locations involved. CNS PNETs are usually solid masses with or without cysts, necrosis, or hemorrhage. Calcification is frequently seen. CSF dissemination is seen in about one-third of cases while bone, lymph node, and liver metastases have been rarely described.

The majority of CNS PNETs belong to a histologic group not otherwise specified, and cases classified as the CNS PNET variants described below are uncommon.[23] They are highly cellular and composed mostly of small, primitive appearing cells with high N/C ratios, often with a predominantly solid component and variably infiltrating peripheral margins.[23] Nuclear molding and mitotic figures are frequently seen. Homer Wright rosettes can be identified but vary in frequency. Anaplastic (increased cell and nuclear size with irregular, pleomorphic hyperchromatic nuclei) and large cell (increased cell and nuclear size with round to oval shaped nuclei and macronucleoli) features as described in MBs are found in about a half of cases. Sarcomatous features are rarely seen.[23] Immunohistochemically, synaptophysin is positive in most cases but varies in extent of expression from focal to extensive (Figure 7-12C). Other neuronal markers (NFP and NeuN) are also immunoreactive in greater than two-thirds of cases.[23] INI-1 expression is retained (Figure 7-12D).

The following four histologic variants are recognized by the current WHO classification on the basis of the distinctive pattern of differentiation: CNS neuroblastoma, CNS ganglioneuroblastoma, medulloepithelioma (MEPL), and ependymoblastoma (EBL). The latter two variants and another unique variant of CNS embryonal tumor in children, embryonal tumor with abundant

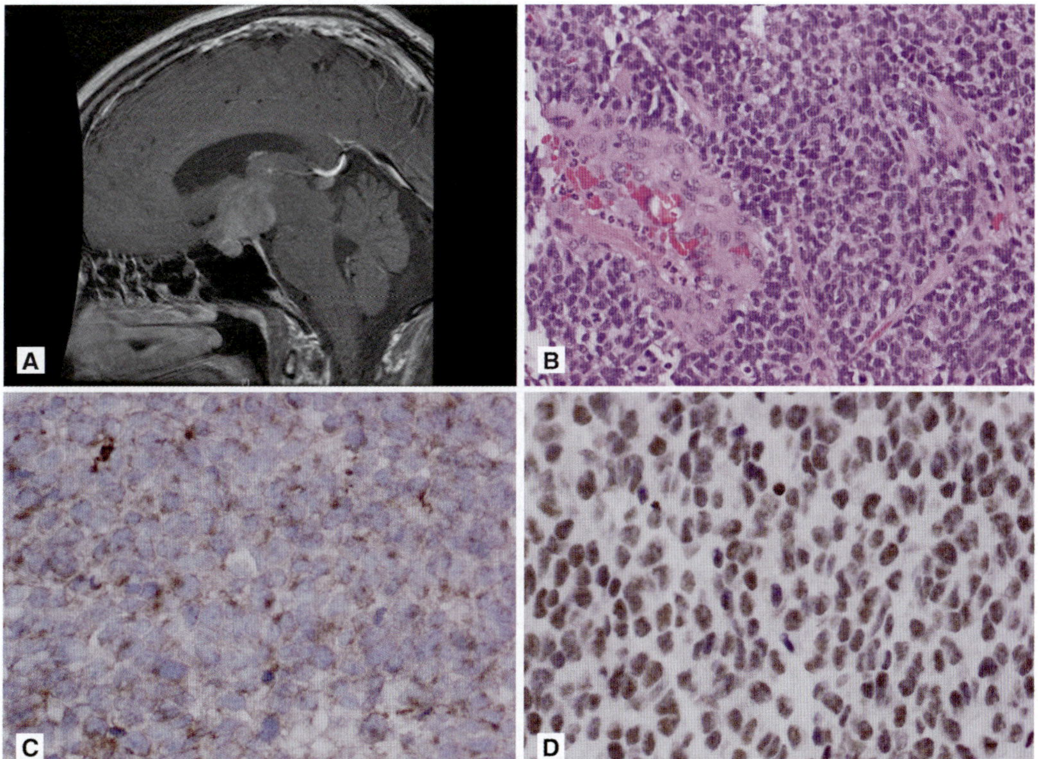

FIGURE 7-12: Suprasellar primitive neuroectodermal tumor (neuroblastoma). MR T1-WI showing a sellar and suprasellar heterogeneously enhancing mass with an extension into the hypothalamus (**A**). Histologic section showing cellular small blue cells with microvascular proliferation (**B**). Synaptophysin immunostain exhibiting positivity in tumor cells (**C**). INI-1 immunostain revealing retained nuclear immunoreactivity in tumor cells (**D**).

neuropil and true rosettes (ETANTR),[24] are known within the family of embryonal rosette-forming neuroepithelial brain tumors. All these three tumors share a uniform molecular signature, characterized by amplification of the *C19MC* microRNA cluster at 19q13.42, similar histologic patterns and clinical features, and are considered to comprise a single biologic entity, for which a generic name of "embryonal tumor with multilayered rosettes (ETMR)" is proposed.[25,26]

CNS PNETs are histologically indistinguishable from MBs but characteristically have more aggressive biologic behavior (Figure 7-12B). Patients with anaplastic or large cell features have even worse overall survival.[23] CNS PNETs have different genetic alterations from MBs (e.g., very rare loss of 17p and isochromosome of 17q; common polysomy 2 and 8 in CNS PNETs), while some molecular resemblance to subsets of MBs (i.e., *MYC/MYCN* amplifications) is also reported in roughly half of pediatric patients.[23,27] Studies of global gene expression signatures revealed the absence of external granular cell layer gene and proneuronal transcripts in CNS PNETs.[28] Peripheral PNET/Ewing sarcoma can rarely occur as a meningeal-based lesion in the intracranial or intraspinal sites and is also histologically indistinguishable from CNS PNET. However, it has a characteristic unique molecular signature with Ewing sarcoma/Friend leukemia virus integration 1 (*EWS/FLI1*) translocation, which is not present in CNS PNETs.[23,29] Peripheral and central PNETs differ in histogenesis, molecular characteristics, and clinical behavior.

The most important differential diagnosis of CNS PNETs is AT/RT especially in young children. Immunohistochemical staining for INI1 is important to resolve this differential diagnosis. In adults, CNS PNETs are very rare, and glioblastoma with PNET-like components (GBM-PNET) and small cell GBM should be considered as differential diagnoses. To differentiate from GBM-PNET, infiltrating glial (astrocytic) components need to be identified histologically. In addition, a combination of immunohistochemical stains for CD56 and vimentin can be of use in diagnosis as well as differential diagnosis.[30] In GBM-PNET, vimentin diffusely and strongly highlights the astrocytic components and is negative in PNET-like components, whereas CD56 is diffusely and strongly positive in both astrocytic and PNET-like components. CNS PNETs are usually positive for CD56 and negative for vimentin. GFAP positivity may be absent or focal. Small cell GBMs are composed of monotonous tumor cells (Figure 7-13A and B), which are strongly and diffusely positive for both CD56 (Figure 7-13C) and vimentin. GFAP is usually positive (Figure 7-13D).[31] Genetically, small cell GBM often exhibits frequent *EGFR* amplification.[31]

CNS Neuroblastoma and Ganglioneuroblastoma

CNS PNET with evidence of predominant neuronal differentiation by immunohistochemistry have been termed CNS neuroblastoma, while those with an additional element of more advanced neuronal differentiation (e.g., ganglion cell component) that is histologically appreciated are termed CNS ganglioneuroblastoma.[21] Neuronal markers such as synaptophysin, class III beta-tubulin, and NFP are usually immunoreactive. Although CNS neuroblastomas are histologically indistinguishable from MBs, genetically they are distinctly different. Chromosome 17 alterations (i.e., 17p loss and isochromosome 17q) that are frequently seen in MBs are very rare in cerebral neuroblastomas. Cerebral neuroblastomas show deletion of 9q21.3 spanning the *CDKN2A* and *CDKN2B*.[27]

Embryonal Tumor with Multilayered Rosettes: Ependymoblastoma, Medulloepithelioma, and Embryonal Tumor with Abundant Neuropil and True Rosettes

ETMR is a rare, newly suggested entity and comprises the following three, histologically similar, embryonal rosette-forming neuroepithelial brain tumors: EBL, MEPL, and ETANTR. ETMR is genetically distinct and is characterized by high-level amplification of the microRNA cluster C19MC at 19q13.42. ETMR almost exclusively affects very young children (median age: 2 to 3 years old) with no significant gender predilection and is associated with a dismal prognosis (median overall survival of about 12 months).[26] Most tumors occur supratentorially, and the frontoparietal region is the most common location.[26] Surgery with adjuvant chemotherapy is the mainstay of

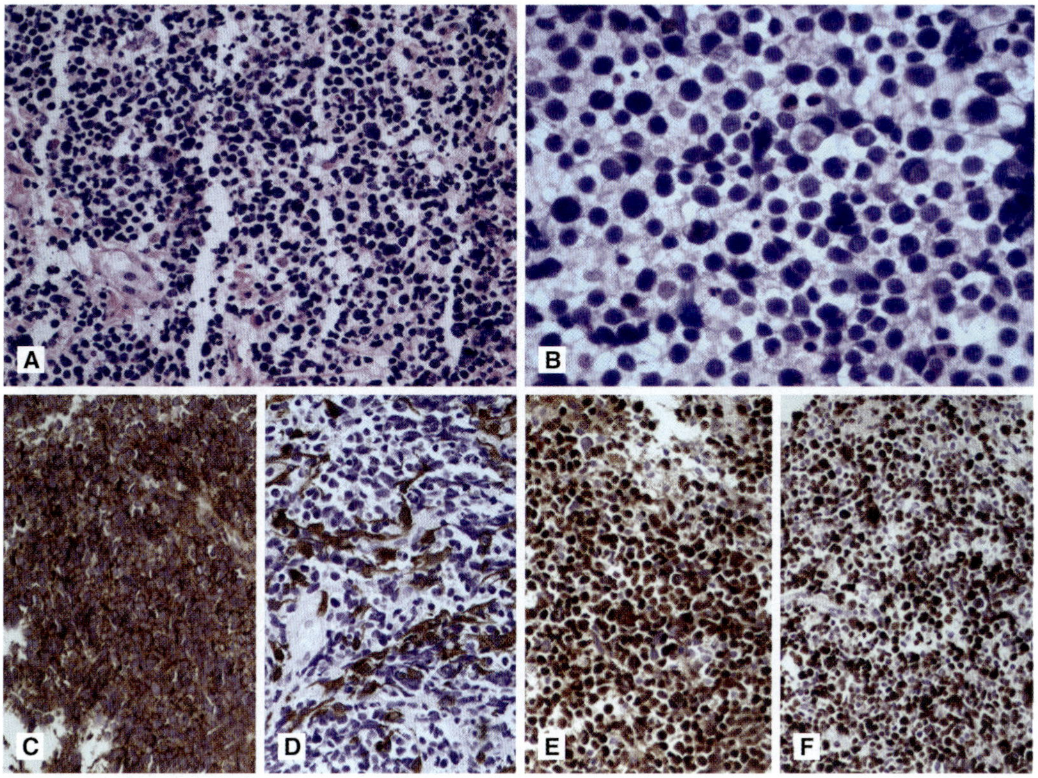

FIGURE 7-13: Small cell glioblastoma. Histologic section showing cellular sheets of relatively monomorphic tumor cells with high N/C ratio (**A**). Cytologic touch imprint showing discohesive tumor cells with hyperchromatic round nuclei and scattered apoptotic bodies (**B**). CD56 immunostain is diffusely and strongly positive in tumor cells (**C**). GFAP immunostain is focally positive (**D**). p53 immunostain is diffusely and strongly positive in tumor cells (**E**). Ki-67 (MIB-1) labeling index is >80% (**F**).

treatment. Histologically, ependymoblastic and/or "medulloepithelial" rosettes are the hallmark (described in detail below). Strong and diffuse LIN28A immunoreactivity is identified as a highly sensitive and specific marker for ETMR, and thus, is of great use in its diagnostic confirmation.[32] Of note is that LIN28A is focally positive in a small proportion of AT/RT cases.[32,33] INI1 immunostain is needed for the differential diagnosis in this setting, especially for small specimens.

Histologically, EBL is characterized by the exclusive presence of nests and clusters of medium sized, poorly differentiated cells forming ependymoblastic rosettes, which are multilayered rosettes containing mitotic figures and a central lumen with an internal limiting membrane and associated cilia and blepharoplasts,[34] without a neuropil-like background (Figure 7-14). These rosettes are intermingled with small- to medium-sized primitive cells with high N/C ratios. ETANTR is briefly described in the current WHO classification,[2] and is typified by a biphasic pattern composed of highly cellular clusters of small- to medium-sized primitive cells with scant cytoplasm, with scattered multilayered rosettes indistinguishable from those of EBL, and characteristic large fibrillar and paucicellular neuropil-like matrix (Figure 7-15), infrequently containing neoplastic neurons and ganglion cells.[24,27] The background of neoplastic neuropil is highlighted with NFP and synaptophysin immunohistochemical stains. MEPL is characterized by tubular, papillary, and trabecular arrangement of pseudostratified primitive tumor cells with an external limiting membrane (ELM), mimicking the embryonic neural tube (Figure 7-16A and B). There are no cilia or blepharoplasts on the inner surfaces in contrast to those of rosettes seen in EBL and ETANTR. The ELM is highlighted with periodic acid–Schiff (PAS) stain (Figure 7-16C) and labeled with type IV collagen immunostain. This tumor often displays multiple lines of differentiation, including neuronal, glial, and mesenchymal elements. The periventricular area is the most common site of occurrence.

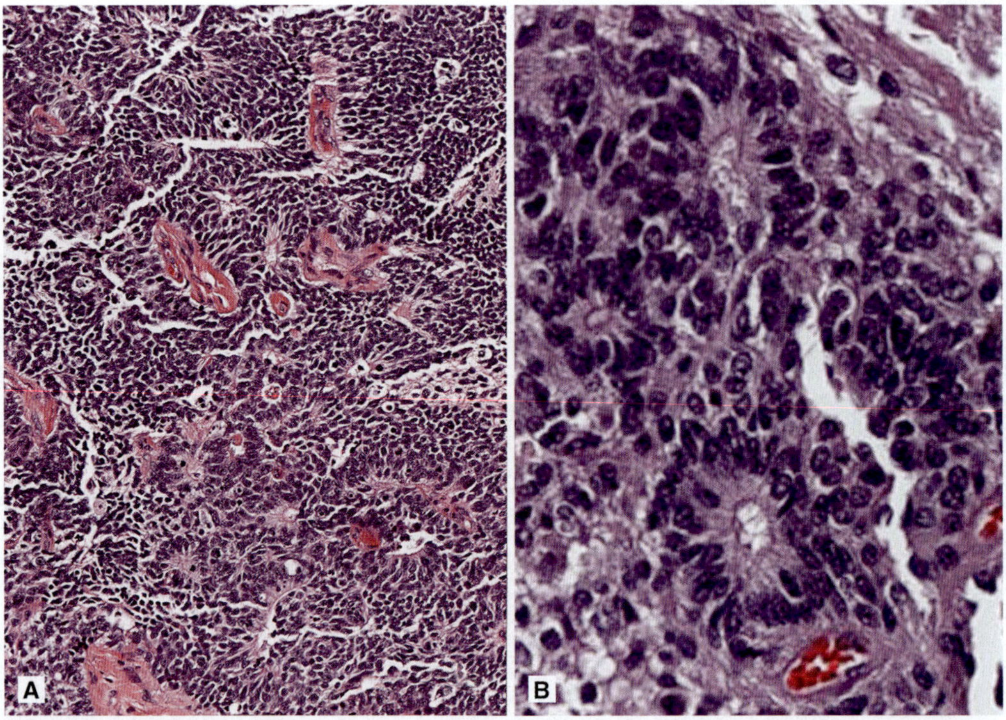

FIGURE 7-14: Ependymoblastoma. Low-power view showing cellular, small- to medium-sized, poorly differentiated tumor cells with prominent multilayered rosette formation (**A**). High-power view showing ependymoblastic rosettes composed of multilayered tumor cells with a central lumen and an internal limiting membrane (**B**).

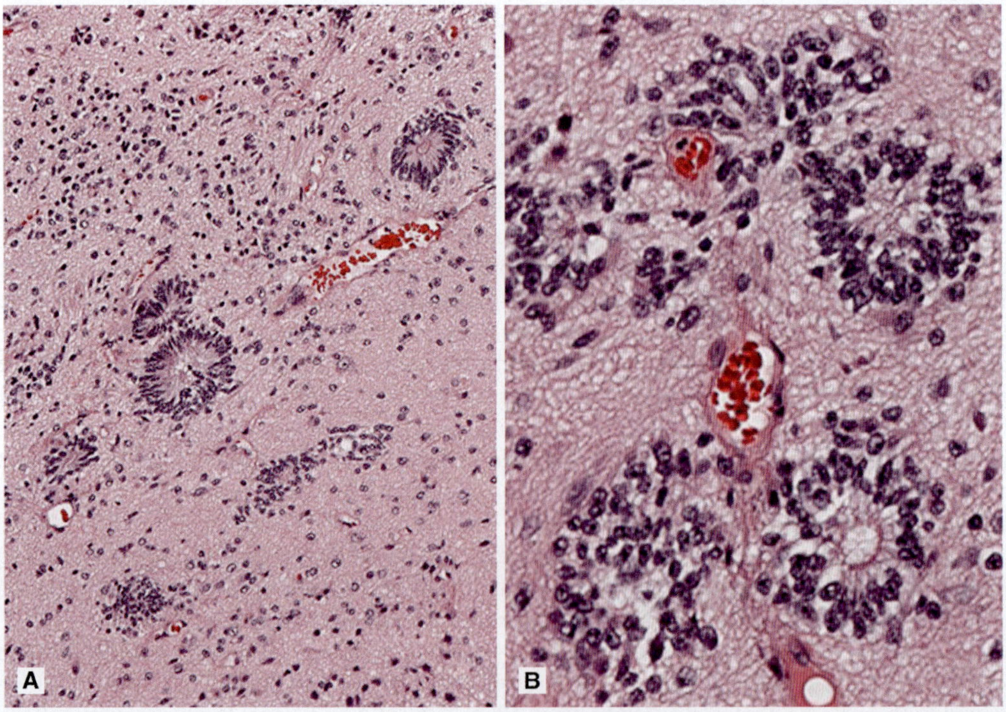

FIGURE 7-15: Embryonal tumor with abundant neuropil and true rosettes (ETANTR). Low-power view showing a biphasic pattern composed of large fibrillary and paucicellular neuropil-like matrix and scattered multilayered rosettes (**A**). High-power view showing multilayered rosettes indistinguishable from ependymoblastic rosettes (**B**).

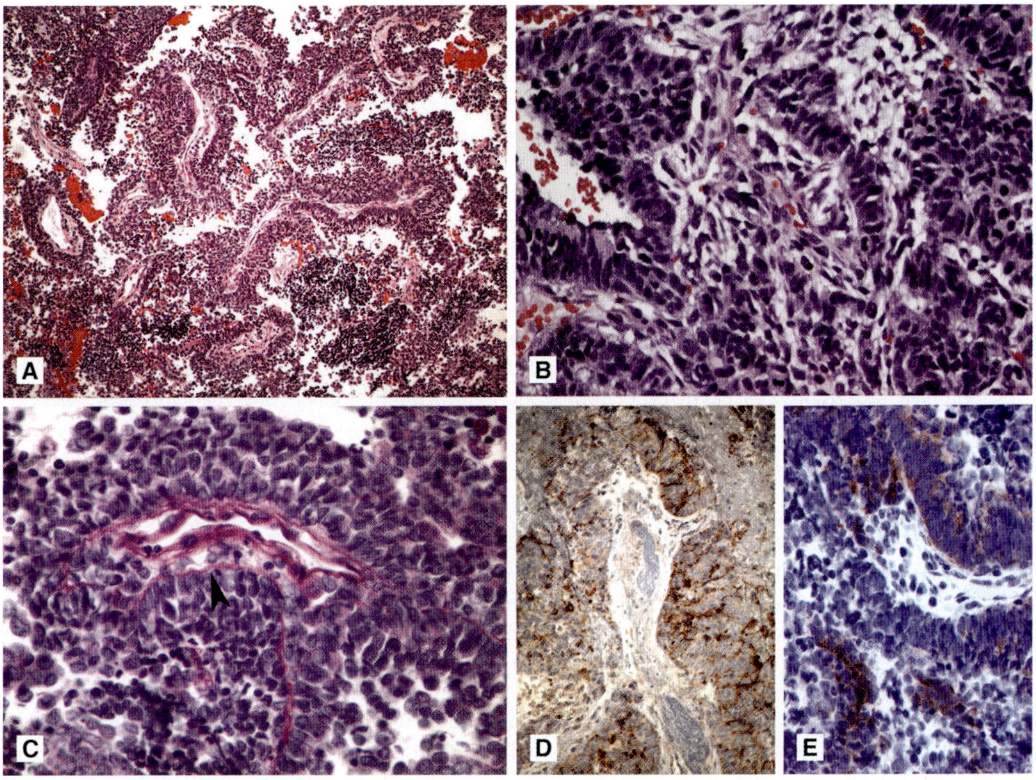

FIGURE 7-16: Medulloepithelioma. Low-power view showing tubular and papillary arrangement of multilayered tumor cells (**A**). Intermediate-power view showing trabecular and tubular arrangement of multilayered tumor cells with hyperchromatic nuclei and high N/C ratio (**B**). PAS stain highlighting an external limiting membrane (*arrowhead*) (**C**). Synaptophysin immunostain is positive in subsets of tumor cells (**D**). Microtubule-associated protein (MAP)-2 immunostain is positive in some of tumor cells (**E**).

References

1. Ostrom QT, Gittleman H, Farah P, et al. CBTRUS statistical report: primary brain and central nervous system tumors diagnosed in the United States in 2006–2010. *Neurooncology* 2013;15:ii1–ii56.
2. Louis DN, Ohgaki H, Wiestler OD, et al. *WHO Classification of Tumors of the Central Nervous System*. 4th ed. Lyon, France: IARC; 2007:131–149.
3. Crawford JR, MacDonald TJ, Packer RJ. Medulloblastoma in childhood: new biological advances. *Lancet Neurol* 2007;6:1073–1085.
4. Lai R. Survival of patients with adult medulloblastoma. A population-based study. *Cancer* 2008;112: 1568–1574.
5. Terterov S, Krieger MD, Bowen I, et al. Evaluation of intracranial cerebrospinal fluid cytology in staging pediatric medulloblastomas, supratentorial primitive neuroectodermal tumors, and ependymomas. *J Neurosurg Pediatr* 2010;6:131–136.
6. Wilne S, Collier J, Kennedy C, et al. Progression from first symptom to diagnosis in childhood brain tumours. *Eur J Pediatr* 2012;171:87–93.
7. National Cancer Institute. *Treatment of Newly Diagnosed Childhood Medulloblastoma*. http://www.cancer.gov/cancertopics/pdq/treatment/childCNSembryonal/healthprofessional/page5#Reference5.17. Accessed August 16, 2014.
8. National Cancer Institute. *Treatment Option Overview for CNS Embryonal Tumors. Risk Stratification for Medulloblastoma*. http://www.cancer.gov/cancertopics/pdq/treatment/childCNSembryonal/healthprofessional/page4. Accessed August 16, 2014.

9. Northcott PA, Korshunov A, Witt H, et al. Medulloblastoma comprises four distinct molecular variants. *J Clin Oncol* 2011;29:1408–1414.
10. de Haas T, Hasselt N, Troost D, et al. Molecular risk stratification of medulloblastoma patients based on immunohistochemical analysis of MYC, LDHB, and CCNB1 expression. *Clin Cancer Res* 2008;14:4154–4160.
11. Taylor MD, Northcott PA, Korshunov A, et al. Molecular subgroups of medulloblastoma: the current consensus. *Acta Neuropathol* 2012;123:465–472.
12. Takei H, Dauser RC, Adesina AM. Cytomorphologic characteristics, differential diagnosis and utility during intraoperative consultation for medulloblastoma. *Acta Cytol* 2007;51:183–192.
13. Takei H, Adesina AM, Mehta V, et al. Atypical teratoid/rhabdoid tumor of the pineal region in an adult. *J Neurosurg* 2010;113:374–379.
14. Rorke LB, Packer RJ, Biegel JA. Central nervous system atypical teratoid/rhabdoid tumors of infancy and childhood: definition of an entity. *J Neurosurg* 1996;85:56–65.
15. National Cancer Institute. *Childhood Central Nervous System Atypical Teratoid/Rhabdoid Tumor Treatment.* http://www.cancer.gov/cancertopics/pdq/treatment/child-CNS-ATRT/patient/page4. Accessed August 23, 2014.
16. Ginn KF, Gajjar A. Atypical teratoid rhabdoid tumor: current therapy and future directions. *Front Oncol* 2012;2:114.
17. Dunham C. Pediatric brain tumors: a histologic and genetic update on commonly encountered entities. *Semin Diagn Pathol* 2010;27:147–150.
18. Parwani AV, Stelow EB, Pambuccian SE, et al. Atypical teratoid/rhabdoid tumor of the brain. Cytologic characteristics and differential diagnosis. *Cancer* 2005;105:65–70.
19. Takei H, Bhattacharjee MB, Rivera A, et al. New immunohistochemical markers in the evaluation of central nervous system tumors: a review of seven selected adult and pediatric brain tumors. *Arch Pathol Lab Med* 2007;131:234–241.
20. Haberler C, Laggner U, Slavc I, et al. Immunohistochemical analysis of INI1 protein in malignant pediatric CNS tumors: lack of INI1 in atypical teratoid/rhabdoid tumors and in a fraction of primitive neuroectodermal tumors without rhabdoid phenotype. *Am J Surg Pathol* 2006;30:1462–1468.
21. Miller S, Ward JH, Rogers HA, et al. Loss of INI1 protein expression defines a subgroup of aggressive central nervous system primitive neuroectodermal tumors. *Brain Pathol* 2013;23:19–27.
22. Hasselblatt M, Oyen F, Gesk S, et al. Cribriform neuroepithelial tumor (CRINET): a nonrhabdoid ventricular tumor with INI1 loss and relatively favorable prognosis. *J Neuropathol Exp Neurol* 2009;12:1249–1255.
23. Behdad A, Perry A. Central nervous system primitive neuroectodermal tumors: a clinicopathologic and genetic study of 33 cases. *Brain Pathol* 2010;20:441–450.
24. Eberhart CG, Brat DJ, Cohen KJ, et al. Pediatric neuroblastic brain tumors containing abundant neuropil and true rosettes. *Pediatr Dev Pathol* 2000;3:346–352.
25. Paulus W, Kleihues P. Genetic profiling of CNS tumors extends histological classification. *Acta Neuropathol* 2010;120:269–270.
26. Korshunov A, Sturm D, Ryzhova M, et al. Embryonal tumor with abundant neuropil and true rosettes (ETANTR), ependymoblastoma, and medulloepithelioma share molecular similarity and comprise a single clinicopathological entity. *Acta Neuropathol* 2014;128:279–289.
27. Pfister SM, Korshunov A, Kool M, et al. Molecular diagnostics of CNS embryonal tumors. *Acta Neuropathol* 2010;120:553–566.
28. Pomeroy SL, Tamayo P, Gaasenbeek M, et al. Prediction of central nervous system embryonal tumour outcome based on gene expression. *Nature* 2002;415:436–442.
29. Vural C, Uloğlu O, Akyürek N, et al. The evaluation of CD99 immunoreactivity and EWS/FLI1 translocation by fluorescence in situ hybridization in central PNETs and Ewing's sarcoma family of tumors. *Pathol Oncol Res* 2011;17:619–625.
30. Song X, Andrew Allen R, Terence Dunn S, et al. Glioblastoma with PNET-like components has a higher frequency of isocitrate dehydrogenase 1 (IDH1) mutation and likely a better prognosis than primary glioblastoma. *Int J Clin Exp Pathol* 2011;4:651–660.
31. Perry A, Aldape KD, George DH, et al. Small cell astrocytoma: an aggressive variant that is clinicopathologically and genetically distinct from anaplastic oligodendroglioma. *Cancer* 2004;101:2318–2326.
32. Korshunov A, Ryzhova M, Jones DT, et al. LIN28A immunoreactivity is a potent diagnostic marker of embryonal tumor with multilayered rosettes (ETMR). *Acta Neuropathol* 2012;124:875–881.
33. Ceccom J, Bourdeaut F, Loukh N, et al. Embryonal tumor with multilayered rosettes: diagnostic tools update and review of the literature. *Clin Neuropathol* 2014;33:15–22.
34. Judkins AR, Ellison DW. Ependymoblastoma: dear, damned, distracting diagnosis, farewell! *Brain Pathol* 2010;20:133–139.

Choroid Plexus Tumors (Choroid Plexus Papilloma, Atypical Choroid Plexus Papilloma, Choroid Plexus Carcinoma, Xanthogranuloma of the Choroid Plexus, and Metastasis)

8

▶ Yasuo Sugita

CHOROID PLEXUS PAPILLOMA AND ATYPICAL CHOROID PLEXUS PAPILLOMA

The choroid plexus is an epithelial–endothelial vascular convolute within the ventricular system.[1] This structure consists of epithelial cells, fenestrated blood vessels, and stroma, and, depending on various physiologic or pathologic conditions, may contain fibroblasts, mast cells, macrophages, granulocytes or other infiltrates, and a rich extracellular matrix. Choroid plexus epithelial tumors are rare intraventricular neoplasms of neuroectodermal origin derived from choroid plexus epithelium, accounting for less than 1% of all intracranial tumors.[2] These tumors are classified as choroid plexus papilloma (CPP) (World Health Organization [WHO] grade I), atypical choroid plexus papilloma (APP) (WHO grade II), and choroid plexus carcinoma (CPC) (WHO grade III). CPP can usually be cured by resection, whereas the prognosis of CPC is poor.[1–9]

CPPs are primarily found in children, but they can also occur in adults and infants. Presenting symptoms are usually related to hydrocephalus. This hydrocephalus is believed to be caused by factors such as direct obstruction of cerebrospinal fluid (CSF) flow, arachnoid granulation blockage due to hemorrhage, and overproduction of CSF.[4,7] Although CPPs are histologically benign and, in general, show a favorable long-term outcome after surgical resection, there is occasional local recurrence. Indeed, cases of benign CPPs with distant seeding have even been reported.[5]

Magnetic resonance imaging (MRI) of CPP shows a T1-weighted image (WI)–isointense and T2-WI–hyperintense, contrast-enhancing mass within the ventricle (Figure 8-1). Associated hydrocephalus is generally seen.[3,7]

Cytologically, CPP exhibits numerous papillary clusters, which are composed of cuboidal cells with ample cytoplasm and regular, round to slightly oval nuclei with evenly dispersed chromatin (Figure 8-2A). In general, these cells show no nuclear molding and no/very rare mitotic figures. In a larger view, CPP appears as cohesive tissue fragments that are composed of regular cuboidal cells with round nuclei, which often occur in papillary fronds.[10,11] Histologically, CPP is

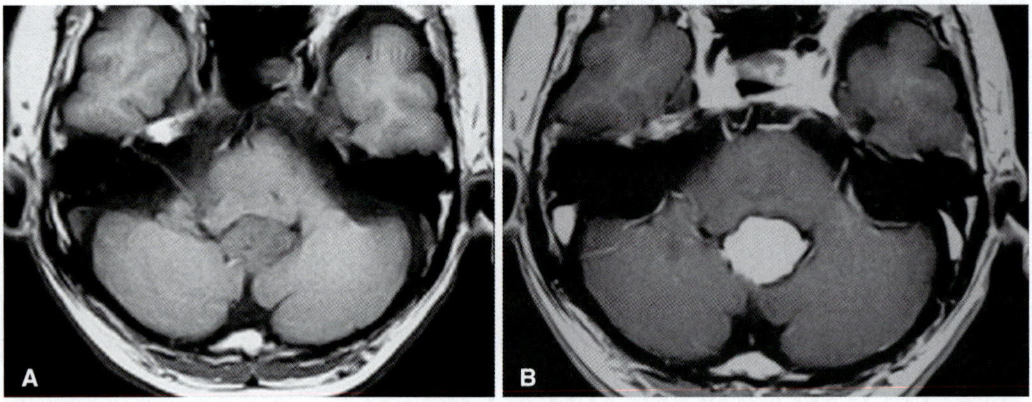

FIGURE 8-1: MRI features of CPP. Axial T1-weighted MRI showing an isointense lesion in the fourth ventricle (**A**). Axial T1-weighted MRI after contrast administration showing an enhancing lesion (**B**).

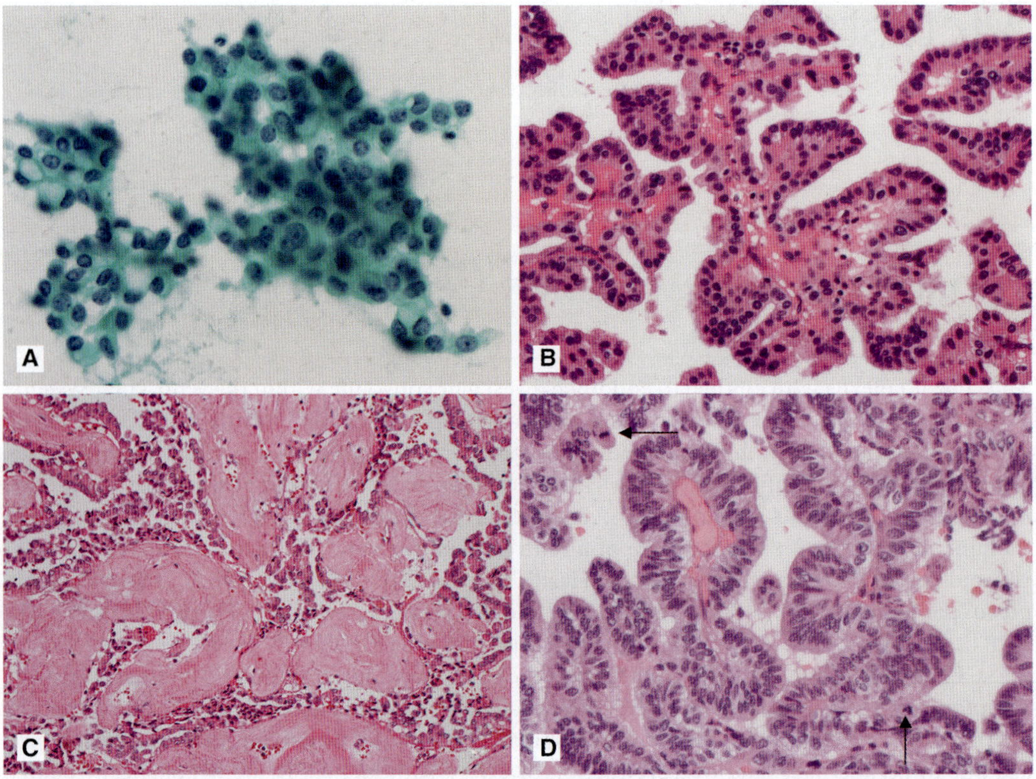

FIGURE 8-2: Choroid plexus papilloma. Cytologic touch smear exhibiting papillary clusters composed of cuboidal cells with regular, round to slightly oval nuclei, evenly dispersed chromatin, and ample cytoplasm (Papanicolaou stain) (**A**). The tumor is composed of papillary structures with a delicate fibrovascular core lined with a layer of columnar, cuboidal to flattened epithelium, which shows low mitotic activity (H&E stain) (**B**). The stroma of papillary cores may show extensive sclerosis (H&E stain) (**C**). Atypical CPP is characterized by increased mitotic activity (*arrows*, H&E stain) (**D**).

composed of papillary structures with a delicate fibrovascular core lined by a layer of columnar, cuboidal to flattened epithelium with no/rare mitoses (Figure 8-2B). The papillary structures have well-formed, continuous basement membranes underneath the epithelial cells. The stroma of papillary cores may show extensive sclerosis (Figure 8-2C), psammoma bodies, and osseous metaplasia in obsolete lesions.[9]

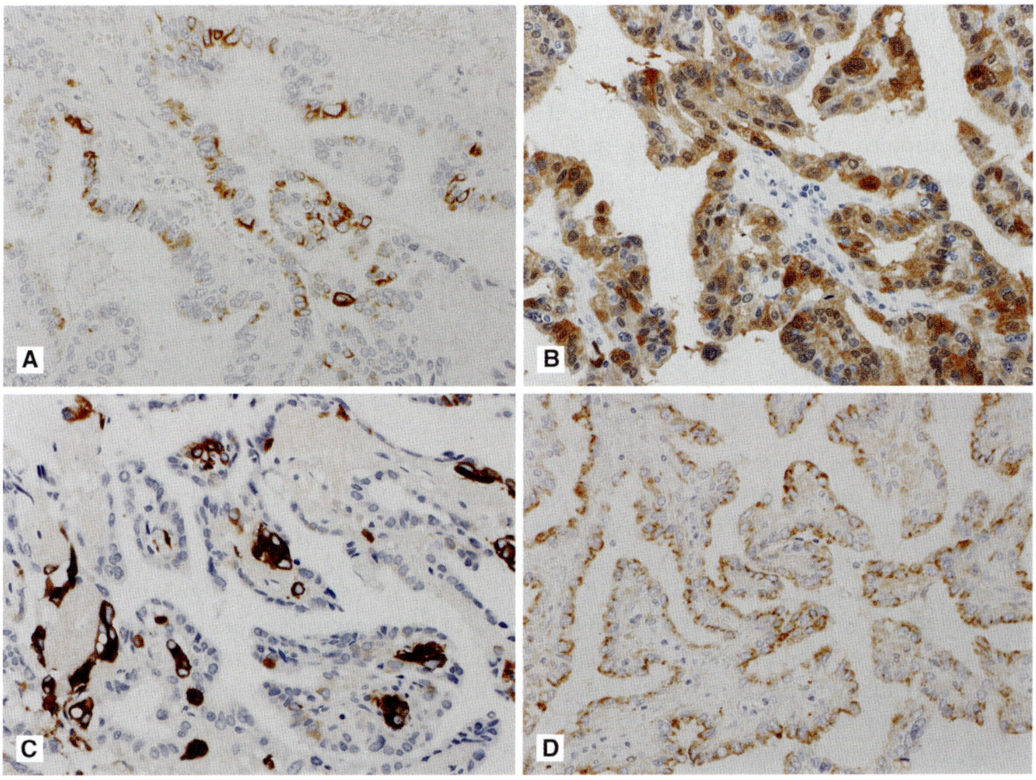

FIGURE 8-3: Immunohistochemical findings of CPP. Tumor cells are positive for cytokeratin 7 (**A**). Tumor cells exhibiting expression of S100 protein (**B**). Tumor cells exhibiting patchy expression of GFAP (**C**). Tumor cells are positive for transthyretin (prealbumin) (**D**).

In 2007, the WHO working group codified APP as an additional entity, an intermediate lesion (WHO grade II).[1–6,9,11–13] Inclusion of this intermediate entity is important because it carries an almost fivefold increase in recurrence at 5 years compared with grade I CPP.[(2–4,6)] APP is characterized by increased mitotic activity compared with CPP (≥2 per 10 high-power fields; HPFs) (Figure 8-2D). Although atypical histopathologic features such as increased cellularity, nuclear pleomorphism, and blurring of the papillary architecture have been described in some reports as diagnostic features of APP, these are not essential for the diagnosis. Therefore, there is still a lack of general consensus regarding the histologic parameters and the minimal criteria required for a diagnosis of APP.[2,9]

Immunohistochemically, the tumor cells of CPP are generally positive for cytokeratin (CK)-7, vimentin, and podoplanin (D2-40) and are negative for CK-20. These cells also show variable expression of S100 protein, glial fibrillary acidic protein (GFAP), transthyretin (prealbumin), and synaptophysin[2,6,9] (Figure 8-3). Novel reliable CPP markers such as Kir7.1 and Stanniocalcin-1 have recently been reported.[14] Kir7.1 is a potassium inwardly rectifying channel that is found in normal choroid plexus and in CPP but not in other primary brain tumors or in metastatic tumors. Stanniocalcin-1 is believed to play a role in calcium homeostasis and has been shown to confer resistance to hypoxic stress. Kir7.1 and Stanniocalcin-1 are both considered as sensitive and specific markers of CPPs.[1,3,4,14] The ultrastructural appearance of CPP is similar to that of choroid plexus tissue.[15] The cells are joined by regular apical junctional complexes, are mainly columnar in shape, and are usually arranged in a pattern with papillary architecture. The outer, apical surfaces give rise to a profusion of microvilli.

It may be difficult to distinguish CPP from villous hypertrophy of the choroid plexus or from papillary ependymoma (WHO grade II). Villous hypertrophy is a benign proliferation of cells that causes enlargement of the choroid plexus in the lateral ventricle.[6] Histologically, this lesion has a cytologic appearance of normal choroid plexus. Proliferation indices assessed by Ki-67/MIB-1 immunostain can be useful in the diagnosis of villous hypertrophy. Papillary ependymoma shows monomorphic cuboidal to columnar cells that have indistinct nucleoli and stippled chromatin, forming papillary structures with smooth external surfaces. In contrast to CPP, the papillary cores are not composed of fibrovascular tissue, without basement membranes underlying tumor cells, and instead contain perivascular pseudorosettes. Immunohistochemically, strong and diffuse GFAP labeling is seen compared to CPP. Additional differential diagnostic considerations may include xanthogranuloma of the choroid plexus and metastatic (papillary) tumors to the choroid plexus. Differential diagnoses from these diseases are discussed below.

CHOROID PLEXUS CARCINOMA

CPCs are rare neoplasms that are most commonly found in children. Approximately 30% of choroid plexus tumors are malignant and are classified by WHO as grade III tumors.[1–5,7–9,16] A case of CPC that developed from a preexisting CPP has also been reported.[17] CPCs are highly aggressive malignant tumors in both adults and infants. They are usually invasive tumors that may appear solid, hemorrhagic, and necrotic. CPCs are associated with obstruction and/or overproduction of CSF, causing manifestations of hydrocephalus, such as increased head circumference, delayed development, bulging fontanelles, separated sutures, and/or vomiting, in infants. Older children and adults present vomiting, headache, neurologic deficits, seizures, and/or lethargy.

In general, maximum surgical resection offers the best chance for long-term survival for patients with CPC.[3,6,8]

MRI of CPCs exhibits a T1-WI large isointense–hyperintense, contrast-enhancing intraventricular mass (Figure 8-4). The tumor is usually associated with hydrocephalus and

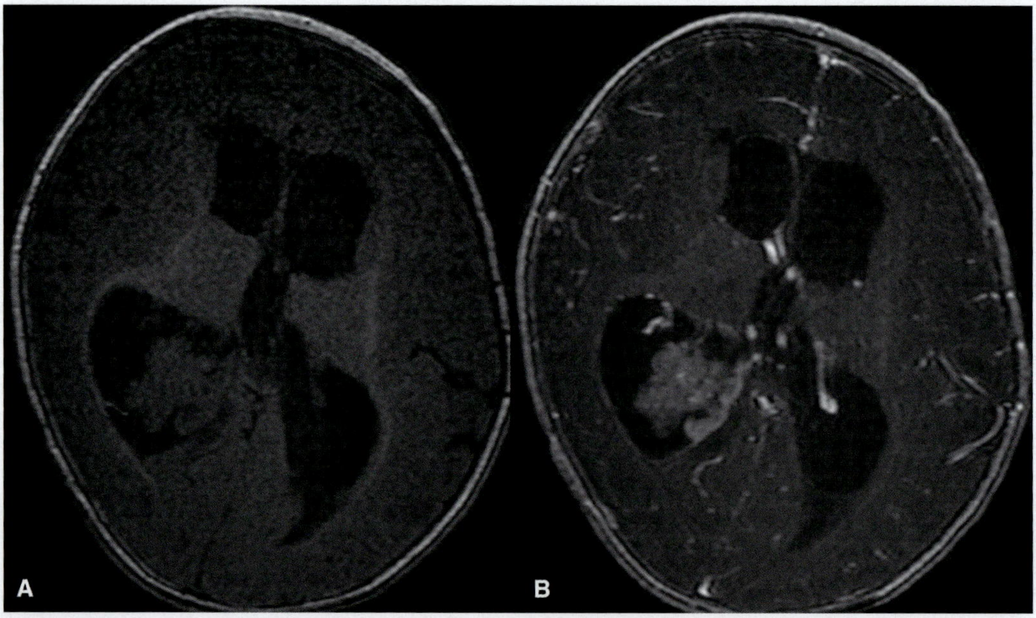

FIGURE 8-4: MRI features of choroid plexus carcinoma. Axial T1-weighted MRI demonstrates a large isointensive intraventricular mass lesion with associated hydrocephalus (**A**). Axial T1-weighted MRI after contrast administration showing a heterogeneous enhancing mass lesion (**B**).

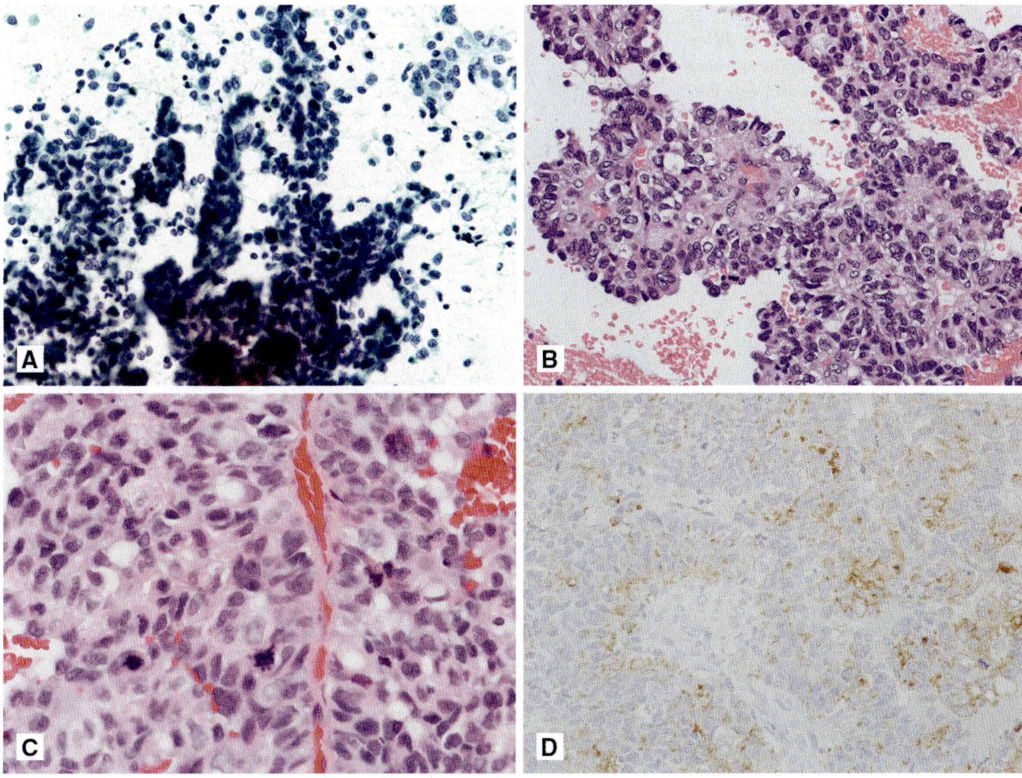

FIGURE 8-5: Choroid plexus carcinoma. Cytologic touch smear showing papillary clusters of markedly atypical cells with a columnar configuration resembling adenocarcinoma (Papanicolaou stain) (**A**). Histologic sections show broad papillary structures characterized by increased cell density and nuclear pleomorphism and hyperchromasia (H&E stain) (**B**). High power view showing frequent mitotic figures (H&E stain) (**C**). Tumor cells exhibiting weak patchy immunoreactivity for transthyretin (prealbumin) (**D**).

may contain focal calcification and hemorrhage. The vascular nature of the neoplasm can be appreciated with multiple flow voids. Distinction of CPPs from CPCs can occasionally be difficult because CPPs sometimes show irregular tumor margins.[18] However, CPPs tend to appear as lobulated, homogeneous-enhancing masses, whereas CPCs appear as more heterogeneous-enhancing masses.[3–5] In addition, CPC may have metastases along the CSF pathways.[3–5,8,18] Therefore, in order to distinguish between CPP and CPC, neuroimaging of the entire neuraxis is essential.

Cytologically, CPC exhibits hypercellular smears composed of cell clusters and singly dispersed cells.[19–21] The cell clusters are mainly three-dimensional and papillary. The individual tumor cells are markedly pleomorphic with nuclear polylobation and hyperchromasia. Clusters of cells with a columnar configuration resemble those of metastatic adenocarcinomas (Figure 8-5A). Histologically, CPC shows obvious malignant features, including increased cell density, nuclear pleomorphism, blurred papillary structures, solid tumor areas, necrosis, and frequent mitoses (>5 per 10 HPFs)[1,4,16] (Figure 8-5B and C). Diffuse invasion of adjacent brain tissue is often seen. Positive immunohistochemical markers for CPC and CPP are approximately the same (Figure 8-5D). However, the intensity of positive staining of such markers as S100 protein and transthyretin (prealbumin) is typically weaker than that of CPP. The MIB-1 labeling index can be useful in the diagnosis of CPC. The mean MIB-1 labeling index of CPP and CPC is 1.9% and 13.8%, respectively.[16]

The differential diagnosis includes papillary meningioma, atypical teratoid rhabdoid tumor (ATRT), and metastasis to the choroid plexus. Papillary meningioma is a high-grade meningioma

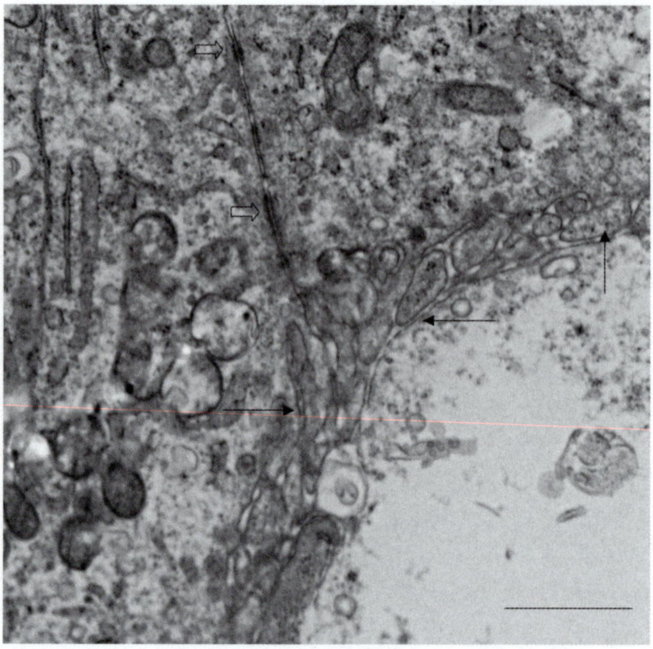

FIGURE 8-6: Ultrastructural features of choroid plexus carcinoma. In better differentiated areas, cells bordering the extracellular space may form microvilli (*arrows*). An apical zonula adherence junction is also present (*open arrows*) (bar = 10 μm).

(WHO grade III) and can arise in the choroid plexus, especially in young patients. Histologically, papillary meningioma is characterized by the presence of a perivascular pseudopapillary pattern of tumor cell growth, which bears some resemblance to CPC. Choroid plexus and neuroglial immunohistochemical markers are supposed to be negative in this tumor.

ATRT is a highly malignant central nervous system tumor, characterized by its predominant occurrence in young children, presence of typical rhabdoid cells and primitive neuroectodermal cells, divergent differentiation along epithelial, mesenchymal, neuronal, and/or glial lines, and inactivation of the *INI1/hSNF5* gene.[1–4,16] Almost all CPCs were reportedly immunoreactive for INI1 whereas the majority of ATRTs were negative. Thus, INI1 staining could potentially assist in distinguishing between CPC and ATRT with epithelial differentiation.[16] On the other hand, Schittenhelm et al.[22] reported cases of ATRT that exhibited membranous staining of Kir7.1, indicating a plexus epithelial differentiation of these tumors. They therefore proposed that a panel of immunohistochemical markers, including INI1, and glial, mesenchymal, and epithelial markers should be performed in such cases to make a reliable distinction between ATRT and CPC. Ultrastructurally, CPCs often retain many features typical of normal choroid plexus[15] (Figure 8-6).

XANTHOGRANULOMA OF THE CHOROID PLEXUS

Xanthogranulomas of the choroid plexus tend to be found relatively frequently at autopsy and their size does not usually exceed 2 cm.[22–27] On the other hand, symptomatic xanthogranulomas are uncommon lesions of the choroid glomus. The most common neurologic symptoms include headache, papilledema, nystagmus, epilepsy, mental retardation, and visual disturbance.[24,25,27] Duration of the symptoms ranges from 1 month to 5 years. Xanthogranulomas are more common in older than in younger patients. Surgical excision is a curative treatment, and the histologic diagnosis is definitive. The etiology is unknown; however, there are many theories regarding the pathogenesis of these lesions, including cellular degeneration, tissue reaction to hemorrhage, and general disturbance of lipid metabolism.[22–27] It is possible that xanthogranuloma of the

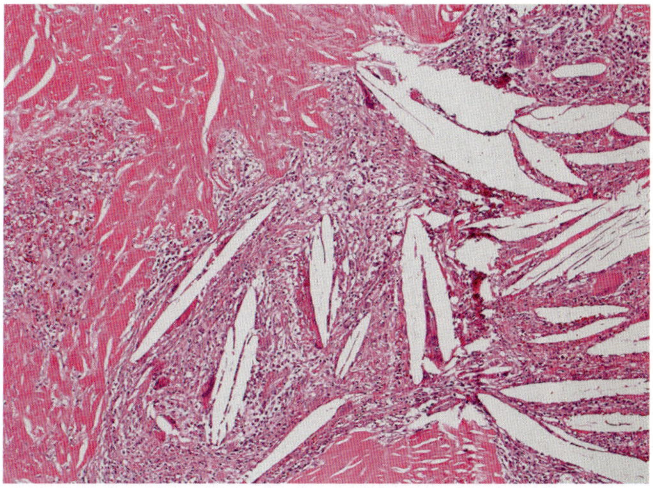

FIGURE 8-7: Xanthogranuloma of the choroid plexus. Xanthogranulomas are composed of xanthoma cells, cholesterol crystals, or foreign body giant cells. In addition, they are embedded in a fibrous stroma (H&E stain). (Courtesy of Dr. T. Hitotsumatsu, Kurume, Fukuoka, Japan.)

choroid plexus might form due to active lipid storage caused by a metabolic derangement of foamy cells.[22]

MRI of xanthogranulomas usually shows homogeneous hypointensity on T2-WI and isointensity on T1-WI with contrast enhancement.[24–28] Several cases of bilateral involvement have been reported.[25,27]

Xanthomas and xanthogranulomas may be distinguished each other based on a histologic basis. Xanthomas are usually small and consist merely of xanthoma cells without cholesterol crystals, foreign body giant cells, or hemorrhage. Xanthogranulomas tend to be larger, and are composed of a mixture of xanthoma cells, cholesterol crystals, and/or foreign body giant cells[22–27] (Figure 8-7). In addition, xanthogranulomas are embedded in a fibrous stroma and in residue of previous hemorrhage. Indeed, Hicks et al.[28] reported that xanthogranuloma is a misnomer for lesions that consist only of foam cells or only of cholesterol deposition with foreign body giant cell reaction. They also commented that in the former type of lesion, features of true xanthogranulomatous process can be inconspicuous, and the latter type of lesion should be classified as cholesterol granuloma.

METASTASIS TO THE CHOROID PLEXUS

Although brain metastases are the most common brain tumors among adults, metastasis to the choroid plexus, especially mass-forming lesions, is uncommon. However, in a diagnostic neurooncology practice, metastasis should be considered first in any tumors involving the choroid plexus in older adults given the rare occurrence of CPP and CPC in this age group. Of note is that the patient's clinical history and radiologic information are crucial.

Virtually any extracranial malignancies can give rise to metastasis to the choroid plexus. Shapira et al.[29] recently reported a high affinity of renal cell carcinoma to the ventricular system with close association to the choroid plexus in their metastatic brain tumor cohort. Differential diagnosis of metastatic carcinomas from primary choroid plexus neoplasms becomes more difficult when the metastasis exhibits papillary features on histologic examination. Although very rare, one of the examples of metastatic papillary neoplasms is metastatic papillary thyroid carcinoma (PTC) (Figure 8-8).[30–33] Characteristic nuclear features of PTC (e.g., ground grass chromatin, intranuclear pseudoinclusions, and nuclear grooves)[34] and immunohistochemistry (TTF-1 and thyroglobulin positivity) are of great help in the differential diagnosis (Figure 8-9).

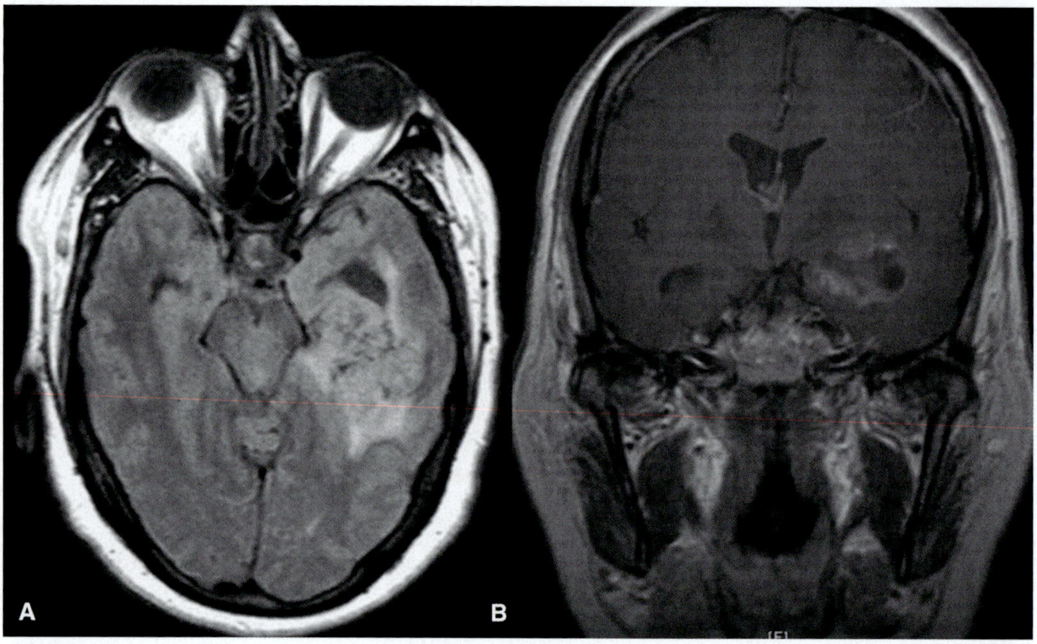

FIGURE 8-8: MRI of metastatic PTC to the choroid plexus (**A**, axial view and **B**, coronal view) T1-weighted MRI after contrast administration showing an irregularly enhancing lesion within and around the left lateral ventricle.

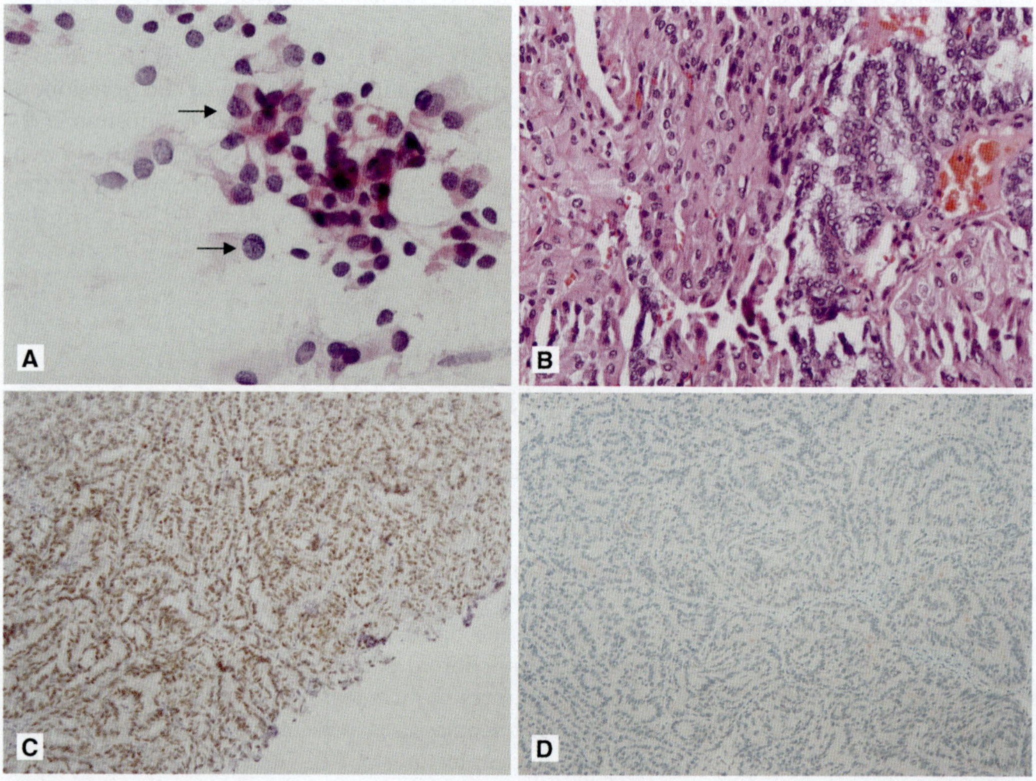

FIGURE 8-9: Metastatic PTC to the choroid plexus. Cytologic touch preparation showing a cellular smear composed of monomorphic cells with ground glass chromatin and occasional nuclear grooves (*arrows*) (H&E stain) (**A**). Histologic section showing papillotubular structures composed of columnar epithelial cells with ground glass chromatin (H&E stain) (**B**). Tumor cells are immunoreactive for TTF-1 (**C**). Tumor cells are immunonegative for transthyretin (prealbumin) (**D**).

References

1. Paulus W, Wolburg H. Choroid plexus: biology and pathology. *Acta Neuropathol* 2010;119:75–88.
2. Paulus W, Brandner S. Choroid plexus tumours. In: Louis DN, Ohgaki H, Wiestler OD, Cavenee WK, eds. *Pathology and Genetics of Tumours of the Nervous System*. 4th ed. Lyon, France: International Agency for Research on Cancer Press; 2007:188–192.
3. Safaee M, Oh MC, Bloch O, et al. Choroid plexus papillomas: advances in molecular biology and understanding of tumorigenesis. *Neuro Oncol* 2013;15:255–267.
4. Jaiswal S, Vij M, Mehrotra A, et al. A clinic-pathological and neuro-radiological study of 23 cases. *Asian J Neurosurg* 2013;8:29–35.
5. Ortega-Martínez M, Cabezudo-Artero JM, Fernández-Portales I, et al. Diffuse leptomeningeal seeding from benign choroid plexus papilloma. *Acta Neurochir (Wien)* 2007;149:1229–1237.
6. Ogiwara H, Dipatri AJ, Alden TD, et al. Choroid plexus tumors in pediatric patients. *Br J Neurosurg* 2012;26:32–37.
7. Paulus W, Jänisch W. Clinicopathologic correlations in epithelial choroid plexus neoplasms: a study of 52 cases. *Acta Neuropathol* 1990;80:635–641.
8. Pencalet P, Sainte-Rose C, Lellouch-Tubiana A, et al. Papillomas and carcinomas of the choroid plexus in children. *J Neurosurg* 1998;88:521–528.
9. Tena-Suck ML, Salinas-Lara C, Rembao-Bojórquez D, et al. Clinicopathologic and immunohistochemical study of choroid plexus tumors: single-institution experience in Mexican population. *J Neurooncol* 2010;98:357–365.
10. Bigner SH, Johnston WW. The cytopathology of cerebrospinal fluid II. Metastatic cancer, meningeal carcinomatosis and primary central nervous system neoplasms. *Acta Cytol* 1981;25:461–479.
11. Buchino JJ, Mason KG. Choroid plexus papilloma report of a case with cytologic differential diagnosis. *Acta Cytol* 1992;36:95–97.
12. Jeibmann A, Hasselblatt M, Gerss J, et al. Prognostic implication of atypical histologic features in choroid plexus papilloma. *J Neuropathol Exp Neurol* 2006;65:1069–1073.
13. Wrede B, Hasselblatt M, Peters O, et al. Atypical choroid plexus papilloma: clinical experience in the CPT-SIOP-2000 Study. *J Neurooncol* 2009;95:383–392.
14. Hasselblatt M, Böhm C, Tatenhorst L, et al. Identification of novel diagnostic markers for choroid plexus tumors. A microarray-based approach. *Am J Surg Pathol* 2006;30:66–74.
15. Moss TH. Choroid plexus tumors. In: *Tumours of the Nervous System: An Ultrastructural Atlas. Springer-Verlag*; 1986:43–56.
16. Gopal P, Parker JR, Debski R, et al. Choroid plexus carcinoma. *Arch Pathol Lab Med* 2008;132:1350–1354.
17. Niikawa S, Ito T, Murakawa T, et al. Recurrence of choroid plexus papilloma with malignant transformation. *Neurol Med Chir* 1993;33:32–35.
18. Meyers SP, Khademian ZP, Chuang SH, et al. Choroid plexus carcinoma in children: MRI features and patient outcomes. *Neuroradiology* 2004;46:770–780.
19. Kim K, Greenblatt SH, Robinson MG. Choroid plexus carcinoma. Report of a case with cytopathologic differential diagnosis. *Acta Cytol* 1985;29:846–849.
20. McCallum S, Cooper K, Franks DN. Choroid plexus carcinoma. Cytologic identification of malignant cells in ascitic fluid. *Acta Cytol* 1988;32:263–266.
21. Savage NM, Crosby JH, Reid-Nicholson MD. The cytologic findings in choroid plexus carcinoma: report of a case with differential diagnosis. *Diagn Cytopathol* 2012;40:1–6.
22. Schittenhelm J, Nagel C, Meyermann R, et al. Atypical teratoid/rhabdoid tumors may show morphological and immunohistochemical features seen in choroid plexus tumors. *Neuropathology* 2011;31:461–467.
23. Shuangshoti S, Netsky MG. Xanthogranuloma (xanthoma) of choroid plexus. The origin of foamy (xanthoma) cells. *Am J Pathol* 1966;48:503–533.
24. Pear BL. Xanthogranuloma of choroid plexus. *AJR Am J Reontgenol* 1984;143:401–402.
25. Rutherfoord GS, Mathew B. Xanthogranuloma of choroid plexus of lateral ventricle, presenting with parosmia and parageusia. *Br J Neurosurg* 1987;1:285–288.
26. Brück W, Sander U, Blanckenberg P, et al. Symptomatic xanthogranuloma of choroid plexus with unilateral hydrocephalus. *J Neurosurg* 1991;75:324–327.
27. Kadota T, Mihara N, Tsuji N, et al. MR of xanthogranuloma of choroid plexus. *AJNR Am J Neuroradiol* 1996;17:1595–1597.

28. Hicks MJ, Albrecht S, Trask T, et al. Symptomatic choroid plexus xanthogranuloma of the lateral ventricle. *Clin Neuropathol* 1993;12:92–96.
29. Shapira Y, Hadelsberg UP, Kanner AA, et al. The ventricular system and choroid plexus as a primary site for renal cell carcinoma metastasis. *Acta Neurochir (Wien)* 2014;156:1469–1474.
30. Zhang YA, Kavar B, Drummond KJ. Thyroid carcinoma metastasis to choroid plexus of lateral ventricle. *J Neurosci* 2009;16:118–121.
31. Wasita B, Sakamoto M, Mizushima M, et al. Choroid plexus metastasis from papillary thyroid carcinoma presenting with intraventricular hemorrhage: case report. *Neurosurgery* 2010;66:E1213–E1214.
32. Heery CR, Engelhard HH, Slavin KV, et al. Unusual CNS presentation of thyroid cancer. *Clin Neurol Neurosurg* 2012;114:1107–1109.
33. Kitagawa Y, Higuchi F, Abe Y, et al. Metastasis to the choroid plexus from thyroid cancer. Case report. *Neurol Med Chir* 2013;53:832–836.
34. Galera-Davidson H, González-Cámpora R. Thyroid. In: Bibbo M, Wilbur D, eds. *Comprehensive Cytopathology*. 3rd ed. Philadelphia, PA: Saunders Elsevier; 2008:650–653.

Pineal Region Tumors

9

Shinya Tanaka
Hiromi Kanno
Tamio Ito

Pineal gland is located posteriorly in the midline of the brain, attached to the posterior end of the roof of the third ventricle, at the quadrigeminal plate cistern. It is one of the circumventricular organs of the brain (i.e., lacking a blood–brain barrier) and is composed primarily of two cellular elements; the main cellular component, pineal parenchyma cells or pineocytes, and stromal supporting glia (astrocytes). The pineocytes are specialized neuroepithelial cells with synthesis and secretion of melatonin, which are arranged into lobules separated by delicate connective tissue septa and thin-walled blood vessels.

Tumors of the pineal gland are uncommon but characteristically show a great variety of histologic types. They can generally be divided into germ cell tumors (GCTs) and non-GCTs. The former tumors are more frequently encountered and are derived presumably from misplaced germ cells. The vast majority of the latter tumors are pineal parenchymal tumors (PPTs), which are rare neoplasms arising from pineocytes and account for less than 1% of primary central nervous system (CNS) tumors. PPTs form a spectrum that spans from benign to high-grade malignancy and can be subdivided into three broad categories: pineocytoma (PC), PPT of intermediate differentiation (PPTID), and pineoblastoma (PB), corresponding to grades I, II or III, and IV, respectively, according to the latest edition of the WHO classification of CNS tumors.[1] The clinical symptoms of pineal tumors are directly related to normal pineal anatomy.

Other tumors occurring in and around the pineal gland include glial tumors (e.g., astrocytomas, ependymomas), papillary tumor of the pineal region (PTPR), meningioma, and choroid plexus tumors. Of these tumors, a very unique tumor in this location, PTPR, is described in this chapter.

PINEOCYTOMA

PC is a slowly growing, well-demarcated, well-differentiated pineal parenchymal neoplasm that is composed of relatively small and mature pineocytes often forming pineocytomatous rosettes. This tumor typically remains localized to the pineal region and compresses adjacent structures such as cerebral aqueduct, brain stem, and cerebellum, sometimes protruded into the posterior third ventricle.

PC mainly occurs in young adults, although it can be encountered at any age, and affects both genders equally. As with other pineal region masses, the clinical symptoms are mostly related to increased intracranial pressure such as headache, nausea, and vomiting, due to aqueduct compression and resultant obstructive hydrocephalus. Compression of the quadrigeminal plate can lead to a characteristic neuro-ophthalmologic dysfunction (a supranuclear vertical gaze disturbance), known as Parinaud syndrome. The 5-year survival rate of PC is 86% to 100%, and there is no report of metastasis or cerebrospinal fluid (CSF) dissemination in PCs.[2,3]

On CT scan, PCs are recognized as a well-demarcated globular mass with intermediate density, similar to adjacent brain. Marked enhancement is seen on postcontrast CT. Peripheral

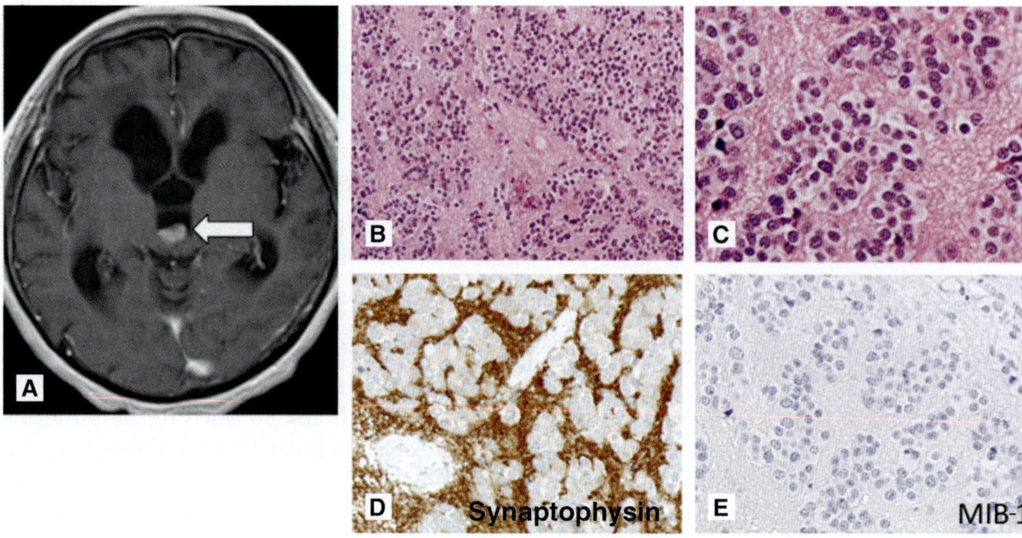

FIGURE 9-1: Pineocytoma. MRI (T1-weighted image) showing a well-demarcated, homogenously enhancing mass with an enlarged ventricular system (tumor is indicated by white arrow) (**A**). Low magnification showing sheets and lobules of tumor cells with pineocytomatous rosettes (H&E stain) (**B**). Intermediate magnification showing vague lobules of small uniform tumor cells (H&E stain) (**C**). Synaptophysin immunostain showing a granular neuropil pattern of reactivity (**D**). Ki-67 (MIB-1) immunostain revealing absent labeling (**E**).

calcification or cystic change is sometimes observed. On MRI, the tumor demonstrates low-to-isointense signal intensity on T1-weighted imaging (WI) and heterogeneous, high-to-isointense signal intensity on T2-WI (Figure 9-1A). Areas of cystic changes are common, while the solid areas show avid homogeneous contrast enhancement.

As molecular pathologic features of PCs, microarray analysis demonstrated the expression of the genes associated with melatonin synthesis such as *TPH1* and *HIOMT* and retinal phototransduction as *OPN4*, *RGS16*, and *CRB3*.[4] Copy number variation study demonstrated few gains of chromosomes in PCs, which appeared to have much fewer chromosomal imbalances compared to higher-grade PPTs.[5]

Histologically, PC is a moderately cellular neoplasm composed of uniform well-differentiated cells with small, rounded nuclei, and ill-defined cytoplasm resembling pineocytes that are arranged in a sheet-like or vague lobular pattern (Figure 9-1B and C). Fibrovascular stroma highlights expansive lobular architecture. Infiltration into the surrounding brain parenchyma or tumor necrosis is not seen. Microcalcifications can be present. Pineocytomatous rosettes, characterized by large, loose, Homer Wright–like rosettes with central fibrillary zone surrounded by neoplastic cells, are sometimes observed. Of note is that pineocytomatous rosettes are different from Homer Wright rosettes in their larger size (i.e., more neuropil at the center of rosettes) as well as their more irregular contours. The size and numbers of those rosettes are usually variable. The tumor cells have inconspicuous nucleoli, fine chromatin, and conspicuous short cytoplasmic processes with no/minimal atypia. Mitotic figures are absent or rare (<1/10 high power fields [HPF]). Interestingly, glial and ganglionic differentiation can occasionally be observed. It should be borne in mind that pleomorphic ganglionic tumor cells in those cases could lead to erroneous interpretation of malignancy, especially in small biopsy samples. Of note is that these pleomorphic tumor cells are usually mitotically inactive.

Immunohistochemically, PC is positive for synaptophysin (Figure 9-1D), neuron-specific enolase (NSE), and neurofilament protein (NFP). Short stubby cytoplasmic processes may be highlighted with NFP. In variable frequency, chromogranin A, class III β-tubulin, PGP9.5, neuropeptide serotonin, and retinal S-antigen, which represents photosensory differentiation, can be immunoreactive.[1] The enzyme for melatonin synthesis such as tryptophan hydroxylase may also be immunoreactive.[6] As reflecting slow tumor growth, the MIB-1/Ki-67 labeling index is usually zero or as low as 0.27% to 3.9%[2,3,7] (Figure 9-1E).

Pineal cysts are usually asymptomatic and frequently encountered at routine autopsy. However, such cysts rarely become large enough to produce a mass effect, requiring surgical excision. Histologically, the cysts are composed of three layers: inner astroglial layer with Rosenthal fibers; middle layer of normally lobulated pineal parenchyma with calcospherites; and outer thin discontinuous fibrous layer. Proper orientation of the surgical specimens is of great importance to avoid misdiagnosis of well-differentiated PPTs (e.g., PC) and low-grade gliomas (e.g., pilocytic astrocytoma).

PINEAL PARENCHYMAL TUMOR OF INTERMEDIATE DIFFERENTIATION

PPTID is a transitional form between PC and PB and consists of at least 20% of pineal tumors. This incidence varies between 0% and 60%, and this wide variation reflects lack of defined criteria of the differential diagnosis of PPTID from PC and PB.[1] PPTIDs occur at all age groups but are mainly seen in young adults. The clinical manifestations are similar to those of PCs, including symptoms related to increased intracranial pressure, Parinaud syndrome, ataxia, and diplopia. PPTID is described as a "potentially aggressive neoplasm" and thus has the potential for CSF dissemination and a higher recurrence rate in contrast to PC. Unlike other histologic subtypes, the optimal management for PPTIDs remains to be determined.

Radiologically, no specific findings that separate PPTID from PC or PB are generally found. In some reports, T2-WI on MRI tends to show a more heterogeneous pattern in comparison to other pineal tumors[8,9] (Figure 9-2A).

Molecular analysis using real-time RT-PCR revealed an increase in the expression of *PRAME*, *CD24*, *POU4F2*, and *HOX13*, and the levels of these transcriptomes may contribute to grading of PPTID.[4] On comparative genomic hybridization (CGH) analysis, chromosomal abnormalities of +4q, +12q, and −22 were noted.[10]

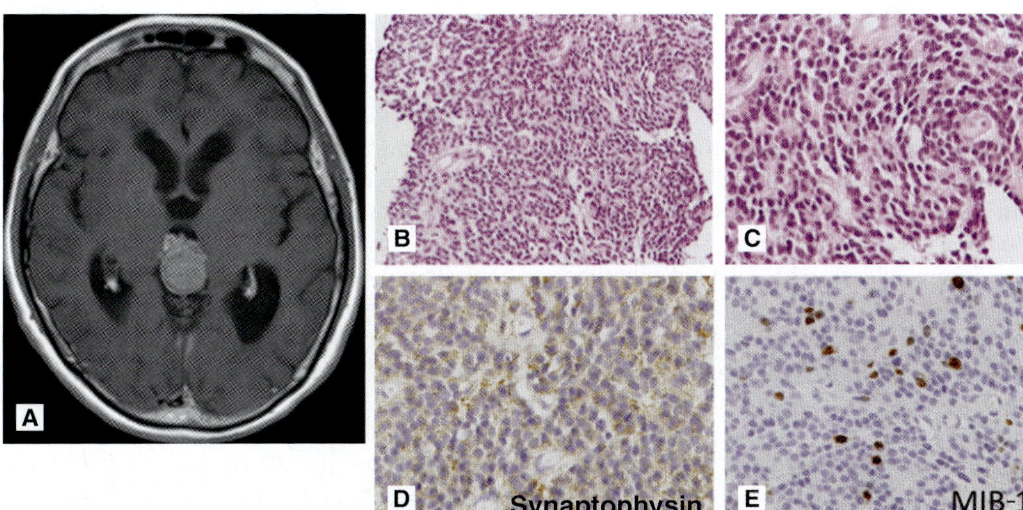

FIGURE 9-2: Pineal parenchymal tumor with intermediate differentiation (PPTID). MRI (T1-weighted image) showing a focally irregular, heterogeneously enhancing mass with enlarged ventricular system (**A**). Low magnification showing a highly cellular lesion with no large rosette formation (H&E stain) (**B**). Intermediate magnification showing a cellular lesion composed of mildly to moderately pleomorphic tumor cells with focal ribbon and rosette-like pattern (H&E stain) (**C**). Synaptophysin immunostain revealing positivity in tumor cells (**D**). Ki-67 (MIB-1) immunostain showing a labeling index of 3.7% (**E**).

Histologically, PPTID is composed of diffuse sheets or vague lobules of tumor cells with mild-to-moderate cytologic atypia and low-to-moderate mitotic activity (Figure 9-2B and C). The tumor cellularity is moderate to high. Reflecting its intermediate differentiation, all these morphologic parameters are intermediate between PC and PB. Occasional giant cells, Homer Wright rosettes, or ganglion cells may be seen.[1] Despite high cellularity, neither microvascular proliferation nor necrosis is found. Rare mixed pineal tumors composed of elements of both PC and PB are difficult to categorize and might be occasionally included in the PPTID category; however, their prognostic and therapeutic significance is uncertain.

PPTIDs are recognized as either grade II or III according to the current WHO classification. Differentiation of grades II and III tumors can be made based on a combination of the mitotic activity and NFP immunoreactivity, although no exact, definite criteria are present. Multicenter study reported that the Ki-67 (MIB-1) labeling indices of PCs, PPTIDs grade II, PPTIDs grade III, and PBs were 0%, 5.2%, 11.2%, and 36%, respectively[11] (Figure 9-2E). Mitotic indices of the reported series of PPTID cases are variable with 0/10 HPF in 58%, 1 to 2/10 HPF in 28%, and 3 to 6/10 HPF in 14%.[1]

In PPTIDs, the immunohistochemical expression of neuronal markers (e.g., NFP, chromogranin A, synaptophysin, and retinal S-antigen) is variable (Figure 9-2D). Correlation of NFP immunoreactivity with good prognosis was previously reported[12,13] but is currently controversial.[7]

PINEOBLASTOMA

PB is a highly malignant, primitive neuroectodermal tumor (PNET) of the pineal gland and is the most aggressive tumor of PPTs, corresponding to WHO grade IV. PBs comprise approximately 40% of all PPTs, and most of cases arise in children and adolescent under 20 years of age (average 18.5 years) without gender predilection.[1] Given its large size, PB almost always manifests itself as symptoms associated with obstructive hydrocephalus. Parinaud syndrome may be seen. PB is a highly malignant tumor with a significant propensity for CSF dissemination, which can be detected at the time of diagnosis. Treatment of PB is usually a combination of surgical resection, chemotherapy, and radiation. Despite the management, the prognosis is poor with a 5-year survival of 62.6%,[14] which is significantly lower than that of medulloblastomas (MBs).

On CT scan, PB is often sizable and tends to be lobulated in contrast to round-shaped tumor seen in PC. The solid component tends to be slightly hyperdense compared to the adjacent brain. Calcification is infrequency seen, but a typical peripherally disperse or "exploded" calcification pattern can be seen. On MRI, T1-heterogeneous, iso-to-hypointense, and T2-isointense pattern with vivid heterogeneous contrast enhancement, representing areas of necrosis and cystic change, is common. Invasion into the adjacent brain is often seen. Screening of the whole neural axis is crucial to identify CSF dissemination. Diffusion-weighted image (DWI) shows restricted diffusion due to dense cellularity.

Some children with bilateral inherited retinoblastomas also develop a PB (with or without retinoblastomatous components), a condition termed trilateral retinoblastoma. This heritable disease is known to typically occur in the setting of germline *RB1* gene mutations. It is not known whether RB1 gene/protein alterations occur in sporadic PBs.[15] As a second susceptibility gene, novel germline mutations in *dicer 1, ribonuclease type III (DICER1)* gene (on chromosome 14q32.13) have recently been reported with accompanying loss of heterozygosity of the wild-type allele within the tumors.[16] Frequent gain of *PCDHGA3* (protocadherin gene) at 5q31.3 and *FAM129A* at 1q25.3 was also reported.[17] Microarray analysis showed an increase in expression of *HOXD19, PITX2, POU4F2, Hist1H3D, Hist1H4E, DSG1*, and *TERT*.[4]

Histologically, PB is characterized by highly cellular, tightly packed, patternless sheets of malignant small round blue cells with scant cytoplasm and brisk mitotic activity (Figure 9-3A and B). Areas of necrosis and hemorrhage are common. Tumor infiltration into the adjacent brain is often noted. Homer Wright rosettes, and less commonly, Flexner-Wintersteiner rosettes and fleurettes (small bouquet-like structures of benign-appearing tumor cells) can be formed.

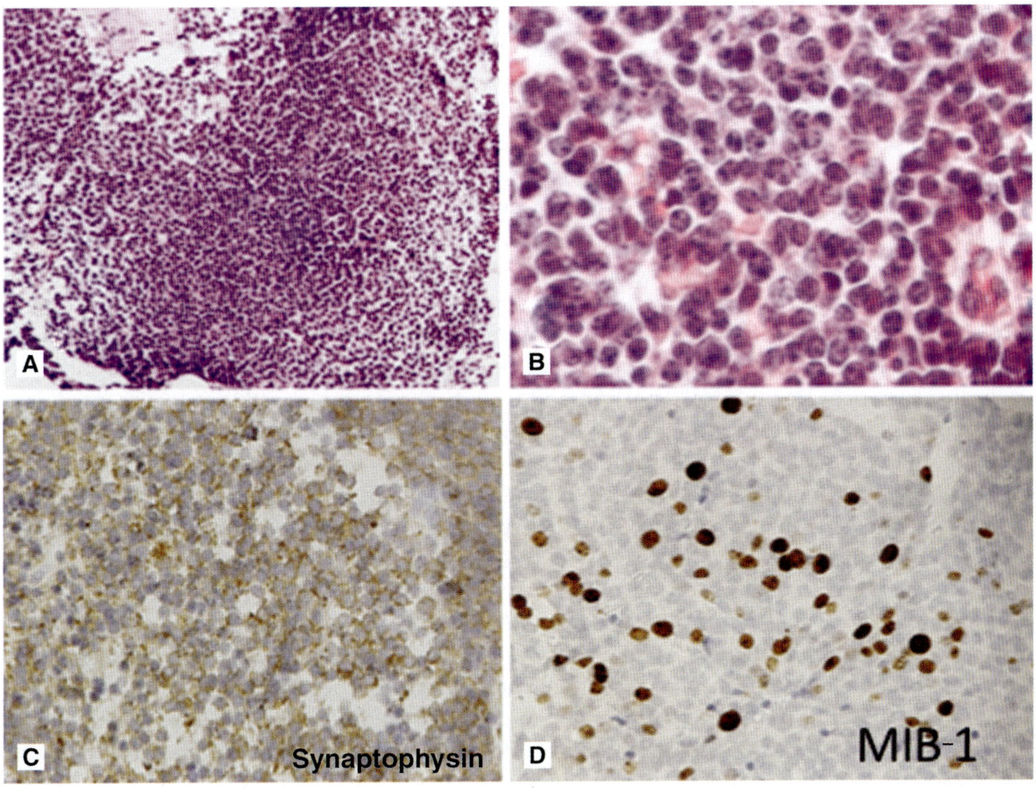

FIGURE 9-3: Pineoblastoma. Low magnification showing highly cellular sheets of malignant small blue cells (H&E stain) (**A**). High magnification showing pleomorphic malignant small blue cells with mitotic activity (H&E staining) (**B**). Synaptophysin immunostain revealing positivity in tumor cells (**C**). Ki-67 (MIB-1) immunostain showing a labeling index of 12.7% (**D**).

Flexner-Wintersteiner rosettes consist of tumor cells surrounding a central lumen that contains cytoplasmic extensions from the tumor cells unlike the center of the Homer Wright rosettes. PBs with Flexner-Wintersteiner rosettes and fleurettes can bear close resemblance to retinoblastoma. Pineocytomatous rosettes are not seen.

Immunohistochemically, PB is positive for neuronal markers such as synaptophysin (Figure 9-3C), NSE, class III β-tubulin, and chromogranin A as well as retinal *S*-antigen indicative of photosensory differentiation. This immunophenotype is very similar to that of PC. It is reported that *O*(6)-methylguanine DNA methyltransferase is highly expressed.[7] The Ki-67 (MIB-1) labeling index is as high as 36%[11] (Figure 9-3D).

Malignant embryonal tumor entities in CNS recognized by the current WHO classification include MB, CNS-PNETs, and atypical teratoid rhabdoid tumor (AT/RT). Since morphology cannot discriminate PB from CNS-PNET and MB, tumor localization (i.e., pineal region) is critical for the diagnosis of PB. Large MB arising from the rostral portion of cerebellar vermis is often difficult to differentiate from PB. PBs appear genetically distinct from MBs; isochromosome 17q (seen in greater than one-third of MBs) and loss of chromosome 6 (seen in WNT subgroup of MB) are not seen in PBs.[17] By array CGH analysis, PBs demonstrated much fewer chromosomal imbalances than CNS-PNETs, in which imbalances involving gain of 2p, amplification of 19q13.41, and loss of CDKN2B (9p21.3) were frequently observed (>20% of cases studied).[17] This observed difference may reflect differences in the cells of origin for these two histologically indistinguishable primitive embryonal tumors. Rare AT/RT cases arising from the pineal region have been reported, and given the overlapping morphologic features, INI-1 immunohistochemistry is of great importance for the differential diagnosis of PB.[18]

PAPILLARY TUMOR OF THE PINEAL REGION

PTPR is a rare neuroepithelial neoplasm that was newly recognized as a distinct entity in the 2007 WHO classification of CNS tumors.[1] This tumor is currently thought to originate from the remnants of the specialized ependymal cells of the subcommissural organ (SCO), which is a part of the circumventricular organs, rather than from the pineal gland itself.

Approximately, 100 cases of PTPR have been reported to date since its first description by Jouvet et al. [19] This tumor occurs in a wide range of ages but is predominantly seen in adults, with an average age of approximately 30 years old. The main clinical symptoms are nonspecific and include headache and visual disturbances secondary to obstructive hydrocephalus related to cerebral aqueduct compression. Because of its rarity, there are no current standard treatment options beyond gross total resection for this tumor. The biologic behavior of PTPR is variable, and cases of local recurrence after surgical resection and CSF dissemination have been documented. It is thus suggested that this tumor may be graded either WHO II or III due to its potential malignant behavior, but pathologic criteria for grading have not yet been formulated.[1]

On MRI, this tumor demonstrates a lobulated lesion with intrinsic high T1 signal and heterogeneous intensity on T2-WI.[8] Screening of the entire neural axis may be required to identify possible CSF dissemination.

Molecular genetic analysis using microarray showed increased expression levels of *SPDF*, *KRF18*, and SCO-related genes such as *ZFH4*, *RFX3*, *TTR*, and *CGRP*.[4] Recently, CGH analysis revealed cytogenetic imbalances in PTPR with −10, +9p, +4, +12p, and +8q being common.[20] These molecular alterations may be useful to classify tumors of the pineal regions.

Grossly, the tumor is well-circumscribed and is indistinguishable from other pineal region tumors. Histologically, PTPR is composed of epithelioid tumor cells with eosinophilic or vacuolated cytoplasm arranged in a multilayered papillary pattern and a diffuse solid growth pattern (Figure 9-4A and B). Within the cellular areas, ependymal differentiation such as true rosettes or tubule formation is often identified.[20] The tumor nuclei are round to oval with stippled chromatin. Mitotic activity is reported to vary (0 to 10/10 HPF). Necrotic foci can be observed. Vascular hyalinization and multiple vascular lumina within the papillary cores are often seen. Cases of PTPR with marked cellular pleomorphism were reported.[21] Given no increase in proliferative activity, cellular pleomorphism in these cases was considered degeneration.

Immunohistochemically, PTPR is very unique in prominent reactivity for cytokeratin (CK) such as AE1/AE3 (Figure 9-4C), CAM5.2, and CK-18 as well as in focal or absent GFAP labeling in contrast to ependymomas. Vimentin, S100 protein, microtubule-associated protein (MAP)-2, neural cell adhesion molecule (NCAM), and NSE are mostly immunoreactive. Variable staining for epithelial membrane antigen (EMA), chromogranin A, and synaptophysin is seen. Focal membrane or dot-like positivity of EMA was previously reported in PTPR as seen in ependymomas, while absence of EMA immunoreactivity was also described.[22]

Histologic differential diagnosis includes papillary tumors occurring in the pineal region, including papillary ependymoma, choroid plexus tumors, papillary meningioma, and metastatic papillary adenocarcinomas. Differentiation from ependymoma is most challenging as PTPR displays histologic ependymal differentiation (i.e., true rosette and pseudorosette formation) and focal EMA immunoreactivity. Striking epithelioid appearance, absent GFAP immunoreactivity, and prominent CK immunoreactivity are not the features of ependymomas. Choroid plexus tumors are rarely located in the third ventricle in adults, and are mostly immunoreactive for Kir7.1 and stanniocalcin-1, which are usually not expressed in PTPRs.[22] Recently, expression of tight junction proteins claudin-1, 2, and 3 was studied immunohistochemically, and claudin-1 and 3, but not claudin-2, were expressed in PTPRs and fetal SCO, while all three claudins were expressed in choroid plexus papillomas.[23] S100 protein, MAP-2, NCAM, NSE, and CK immunoreactivity is not seen in meningiomas. An immunohistochemical panel of CK-7, CK-20, and TTF-1 (positive for metastatic cancers) and MAP-2, NCAM, and S100 protein (positive for PTPR) is of help for differential from metastatic carcinomas, although clinical and radiologic information for the primary tumor is critical.

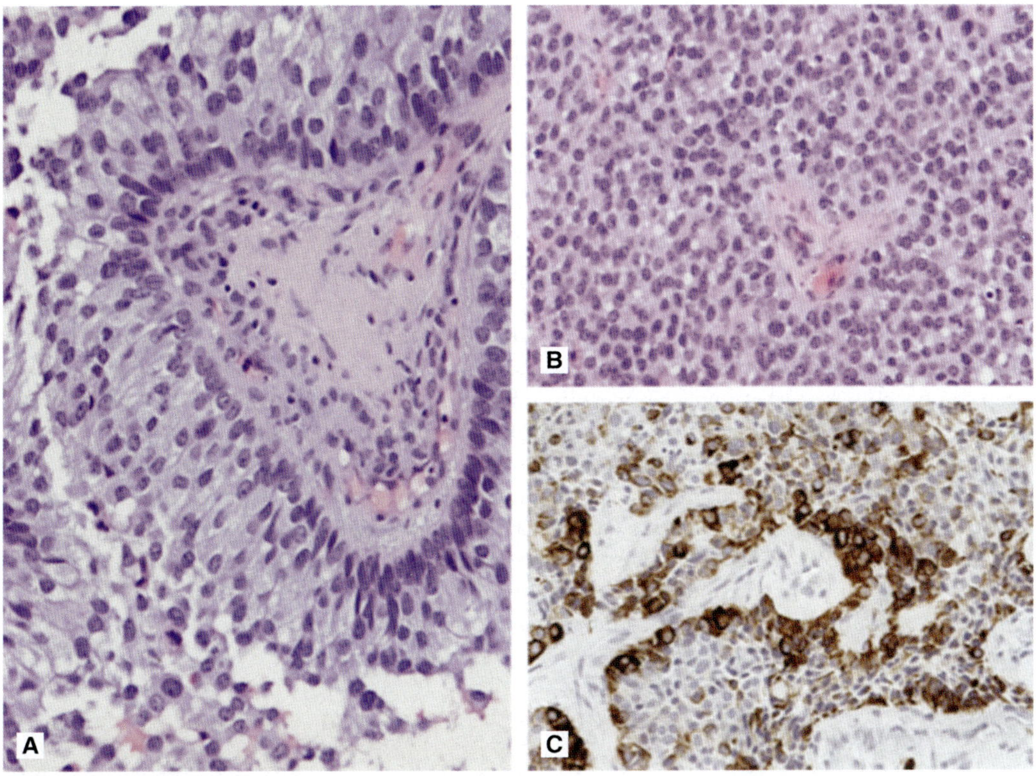

FIGURE 9-4: Papillary tumor of the pineal region (PTPR). Histologic section showing epithelial tumor cells arranged in (**A**) a multilayered papillary pattern and (**B**) a diffuse solid pattern. The tumor cells have round to oval nuclei with stippled chromatin and eosinophilic and vacuolated cytoplasm. Pancytokeratin (AE1/AE3) immunostain-labeling tumor cells (**C**).

GERM CELL TUMORS

Extragonadal GCTs typically arise in midline locations and specific sites vary with age. Primary intracranial GCTs (P-ICGCTs) are a group of uncommon heterogeneous brain tumors with a variety of different histologic types, which carry different prognoses. P-ICGCTs are characteristically located in the pineal and suprasellar regions, with the former location being more frequently affected. Rare GCTs involving both of these locations simultaneously or sequentially are known to be present. Some GCTs arise from unusual locations in the CNS, including basal ganglia, thalamus, and fourth ventricle. Most of GCTs occur before the age of 25 years, and males are much more frequently affected than females, which is more evident in pineal GCTs. In contrast, suprasellar tumors have a fairly even distribution between genders. P-ICGCTs vary in their geographic incidence; the reported incidence is substantially higher in Japan and East Asia than in Western countries as is the incidence of testicular tumors.

P-ICGCTs encompass a wide histopathologic spectrum and are classified by the WHO into the following major entities: germinoma, teratoma (mature, immature, and teratoma with malignant transformation), yolk sac tumor, embryonal carcinoma, and choriocarcinoma. These P-ICGCTs are histologically identical to gonadal GCTs. Germinomas and teratomas are frequently encountered as pure tumors, whereas other types are mostly parts of mixed GCTs. Of P-ICGCTs, the most common subtypes are pure germinomas, followed by teratomas and mixed GCTs. It is known that GCTs, especially germinomas, can disseminate the neuraxis at the time of diagnosis or early in the course of the disease. In the majority of clinical settings, biopsy is usually required for the specific diagnosis and treatment. Evaluation of serum and CSF tumor markers, which are specific for secreting GCT elements (e.g., alpha fetoprotein [AFP] for yolk sac tumor and beta human chorionic gonadotropin [hCG] for choriocarcinoma), is now routine in preoperative assessment for suspected GCTs and is useful for prognostication and monitoring following treatment. Given that the pathologic diagnosis is highly dependent on tumor sampling, especially for small biopsies, it should be correlated with the tumor marker levels.

The clinical presentation depends on the location of tumor; the pineal GCTs, independent of histologic subtypes, most commonly present with signs of obstructive hydrocephalus and Parinaud syndrome, while the suprasellar GCTs present with hypothalamic/pituitary dysfunction (e.g., diabetes insipidus). Germinomas are exquisitely radiosensitive and thus, localized primary germinomas are treated effectively with radiation therapy, with an excellent prognosis/high cure rate. Chemotherapy is reserved for disseminated germinomas. Mature teratomas are treated surgically with an excellent prognosis. The rest of P-ICGCTs are managed with various combinations of surgery, radiation, and chemotherapy, depending on the tumor type, although radiation has been the backbone of treatment. Nongerminomatous GCTs including mixed GCTs, embryonal carcinoma, choriocarcinoma, and yolk sac tumor, carry a poor prognosis.

Radiologically, CT scan and MRI exhibit a mass with vivid contrast enhancement in general but cannot reliably differentiate between different types of ICGCTs, with the exception of mature teratomas, which demonstrate fat density. Germinomas tend to show vivid homogeneous enhancement on MRI and commonly show restriction due to high cellularity on DWI. A pattern of calcification on CT scan is helpful in distinguishing between PPTs (calcifications exploded to periphery) and pineal GCTs (engulfed pineal calcification) (Figure 9-5A).

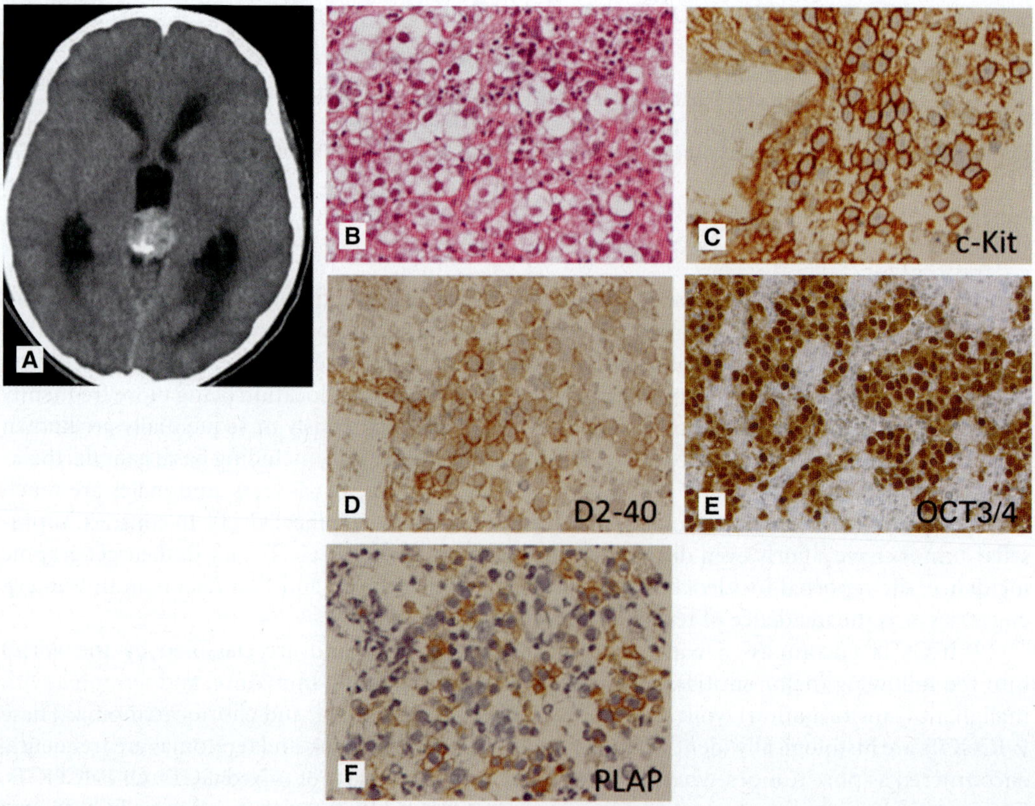

FIGURE 9-5: Germinoma. CT scan showing a nodular mass with focal calcification (**A**). Histologic section showing nests of large tumor cells with clear cytoplasm and prominent nucleoli, admixed with lymphocytes (H&E stain, ×160) (**B**). c-Kit immunostain revealing membranous positivity (**C**). D2-40 immunostain exhibiting membranous positivity (**D**). OCT3/4 immunostain revealing nuclear positivity (**E**). PLAP immunostain revealing heterogeneous reactivity in tumor cytoplasm (**F**).

1. *Germinoma*: Pure form of germinoma is the most commonly encountered P-ICGCT, and is the most common tumor of the pineal region. Molecular genetic analysis discloses a high frequency of somatic mutations in *KIT* or *RAS* genes, which are mutually exclusive, while these mutations are rare in nongerminomatous GCTs.[24] In addition, these mutations are associated with high *KIT* mRNA expression levels, regardless of *Kit* or *Ras* mutations, as well as with chromosomal instability in germinomas.[24] Interestingly, regardless of the mutation status or mRNA expression, KIT protein is expressed immunohistochemically in germinomas. It is reported that the somatic alterations in the AKT/mTOR pathway with corresponding AKT expression is found in 19% of germinomas in addition to mutations in the *KIT/RAS* signaling pathway seen in >50% of cases.[25] These findings suggest that those two signaling pathways can be potentially promising therapeutic targets.

   Histologically, germinoma is composed of lobules or sheets of uniform cells with large vesicular nuclei, prominent nucleoli, well-defined cell boundaries, and abundant clear cytoplasm due to glycogen accumulation, admixed with lymphoplasmacytic infiltrates (Figure 9-5B). Mitotic figures are usually identified without difficulty, but necrosis is uncommon. Noncaseating granulomata are often seen and are sometimes so florid that they obscure the tumor cells. Syncytiotrophoblastic giant cells are occasionally present and are associated with elevation of hCG level in CSF.

   Immunohistochemically, germinoma exhibits membranous positivity for c-kit (Figure 9-5C), diffuse membranous positivity for D2-40 (Figure 9-5D), and nuclear positivity for octamer-binding transcription factor (OCT) 3/4 (Figure 9-5E). Placental alkaline phosphatase (PLAP) labeling is present, but it is not a constant feature with variable sensitivity, intensity, and extent of reactivity (Figure 9-5F). Sal-like protein (SALL)-4 is a helpful marker for confirmation of the germ cell nature of an intracranial tumor, and is positive in germinomas with no discriminative value of GCT subtypes.
2. *Teratoma*: Teratoma is composed of an admixture of different tissue types derived from at least two and usually all three embryonic germ layers: ectoderm, mesoderm, and endoderm. Congenital examples are also well recognized. Mature and immature variants require distinction given the difference in prognosis (a good prognosis with a very low recurrence rate after gross total resection vs. less favorable prognosis with frequent recurrence, respectively).
   (i) *Mature teratoma*: This tumor is composed exclusively of fully differentiated tissue elements. Microscopically, teratomas can contain skin, brain, and choroid plexus as ectodermal components; bone, cartilage, fatty tissue, and muscle as mesodermal; and cystic areas often lined by squamous, respiratory, and/or enterogenous epithelium as endodermal (Figure 9-6). When mature teratoma contains an additional somatic malignant tumor of conventional type such as carcinoma and sarcoma, it should be classified as a "mature teratoma with malignant transformation."
   (ii) *Immature teratoma*: The hallmark of this tumor is the presence of undifferentiated/incompletely differentiated components exhibiting embryonal or fetal appearances. The immature components frequently encountered include primitive neuroepithelial and hypercellular mitotically active mesenchymal elements. The former element may contain neuroepithelial rosettes and canalicular arrangements resembling embryonal neural tubes. Mature tissue components identical to those seen in pure mature teratomas are usually present.
3. *Yolk sac tumor (endodermal sinus tumor)*: This tumor is composed of primitive epithelial cells in a loose, variably cellular, myxoid matrix resembling extraembryonic mesoblasts, and is characterized by the presence of embryonic structures reminiscent of the normal fetal yolk sac, Schiller-Duval bodies, and periodic acid–Schiff-positive intracellular and extracellular hyaline globules. Immunohistochemically, yolk sac tumor is positive for AFP, glypican 3, and SALL-4, and is negative for c-kit and OCT3/4. Solid variant of yolk sac tumor may resemble embryonal carcinoma and germinoma. Immunohistochemistry is of help for this differential.

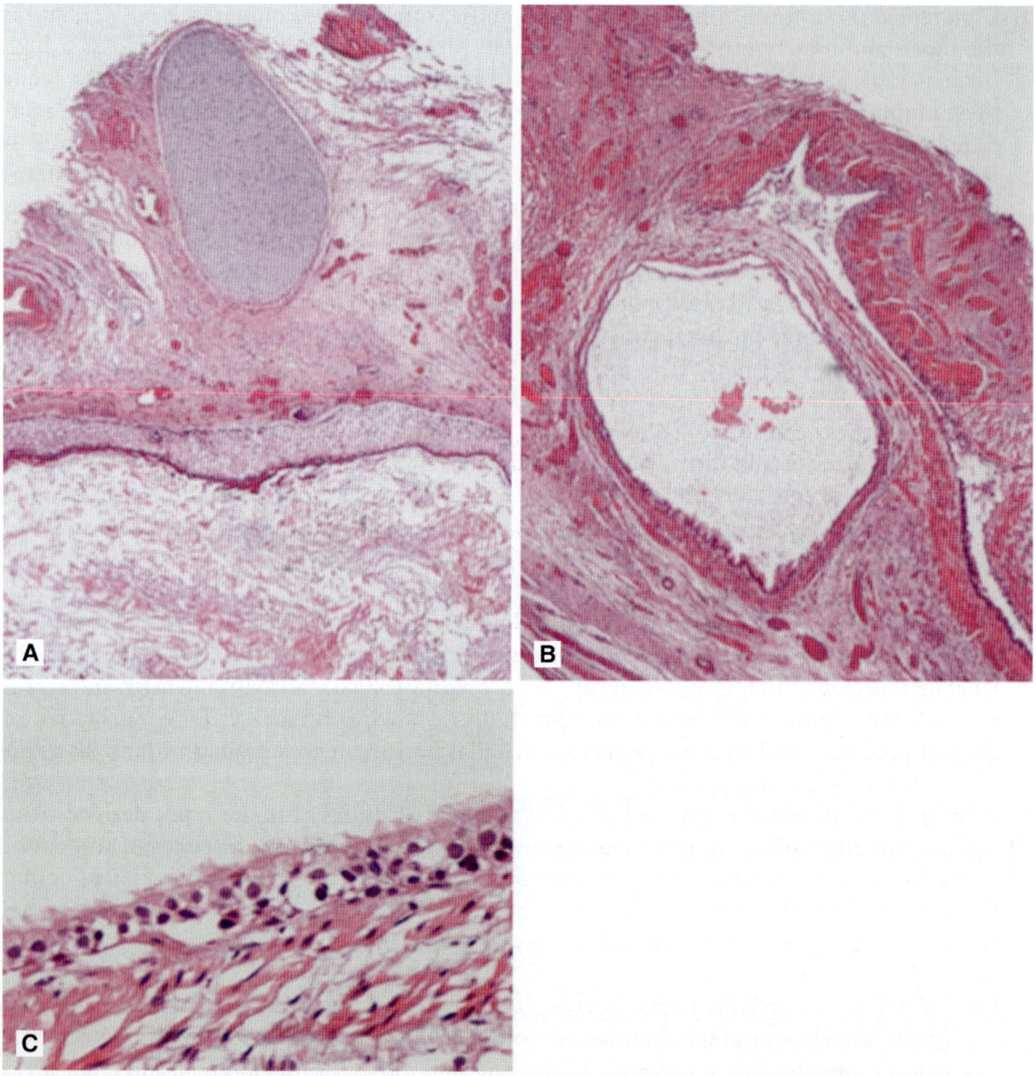

FIGURE 9-6: Mature teratoma. Histologic section showing (**A**) a nodule of cartilage, a cyst lined by stratified squamous epithelium with a granular layer and filled with lamellated keratinous debris and (**B**) a cyst lined by respiratory epithelium surrounded by smooth muscle (H&E stain). High magnification of ciliated epithelium in (**B**) (H&E stain) (**C**).

4. *Embryonal carcinoma*: This tumor component is often seen in mixed GCTs and usually represents the most aggressive component of the tumor. Intratumoral hemorrhage and CNS dissemination/extraneural metastasis can occur. Microscopically, the tumor is composed of large, markedly atypical cells forming nests and sheets, abortive papillae or gland-like structures. Brisk mitotic activity and coagulative necrosis is noted. Immunohistochemically, embryonal carcinoma is CK, OCT3/4, CD30, and SALL-4 positive and c-kit and glypican 3 negative.
5. *Choriocarcinoma*: This tumor is a highly malignant tumor with high risk for intratumoral hemorrhage and propensity for CNS dissemination/extraneural metastasis. The prognosis is very poor. Choriocarcinoma exhibits extraembryonic differentiation along trophoblastic lines and is characterized by intimately admixed dimorphic tumor cells (i.e., mononucleated cytotrophoblastic cells and multinucleated large syncytiotrophoblastic cells). Immunohistochemically, the syncytiotrophoblastic tumor cells are positive for hCG and inhibin, whereas the cytotrophoblastic cells are negative. SALL-4 exhibits variable positivity. OCT3/4, c-kit, and CD30 are negative.

References

1. Louis DN, Ohgaki H, Wiestler OT, et al. *WHO Classification of Tumours of the Central Nervous System*. Lyon, France: IARC; 2007.
2. Schild SE, Scheithauer BW, Haddock MG, et al. Histologically confirmed pineal tumors and other germ cell tumors of the brain. *Cancer* 1996;78:2564–2571.
3. Fauchon F, Jouvet A, Paquis P, et al. Parenchymal pineal tumors: a clinicopathological study of 76 cases. *Int J Radiat Oncol Biol Phys* 2000;46:959–968.
4. Fevre-Montange M, Champier J, Szathmari A, et al. Microarray analysis reveals differential gene expression patterns in tumors of the pineal region. *J Neuropathol Exp Neurol* 2006;65:675–684.
5. von Bueren AO, Gerss J, Hagel C, et al. DNA copy number alterations in central primitive neuroectodermal tumors and tumors of the pineal region: an international individual patient data meta-analysis. *J Neurooncol* 2012;109:415–423.
6. Fevre-Montange M, Jouvet A, Privat K, et al. Immunohistochemical, ultrastructural, biochemical and in vitro studies of a pineocytoma. *Acta Neuropathol* 1998;95:532–539.
7. Kanno H, Nishihara H, Oikawa M, et al. Expression of *O*(6)-methylguanine DNA methyltransferase (MGMT) and immunohistochemical analysis of 12 pineal parenchymal tumors. *Neuropathology* 2012;32:647–653.
8. Fang AS, Meyers SP. Magnetic resonance imaging of pineal region tumours. *Insights Imaging* 2013;4:369–382.
9. Ito T, Kanno H, Sato K, et al. Clinicopathologic study of pineal parenchymal tumors of intermediate differentiation. *World Neurosurg* 2014;81:783–789.
10. Rickert CH, Simon R, Bergmann M, et al. Comparative genomic hybridization in pineal parenchymal tumors. *Genes Chromosomes Cancer* 2001;30:99–104.
11. Fevre-Montange M, Vasiljevic A, Frappaz D, et al. Utility of Ki67 immunostaining in the grading of pineal parenchymal tumours: a multicentre study. *Neuropathol Appl Neurobiol* 2012;38:87–94.
12. Jouvet A, Saint-Pierre G, Fauchon F, et al. Pineal parenchymal tumors: a correlation of histological features with prognosis in 66 cases. *Brain Pathol* 2000;10:49–60.
13. Arivazhagan A, Anandh B, Santosh V, et al. Pineal parenchymal tumors—utility of immunohistochemical markers in prognostication. *Clin Neuropathol* 2008;27:325–333.
14. Farnia B, Allen PK, Brown PD, et al. Clinical outcomes and patterns of failure in pineoblastoma: a 30-year single institution retrospective review. *World Neurosurg* 2014;82:1232–1241.
15. Li MH, Bouffet E, Hawkins CE, et al. Molecular genetics of supratentorial primitive neuroectodermal tumors and pineoblastoma. *Neurosurg Focus* 2005;19:E3.
16. de Kock L, Sabbaghian N, Druker H, et al. Germ-line and somatic DICER1 mutations in pineoblastoma. *Acta Neuropathol* 2014;128:583–595.
17. Miller S, Rogers HA, Lyon P, et al. Genome-wide molecular characterization of central nervous system primitive neuroectodermal tumor and pineoblastoma. *Neuro Oncol* 2011;13:866–879.
18. Takei H, Adesina AM, Mehta V, et al. Atypical teratoid/rhabdoid tumor of the pineal region in an adult. *J Neurosurg* 2010;113:374–379.
19. Jouvet A, Fauchon F, Liberski P, et al. Papillary tumor of the pineal region. *Am J Surg Pathol* 2003;27:505–512.
20. Gutenberg A, Brandis A, Hong B, et al. Common molecular cytogenetic pathway in papillary tumors of the pineal region (PTPR). *Brain Pathol* 2011;21:672–677.
21. Magalhaes J, Rostad S, Foltz G, et al. Cellular pleomorphism in papillary tumors of the pineal region. *Brain Tumor Pathol* 2013;30:93–98.
22. Hasselblatt M, Blumcke I, Jeibmann A, et al. Immunohistochemical profile and chromosomal imbalances in papillary tumours of the pineal region. *Neuropathol Appl Neurobiol* 2006;32:278–283.
23. Fevre Montange M, Vasiljevic A, Bergemer Fouquet AM, et al. Histopathologic and ultrastructural features and claudin expression in papillary tumors of the pineal region: a multicenter analysis. *Am J Surg Pathol* 2012;36:916–928.
24. Fukushima S, Otsuka A, Suzuki T, et al. Mutually exclusive mutations of KIT and RAS are associated with KIT mRNA expression and chromosomal instability in primary intracranial pure germinomas. *Acta Neuropathol* 2014;127:911–925.
25. Wang L, Yamaguchi S, Burstein MD, et al. Novel somatic and germline mutations in intracranial germ cell tumours. *Nature* 2014;511:241–245.

10 Sellar and Suprasellar Region Tumors

▶ Nishant Tiwari
▶ Hidehiro Takei

INTRODUCTION

Sellar and suprasellar tumors are commonly seen in diagnostic neuropathology practice, and pituitary adenoma and craniopharyngioma (CP) are the most common lesions.[1] Sellar and suprasellar lesions encountered in a practice are listed in Table 10-1. Of note is that the clinical pictures and radiologic features can be essentially the same among these lesions.[2]

RATHKE CLEFT CYST

Rathke cleft cyst (RCC) is not a true neoplasm but is believed to derive from remnants of the embryologic Rathke pouch. The Rathke pouch arises as an epithelialized rostral diverticulum of the stomodeum (stomatodeum) and is composed of an anterior and posterior wall with a central embryonic cleft. The adenohypophysis and the pars tuberalis arise from the anterior wall, while the posterior wall develops into the pars intermedia. The central cleft generally regresses; however, it is believed that this structure may persist and enlarge, resulting in a formation of RCC. Uncommon cases of a pituitary adenoma in combination of components of RCC have been documented.[3] These cases can be explained by the common embryologic ancestry of both lesions.[4,5]

Clinical and Radiologic Features

RCCs are usually asymptomatic and discovered incidentally by radiologic study or at autopsy. Symptomatic RCCs are uncommon, and the presenting symptoms include headache, visual disturbance, and pituitary hypofunction with multiple endocrinopathies. Most symptomatic lesions are intrasellar with suprasellar extension.[1] The MRI features often show a cystic lesion with variable signal intensity based on the cyst contents (Figure 10-1A). Clear serous fluid is T2 hyperintense, and mucinous contents can be hyperintense on T1 due to the high protein content.[6–9] No calcifications are usually identified.

Histopathology

On cytologic examination, the lesion shows a background of abundant extracellular colloidal material. Scattered cuboidal to columnar epithelial cells with bland nuclei and cilia/terminal bar appear singly and/or in clusters (Figure 10-1B). Lymphocytes and macrophages can also be seen as reaction to mucinous material. The overall cellularity is usually very low.

Histologically, the cyst fluid often forms a dominant component of the surgical specimens. The cyst is lined often by flattened/attenuated epithelium. Variable numbers of well-differentiated columnar to cuboidal epithelium with cilia and goblet cells are present (Figure 10-1C). The cyst is surrounded by a collagenous wall with chronic inflammation and histiocytes. Identification of ciliated epithelium with a terminal bar is almost pathognomonic of RCC in appropriate clinical

Table 10-1 Sellar and Suprasellar Lesions

<table>
<tr><th colspan="2">Neoplastic Lesions</th><th colspan="2">Nonneoplastic Lesions</th></tr>
<tr><td rowspan="6">Benign</td><td rowspan="6">Pituitary adenoma[a]
Craniopharyngioma[a]
Gangliocytoma
Granular cell tumor
Spindle cell oncocytoma
Pituicytoma
Meningioma
Schwannoma
Langerhans cell histiocytosis</td><td colspan="2">Pituitary hyperplasia</td></tr>
<tr><td rowspan="2">Inflammatory lesions</td><td>Infections (abscess)</td></tr>
<tr><td>Lymphocytic hypophysitis</td></tr>
<tr><td rowspan="3">Cysts</td><td>Rathke cleft cyst[a]</td></tr>
<tr><td>Arachnoid cyst</td></tr>
<tr><td>Dermoid/epidermoid cyst</td></tr>
<tr><td>Malignant</td><td>Pituitary carcinoma
Germ cell tumor
Chordoma
Lymphoma/leukemia
Metastasis</td><td></td><td></td></tr>
</table>

[a]Commonly encountered lesions.

radiologic settings. Occasional goblet cells and squamous metaplastic cells are seen in some examples.[10,11] Normal pituitary gland tissue is usually present in the vicinity.

Differential Diagnosis

Cases of RCC with extensive squamous metaplasia can be difficult to distinguish from a papillary CP (refer to "Differential Diagnosis" of "Papillary Craniopharyngioma"); a surgical pickup of normal intermediate lobe cysts can show ciliated epithelium, which is indistinguishable from that of RCC. Clinical and radiologic information (i.e., no mass-forming lesion seen in intermediate lobe cysts) is important.

CRANIOPHARYNGIOMA

CP is a solid to cystic lesion occurring in the sellar/suprasellar region and characterized by its benign histology with aggressive (malignant) behavior. There are two known histologic subtypes: adamantinomatous and papillary.[1,2,12] The former subtype predominantly occurs in children and adolescence, and the latter occurs exclusively in adults.

It is recently reported that the vast majority of adamantinomatous CP have mutations in *CTNNB1* (β-catenin), and most of papillary CP have recurrent mutations in *BRAF* (p.V600E).[13,14]

Adamantinomatous Craniopharyngioma

This is a prototypical subtype of CP. Given its histologic resemblance to the "adamantinoma of the jaw" (ameloblastoma) and calcifying odontogenic cyst, adamantinomatous CP is believed to arise from misplaced embryonic rest of enamel-producing epithelium.[12,15]

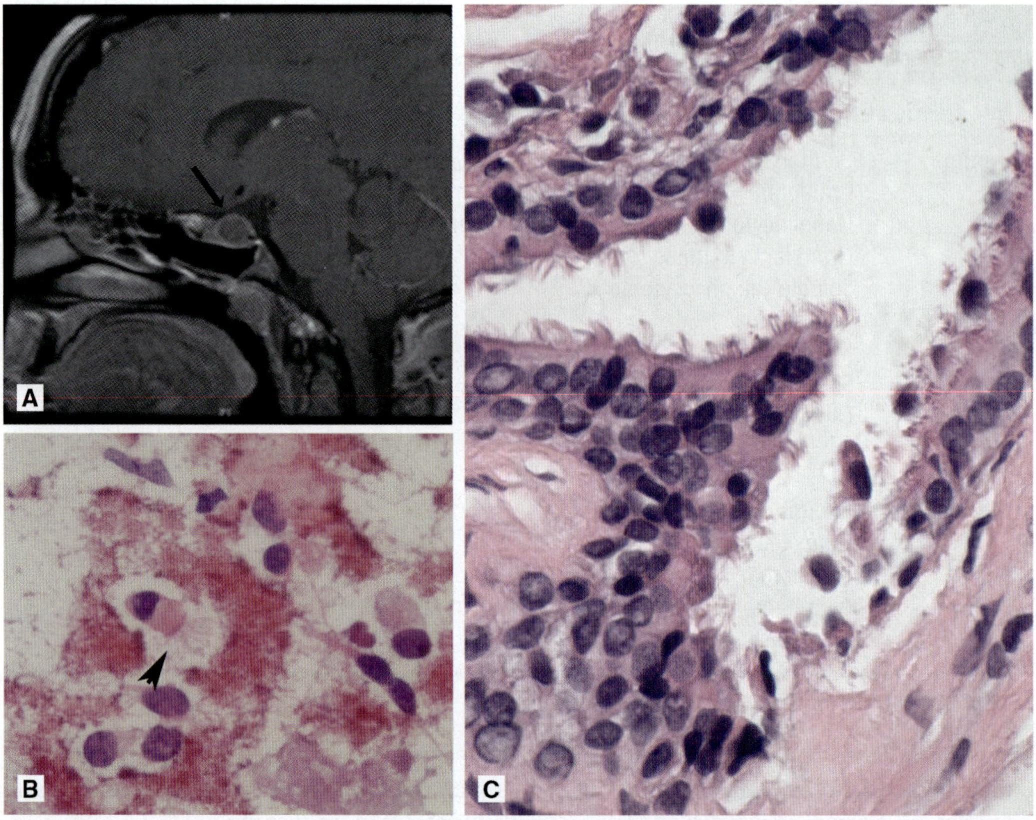

FIGURE 10-1: Rathke cleft cyst. MRI (T1-weighted image with contrast enhancement) showing a cystic mass predominantly located in the sella (*arrow*) (**A**). Cytologic touch imprint showing single columnar cells, one of which has cilia with a terminal bar (*arrowhead*) (**B**). Histologic section showing a cyst lined by a single layer of columnar epithelium with cilia (**C**).

Clinical Features and Imaging

The patients usually present with symptoms of endocrine, visual, and psychological abnormalities. On imaging, the mass is most often suprasellar; however, unusual locations of sphenoid sinus, paranasal sinuses/nasopharynx, cerebellopontine angle, corpus callosum, pineal region, and posterior fossa have been described in the literature.[1,2] The tumor mass is lobulated, solid cystic, and contrast enhancing (Figure 10-2A). The cyst fluid is usually T1 bright. Peripheral calcifications are often seen on plain radiography and CT imaging.[6,7,9] The tumors have significant growth potential with degeneration and accumulation of debris.

Histopathology

Adamantinomatous CP is a complex epithelial lesion with cysts and calcified "wet keratin." The epithelial component shows irregular cords or islands composed of a single layer of small basaloid cells with peripheral palisading, squamous/squamoid cells, and stellate cells in loose connective matrix (stellate reticulum). The "wet keratin" consists of variably sized nests of plump keratinized squamous cells with nuclear shadows and is often calcified (Figure 10-2B).[16,17]

Xanthogranulomatous change is also commonly seen with a fibrohistiocytic response. The cyst fluid is turbid, proteinaceous, and brownish yellow with floating cholesterol crystals, imparting a "machinery oil" appearance. Abundant cholesterol crystals often present are best appreciated on unfixed smears viewed with polarized light. This is dissolved after fixation and during processing with xylene and shows up as cholesterol clefts. The surrounding brain tissue is often gliotic with variable numbers of Rosenthal fibers due to chronic compression by a cystic structure and/or to irritation of cyst content to the surrounding brain (Figure 10-2C).

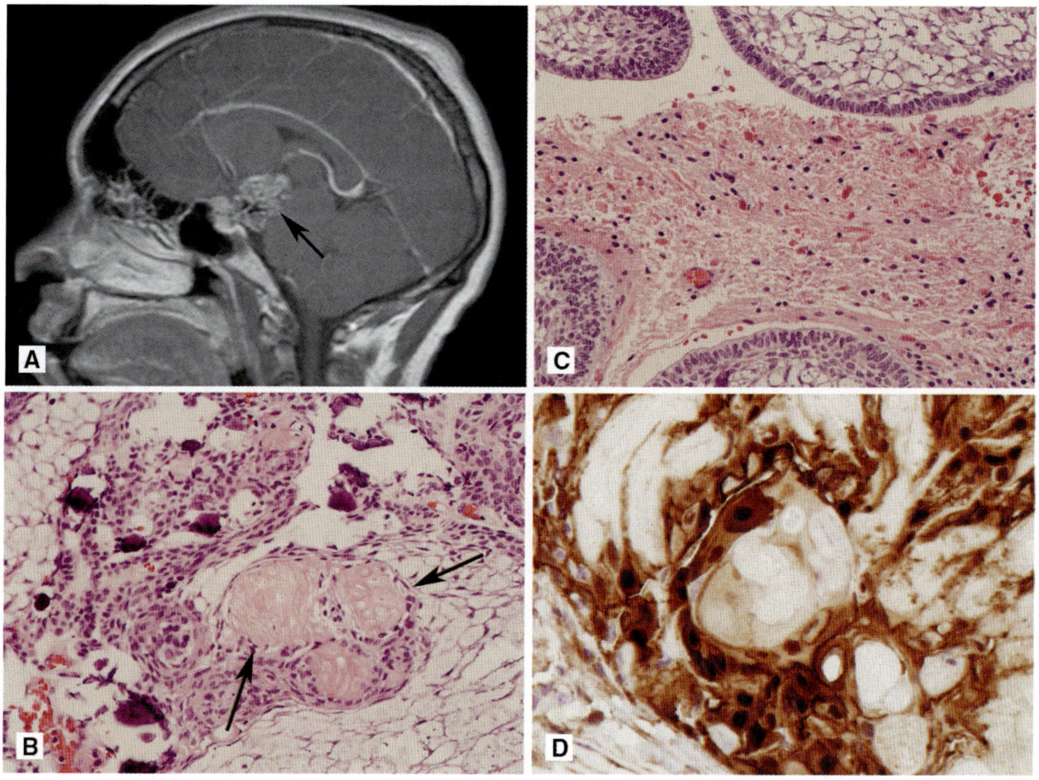

FIGURE 10-2: Craniopharyngioma (adamantinomatous type). MRI (T1-weighted image with contrast enhancement) showing an irregularly shaped, irregularly enhancing mass extending into the suprasellar region (*arrow*) (**A**). Histologic section showing sheets of squamous/squamoid cells with nodules of "wet keratin" (*arrows*) and multiple microcalcifications, surrounded by areas of stellate cells in loose connective matrix (stellate reticulum) (**B**). Multiple cell clusters with prominent basal palisading are surrounded by gliotic brain tissue with many Rosenthal fibers (**C**). β-Catenin immunohistochemical stain demonstrating nuclear positivity in tumor cells (**D**).

Immunohistochemically, translocation of β-catenin expression from the membrane to cytoplasm/nucleus is documented (Figure 10-2D).

Differential Diagnosis

Adamantinomatous CP with dominant cystic areas and extensive squamous component can be difficult to distinguish from RCC. Identification of small foci of characteristic features such as stellate reticulin and "wet keratin" is crucial. Mutation analysis of the *CTNNB1* (β-catenin) gene is of help. Differential diagnosis from papillary CP is described in the "Papillary Craniopharyngioma" section below.

The most common pitfall, especially on intraoperative consultation, is a misinterpretation of gliosis with abundant Rosenthal fibers surrounding CP as a low-grade glioma, especially a pilocytic astrocytoma. Clinical–radiologic correlation is essential to recognize this sampling error.

Papillary Craniopharyngioma

Papillary CP is suggested to originate from Rathke pouch remnants and can have marked histologic overlap with RCC with significant squamous metaplasia.[10,18] It is often considered as a separate entity from adamantinomatous CP even though coexistent lesions have been documented.[17]

Clinical Features and Imaging

The patients are most often adults/elderly presenting with visual abnormalities and mental/personality changes. Imaging shows a solid suprasellar lesion with minor cystic component and no calcifications. The tumor is generally better circumscribed than adamantinomatous CP. MRI shows a T1-hypointense (contrast enhancing) and T2-hyperintense lesion. Cyst fluid when present is often T1 hypointense.[6,7,9]

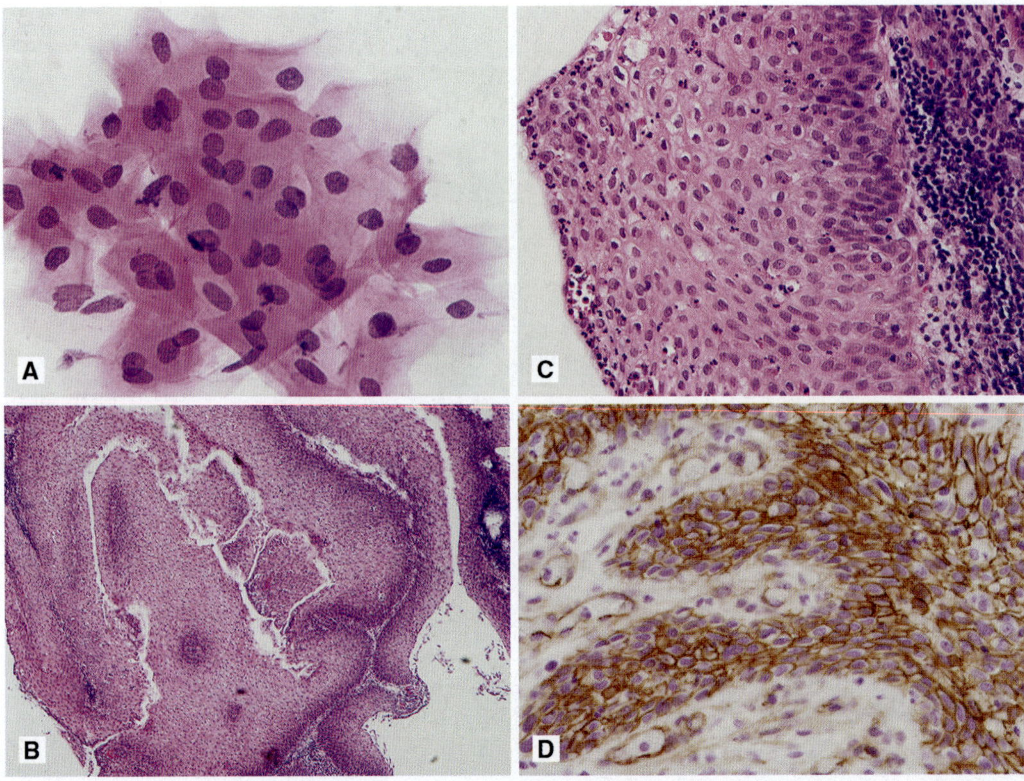

FIGURE 10-3: Craniopharyngioma (papillary type). Cytologic touch imprint showing a cluster of bland squamous cells with monomorphic nuclei and abundant cytoplasm (**A**). Low-power view showing multilayered sheets of squamous cells (**B**). Higher-power view showing multilayered bland squamous epithelium with underlying lymphoplasmacytic infiltrate (**C**). β-Catenin immunohistochemical stain demonstrating membranous positivity in tumor cells (**D**).

Histopathology

Papillary CP is composed of a well-circumscribed mass of multilayered, sheet-like simple squamous epithelium with no atypia (Figure 10-3B and C). Tissue degeneration results in a pseudopapillary architecture (Figure 10-3B). Small epithelial whorls may be present, but no keratinization is present. Focally, the cystic spaces can be lined by goblet cells and ciliated epithelium displaying features similar to RCC. Characteristically, no "wet keratin," stellate reticulum, "machinery oil" fluid, or calcification is seen. Chronic inflammatory cell infiltrate is frequently seen.[12,15,16]

Differential Diagnosis

Adamantinomatous CP, epidermoid cyst, and RCC with squamous metaplasia are included in the differential diagnosis. Small specimens from adamantinomatous CP composed exclusively of squamoid/squamous areas may mimic papillary CP. Immunohistochemical stain for β-catenin is helpful: membranous expression in papillary CP (Figure 10-3D) versus cytoplasm and nuclear expression in adamantinomatous CP. Molecular analysis of *CTNNB1* (β-catenin) and *BRAF* is also useful.

Laminated keratinous debris from cyst content of epidermoid cyst is not seen in papillary CP.

RCC is virtually excluded based on the presence of prominent solid squamous component and absence of ciliated epithelium.

As with adamantinomatous CP, pericystic gliosis accompanied by variable numbers of Rosenthal fibers is noted in this variant, and thus in cases of misdirected sampling, pilocytic astrocytoma can be a histologic differential.

PITUICYTOMA

Pituicytoma is a rare WHO grade I glial tumor arising in the neurohypophysis or infundibulum. It is suggested to develop from specialized glia or native pituicytes in the neurohypophysis. Normal pituicytes can be ultrastructurally separated into five distinct variants: light, dark, ependymal, granular, and oncocytic.[19] Based on this ultrastructural finding, variable tumor cytology can be expected. Normal pituicytes are thyroid transcript ion factor-1 (TTF-1) immunoreactive, and this seems to be preserved in their neoplastic counterpart, pituicytoma.[20]

Clinical Presentation and Imaging

The patients reported are adults with slight male preponderance (1.6:1).[1] They often present with headache and local mass effect causing hypopituitarism or stalk effect.[1,2] MRI shows a well-circumscribed T1 hypo/isointense lesion with marked homogenous enhancement, which is typically clearly separate from the pituitary gland. It is either completely sellar, sellar and suprasellar, or purely suprasellar.[21,22] Surgeons usually identify it as an unusually firm circumscribed and separate lesion from the anterior pituitary. Surgical resection is the mainstay of treatment. Hypervascularity of the tumor may preclude complete resection. Pituicytomas have a tendency to recur locally if not completely excised.[23]

Histopathology

This is a uniform solid compact tumor that is composed of variably lobulated sheets of elongated spindled cells forming short fascicles and swirling architecture (Figure 10-4A). The tumor cells have oval to elongate nuclei with little atypia and eosinophilic nongranular cytoplasm (Figure 10-4B). Mitoses are rare to absent. No Rosenthal fibers or eosinophilic granular bodies are present. Reticulin deposition is scant in between tumor cells and mainly limited to perivascular location.[2] Immunohistochemically, vimentin, TTF-1, and S100 protein are positive in pituicytomas.

Differential Diagnosis

Spindle cell oncocytoma (SCO) and granular cell tumor (GCT) are included in the differential diagnosis. The immunologic profile is compared for this differential in Table 10-2. Due to similar histologic–immunologic features and prognosis, some proposed that SCO and GCT might be pituicytoma variants.[19,21]

Pituicytoma can be differentiated from normal cellular posterior pituitary and infundibulum based on the absence of the "herring bodies." Negative immunostains for synaptophysin and neurofilament protein (for axons) allow pituicytoma to be distinguished from the neurohypophysis.

SPINDLE CELL ONCOCYTOMA

SCO is a rare solid WHO grade I tumor of the adenohypophysis. The cell of origin has been proposed to be folliculostellate cells of the adenohypophysis.[1,2] However, due to consistent TTF-1 immunoreactivity in these tumors,[24,25] the likelihood of derivation from pituicytes has recently been proposed.

Clinical Presentation and Imaging

SCO is a rare tumor, and the patients are adults presenting with symptoms indistinguishable from those of nonfunctional pituitary adenoma (e.g., headache, visual disturbances, and hypopituitarism). The tumor often arises in the anterior pituitary with a suprasellar extension in most cases. MRI features are essentially similar to that for pituicytomas showing a contrast enhancing lesion; however, no separation from adeno- or neurohypophysis is seen.[21,22]

Surgical resection is the mainstay of treatment. Hypervascularity of the tumor may preclude complete resection. SCOs have a tendency to recur locally if not completely excised.[23]

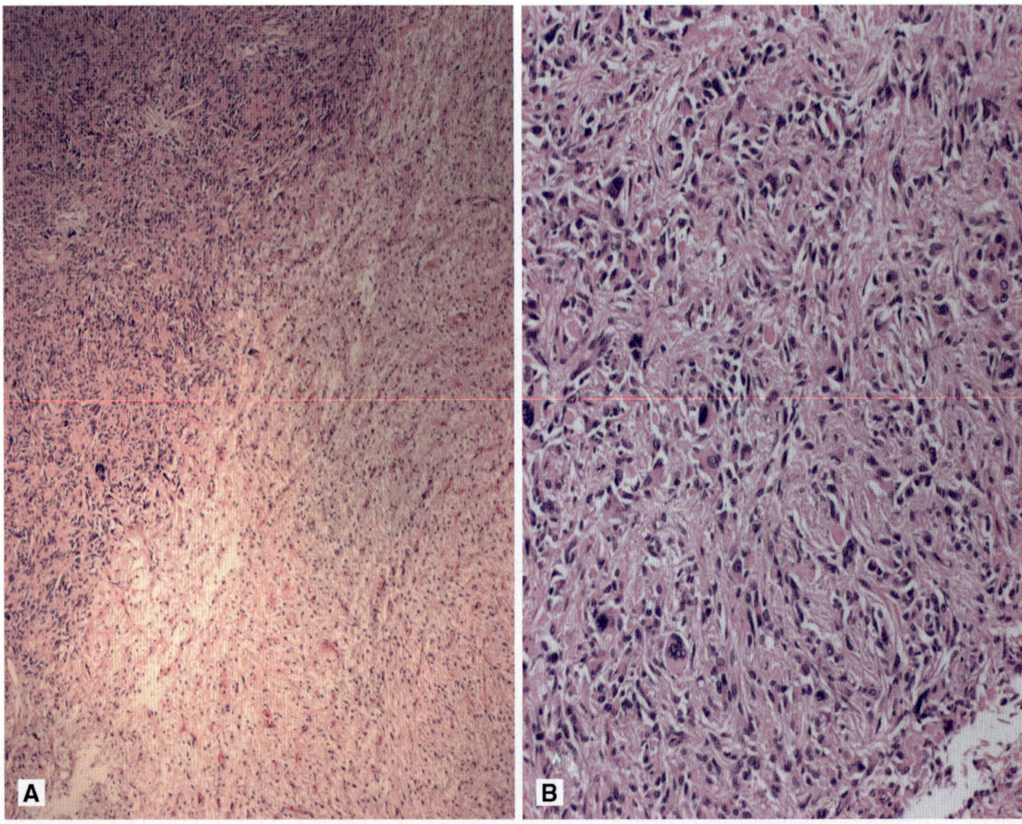

FIGURE 10-4: Pituicytoma. Low-power view showing a solid compact tumor (*upper left*) is surrounded by normal neurohypophysis (*right*) (**A**). Higher-power view showing spindled tumor cells with scattered large pleomorphic cells (**B**).

Table 10-2 Differentiating Immunohistochemical Profile of Pituicytoma, Spindle Cell Oncocytoma (SCO), and Granular Cell Tumor of the Sellar–Suprasellar Region (GCT)[19,21,23–25]

Immunohistochemical Stains	Pituicytoma	SCO	GCT
S100 protein	(+)	(+)	(+) variable
Vimentin	(+)	(+)	(+)
TTF-1	(+)	(+)	(+)
Epithelial membrane antigen	(+) Variable, cytoplasmic	(+)	(+) Variable
Glial fibrillary acidic protein	(+) Variable	(+) Variable	(+) Variable
Galectin-3	(+) Variable	(+)	(+) Variable
CD56	(+) Variable	(+) Variable	(–)
bcl-2	(+) Variable	(+) Variable	(–)
CD68	(+) Variable	(+) Variable	(+) Variable
MU213-UC[a]	(–)	(+)	(–)
Synaptophysin,[b] chromogranin,[c] neurofilament protein[c]	(–)	(–)	(–)

[a]MU213-UC clone 131-1 is antimitochondrial antibody.[25]

[b]Given the constant expression in pituitary adenomas, these markers are used to distinguish from pituitary adenoma.

[c]This is a marker for normal neurohypophysis (axons are stained).

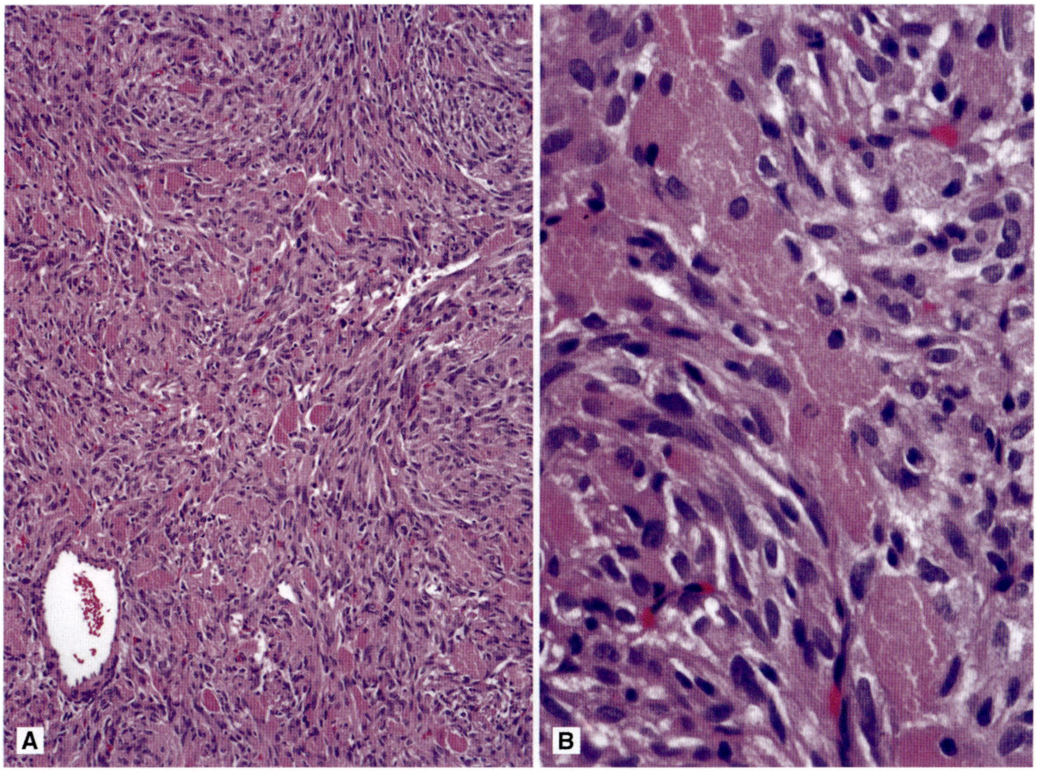

FIGURE 10-5: Spindle cell oncocytoma. Low-power view showing spindled tumor cells in a fascicular growth pattern (**A**). High-power view showing tumor cells with characteristic eosinophilic granular cytoplasm and bland nuclei (**B**).

Histopathology

SCO is composed of epithelioid to spindled cells in a fascicular to sheet-like growth pattern (Figure 10-5A). The tumor cells characteristically have eosinophilic granular cytoplasm with a round central monomorphic nucleus (Figure 10-5B). The cytoplasmic accumulation of mitochondria is responsible for the characteristic oncocytic morphology. Nuclear atypia and focal pleomorphism may be seen with minimal mitotic activity. SCO also has a distinctively infiltrative growth pattern often with no identifiable separate normal pituitary.[24,25] Immunohistochemically, vimentin, TTF-1, and S100 protein are positive in SCO. Electron microscopy can be used in instances to show increased mitochondrial accumulation in the cytoplasm with variable well-formed desmosomes and intermediate fillaments.[19,20]

Differential Diagnosis

The histologic differential diagnoses include pituicytoma and GCT. Immunohistochemical profile used in the differentials is listed in Table 10-2. Ultrastructural or immunohistochemical identification of abundant mitochondria within the cytoplasm is useful for the diagnosis of SCO. Meningioma could also be considered given that both tumors are EMA immunoreactive.

GRANULAR CELL TUMOR OF THE INFUNDIBULUM

GCT is a lysosome-rich tumor, WHO grade I, arising from the neurohypophysis or infundibulum.[1,2] Asymptomatic microscopic clusters of granular cells are referred to as granular cell tumorettes, which were reportedly seen in 5.7% to 6.5% of large postmortem series. Symptomatic GCTs are presumed to develop from enlargement of these tumorettes.[1,2]

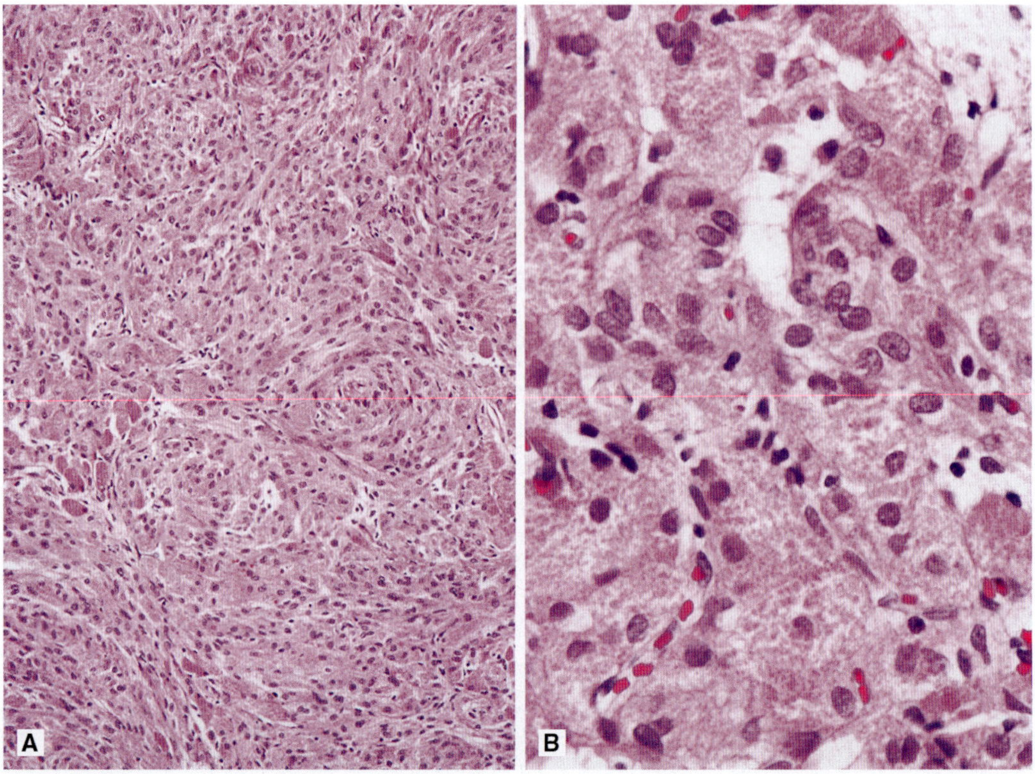

FIGURE 10-6: Granular cell tumor. Low-power view showing spindled tumor cells with a vague storiform pattern (**A**). High-power view showing tumor cells with abundant granular cytoplasm and bland nuclei (**B**).

Clinical Features and Imaging

They are predominantly suprasellar with a highly contrast enhancing tumor on imaging. Purely sellar localization is not a feature.[21] Symptomatic GCT is usually present in adults with visual defects and rarely with hormonal imbalances. A female predilection is often observed for symptomatic lesions.[19,21,22]

Histopathology

GCT is histologically indistinguishable from a tumorette. The tumor is composed of nests of large bland cells with abundant granular, eosinophilic cytoplasm due to intracytoplasmic lysosomes (Figure 10-6A and B), which are periodic acid–Schiff stain positive (diastase resistant). The nuclei are round, eccentric with delicate chromatin. The cells are spaced by dense vasculature with occasional perivascular lymphocytes.[1,2,21,22] Mitosis is usually not seen. Ultrastructural examination of the cells shows abundant lysosomes and variable amounts of intermediate filaments and desmosomes. Immunohistochemically, CD68 and S100 protein are variably positive. Unlike granular cell tumors found elsewhere in the body, the tumors of the infundibulum and neurohypophysis are consistently TTF-1 positive.

Differential Diagnosis

Histologic differential diagnosis includes pituicytoma, spindle cell oncocytoma, and pituitary adenoma. A panel of immunohistochemistry is of help in differential diagnosis (Table 10-2).

Macrophage-rich lesions (xanthomatous lesions) in the pituitary gland such as lymphocytic hypophysitis with abundant foamy macrophages, chronic infarct, and demyelination may be differential diagnoses. Of note is that cells of GCT are significantly larger than macrophages.

METASTASIS TO THE SELLAR/SUPRASELLAR REGION

Metastasis to the sellar/suprasellar region is uncommon and constitutes up to 4% of nonadenomatous surgical cases of the sellar lesions.[26] Elderly patients are most commonly affected. The most common primary malignancies are lung and breast cancers,[27,28] presumably merely due to the large number of cerebral metastasis from these two cancers. However, lesions from the head/neck, thyroid,[29] gastrointestinal tract, liver/pancreas, kidney, prostate, and unknown primaries[26,30] have been reported in the literature.[26] Rare instances of tumor-to-tumor metastasis (e.g., metastatic carcinoma to tuberculum sellae meningioma[31] and pituitary adenoma[32]) have also been documented. In pituitary metastasis, neurohypophysis and infundibulum are more frequently involved than adenohypophysis, which may explain that diabetes insipidus is the most common clinical presentation.

References

1. Louis DN, Ohgaki H, Wiestler OD, et al., eds. *WHO Classification of Tumours of the Central Nervous System*. Lyon, France: IARC; 2007.
2. Burger PC, Scheithauer BW. *Tumors of the Central Nervous System (AFIP Atlas of Tumor Pathology)*. Washington D.C.: American Registry of Pathology; 2007.
3. Ikeda H, Yoshimoto T, Katakura R. A case of Rathke's cleft cyst within a pituitary adenoma presenting with acromegaly—do "transitional cell tumors of the pituitary gland" really exist? *Acta Neuropathol* 1992;83(2):211–215.
4. Mollard P, Hodson DJ, Lafont C, et al. A tridimensional view of pituitary development and function. *Trends Endocrinol Metab* 2012;23(6):261–269.
5. Voelker JL, Campbell RL, Muller J. Clinical, radiographic, and pathological features of symptomatic Rathke's cleft cysts. *J Neurosurg* 1991;74(4):535–544.
6. Gaddikeri S, Vattoth S, Riley KO. Rathke cleft cyst. MRI criteria for presumptive diagnosis. *Neurosciences (Riyadh)* 2013;18(3):258–263.
7. Zada G, Lin N, Ojerholm E, et al. Craniopharyngioma and other cystic epithelial lesions of the sellar region: a review of clinical, imaging, and histopathological relationships. *Neurosurg Focus* 2010;28(4):E4.
8. Riva G, Meli GA, Chiaramonte R, et al. Imaging of Rathke's cleft cysts: criteria for a differential diagnosis. *Neuroradiol J* 2007;20(6):617–621.
9. Choi SH, Kwon BJ, Na DG. Pituitary adenoma, craniopharyngioma, and Rathke cleft cyst involving both intrasellar and suprasellar regions: differentiation using MRI. *Clin Radiol* 2007;62(5):453–462.
10. Wolfe SQ, Heros RC. A Rathke cleft cyst to craniopharyngioma: is there a spectrum? *J Neurosurg* 2010;112(6):1322–1323.
11. Okada T, Fujitsu K, Miyahara K, et al. Ciliated craniopharyngioma—case report and pathological study. *Acta Neurochir (Wien)* 2010;152(2):303–306.
12. Larkin SJ, Ansorge O. Pathology and pathogenesis of craniopharyngiomas. *Pituitary* 2013;16(1):9–17.
13. Larkin SJ, Preda V, Karavitaki N. BRAF V600E mutations are characteristic for papillary craniopharyngioma and may coexist with CTNNB1-mutated adamantinomatous craniopharyngioma. *Acta Neuropathol* 2014;127(6):927–929.
14. Brastianos PK, Taylor-Weiner A, Manley PE, et al. Exome sequencing identifies BRAF mutations in papillary craniopharyngiomas. *Nat Genet* 2014;46(2):161–165.
15. Muller C, Adroos N, Lockhat Z. Toothy craniopharyngioma: a literature review and case report of craniopharyngioma with extensive odontogenic differentiation and tooth formation. *Childs Nerv Syst* 2011;27(2):323–326.
16. Tavangar SM, Larijani B, Mahta A. Craniopharyngioma: a clinicopathological study of 141 cases. *Endocr Pathol* 2004;15(4):339–344.
17. Okada T, Fujitsu K, Ichikawa T, et al. Coexistence of adamantinomatous and squamous-papillary type craniopharyngioma: case report and discussion of etiology and pathology. *Neuropathology* 2012;32(2):171–173.

18. Ogawa Y, Watanabe M, Tominaga T. Rathke's cleft cysts with significant squamous metaplasia—high risk of postoperative deterioration and close origins to craniopharyngioma. *Acta Neurochir (Wien)* 2013;155(6):1069–1075.
19. Mete O, Beatriz Lopes M, Asa LS. Spindle cell oncocytomas and granular cell tumors of the pituitary are variants of pituicytoma. *Am J Surg Pathol* 2013;37:1694–1699.
20. Takei Y, Seyama S, Pearl GS. Ultrastructural study of the human neurohypophysis. II. Cellular elements of neural parenchyma, the pituicytes. *Cell Tissue Res* 1980;205:273–287.
21. Covington MF, Chin SS, Osborn AG. Pituicytoma, spindle cell oncocytoma, and granular cell tumor: clarification and meta-analysis of the world literature since 1893. *AJNR Am J Neuroradiol* 2011;32(11):2067–2072.
22. Hammoud DA, Munter FM, Brat DJ, et al. Magnetic resonance imaging features of pituicytomas: analysis of 10 cases. *J Comput Assist Tomogr* 2010;34(5):757–761.
23. Ogiwara H, Dubner S, Shafizadeh S, et al. Spindle cell oncocytoma of the pituitary and pituicytoma: two tumors mimicking pituitary adenoma. *Surg Neurol Int* 2011;2:116.
24. Zygourakis CC, Rolston JD, Lee HS, et al. Pituicytomas and spindle cell oncocytomas: modern case series from the University of California, San Francisco. *Pituitary* 2015;18(1):150–158.
25. Romero-Rojas AE, Melo-Uribe MA, Barajas-Solano PA, et al. Spindle cell oncocytoma of the adenohypophysis. *Brain Tumor Pathol* 2011;28(4):359–364.
26. Valassi E, Biller BM, Klibanski A, et al. Clinical features of nonpituitary sellar lesions in a large surgical series. *Clin Endocrinol (Oxf)* 2010;73(6):798–807.
27. Mao JF, Zhang JL, Nie M, et al. Diabetes insipidus as the first symptom caused by lung cancer metastasis to the pituitary glands: clinical presentations, diagnosis, and management. *J Postgrad Med* 2011;57(4):302–306.
28. Gormally JF, Izard MA, Robinson BG, et al. Pituitary metastasis from breast cancer presenting as diabetes insipidus. *BMJ Case Rep* 2014; doi:10.1136/bcr-2014-203683.
29. Madronio EB, Lantion-Ang FL. The tale of two tumours: an undiagnosed case of papillary thyroid carcinoma. *BMJ Case Rep* 2011; doi:10.1136/bcr.08.2011.4604.
30. Dutta P, Bhansali A, Shah VN, et al. Pituitary metastasis as a presenting manifestation of silent systemic malignancy: a retrospective analysis of four cases. *Indian J Endocrinol Metab* 2011;15(suppl 3): S242–S245.
31. Dadlani R, Ghosal N, Hegde AS. An unusual metastasis from a breast carcinoma to a psammomatous tuberculum sella meningioma. *J Neurosci Rural Pract* 2013;4(2):233–234.
32. Sogani J, Yang W, Lavi E, et al. Sellar collision tumor involving metastatic lung cancer and pituitary adenoma: radiologic–pathologic correlation and review of the literature. *Clin Imaging* 2014;38(3):318–321.

11 Meningeal Tumors

Junjeong Choi
Se Hoon Kim

MENINGIOMAS

Introduction

Meningiomas originate from meningothelial (arachnoid) cells. Because of their origin, meningiomas are attached to the inner surface of dura mater, and therefore, are considered typical "extra-axial" tumors of the central nervous system (CNS). This is in contrast to gliomas, which are classified as "intra-axial" tumors.

The arachnoid membrane, which lies between the superficial dura mater and the inner pia mater, is composed of a delicate network of bundles of fibrous and elastic tissue that are intimately blended together (Figure 11-1A). Its outer surface is intermittently covered with nests of elongated cells, termed the arachnoid cap cells, which are thought to give rise to meningiomas and share their immunohistochemical features[1] (Figure 11-1B).

Incidence and Epidemiology

According to the recent Central Brain Tumor Registry of the United States (CBTRUS),[2] between 2006 and 2010, histologically diagnosed meningiomas accounted for about 35.8% of all primary CNS tumors in the United States. The incidence of meningiomas in other countries is similar to that of the United States: In Korea, for example, its incidence is about 31.8%.[3] It is well known that meningiomas occur more commonly in females than in males, with the male-to-female ratio of benign meningiomas around 0.44 (M/F = 1.00/2.27) and 0.77 (1.00/1.30) in malignant meningiomas.[2] In cases of sporadic meningioma, multiplicity is less than 10%,[4] and spinal meningiomas account for about 10% of all meningioma cases.[4]

Risk Factors

A number of risk factors are attributed to the development of meningiomas, such as neurofibromatosis type 2 (NF2), exposure to ionizing radiation, and certain hormonal factors.

Neurofibromatosis Type 2

NF2 is an autosomal dominant disorder characterized by neoplastic and dysplastic lesions that primarily affect the nervous system.[5] This disorder is caused by mutations of the *NF2* gene, which is located on chromosome 22q12 and encodes merlin protein, also known as schwannomin protein. Although the precise function of the *NF2* gene is still not fully understood, it is thought to act as a tumor suppressor that is involved in organization of the actin cytoskeleton and regulation of cell motility.[6] The NF2 disorder manifests itself by cutaneous schwannomas, schwannomas of the central or peripheral nervous systems, meningiomas, gliomas, meningoangiomatosis, and glial hamartomas. Of these, multiple meningiomas arise in around 50% of NF2 patients. Moreover, compared to sporadic meningiomas, these tumors are diagnosed in NF2 patients at an earlier age and tend to exhibit a more aggressive biologic behavior and high-grade histology.[7,8] Finally, *NF2* is

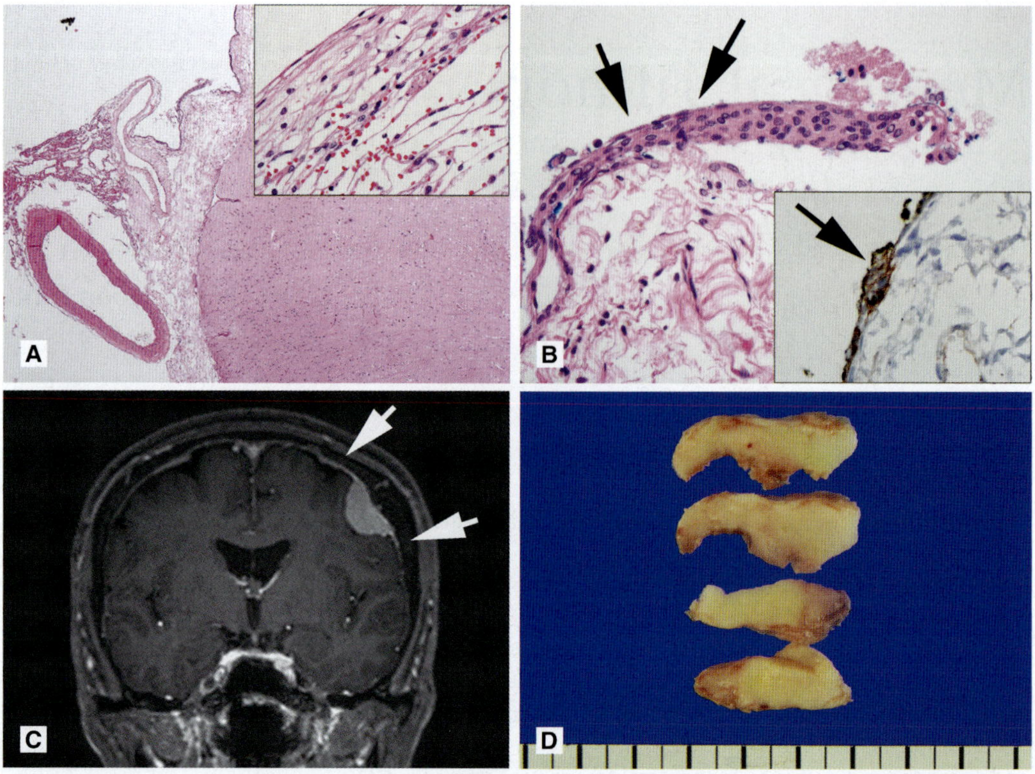

FIGURE 11-1: Normal arachnoid tissue shows arachnoid space with a large blood vessel on the left side (**A**, H&E ×40). Higher magnification reveals long, slender, spindle-shaped arachnoid cells (**A**, **inset**, H&E ×600), and epithelioid arachnoid cap cells with syncytial pattern (**B**, *arrows*, H&E ×400). EMA is expressed in the arachnoid cap cells (**B**, inset, EMA immunostain, ×600). MRI findings indicate an attached dural mass marked by high signal intensity and dural tails (**C**, *white arrows*). A gross pathologic examination reveals a protruding, rubbery white mass with dural attachment (**D**).

also involved in the development of sporadic meningiomas, which develop following its biallelic inactivation, leading to a complete loss of *NF2* expression.[9]

Radiation

Radiation, either therapeutic or due to accidental exposure, is associated with the development of meningiomas.[10] Some reports indicate a 6- to 10-fold increase in the development of meningiomas following radiation exposure.[11] For example, childhood cancer survivors who undergone radiotherapy have a higher propensity for developing meningiomas later in life, with meningioma incidence peaking as late as 30 years after the original diagnosis.[12] Moreover, an increased meningioma incidence had also been observed in survivors of the atomic explosions in Japan.[13]

Hormones

Some evidence exists to suggest a causal relationship between the development and progression of meningiomas and certain hormonal factors.[10] This includes predominance of meningiomas in females, especially those of the reproductive age; expression of estrogen, androgen, and progesterone hormonal receptors on meningioma cells; and changes in the size of meningiomas observed during the luteal phase of the menstrual cycle or during pregnancy. Subsequently, some studies investigated the possibility of treating inoperable recurrent meningiomas with hormonal therapies. However, these studies produced only limited statistical value, and further investigation is needed. In summary, while these are indications of hormonal involvement in the development and progression of meningiomas, data show that these tumors do not behave in a typical "hormone-fed" manner.[10]

Location

Meningiomas occur throughout the CNS, but exhibit an increased propensity for cerebral convexities, parasagittal area, sphenoid ridge, para/suprasellar regions, optic nerve sheath, petrous ridge, tentorium, and posterior fossa. Most spinal meningiomas occur in the thoracic region.[4] In rare instances, meningiomas had also been detected in intraventricular and epidural spaces.

Radiologic Findings

The computer tomography (CT) and magnetic resonance imaging (MRI) are common radiologic modalities used to diagnose meningioma. On CT, meningiomas can be seen as sharply circumscribed lesions that are characterized by a well-defined tumor–brain interface, indicative of their extra-axial localization.[14] CT analysis can also detect occasional calcification of the tumor. Conversely, the MRI analysis displays meningiomas as isointense, contrast-enhancing, dural-based masses that exhibit the so-called dural tails surrounding the dural perimeter of the mass[4] (Figure 11-1C). Occasionally, a radiologic examination also reveals cystic changes in the mass itself or in its periphery. Finally, certain subtypes of meningioma can be accompanied by peritumoral cerebral edema.[15,16]

Macroscopic Features

The most common macroscopic findings associated with a meningioma include a rubbery, firm (could be soft), well-demarcated, lobulated, round mass arising in the dura matter (Figure 11-2D). During dissection, the mass may feel gritty due to tumor calcification. On occasion, meningiomas can grow on the sphenoid ridge as a flat, carpet-like mass, also called "en plaque meningioma." Meningiomas can invade the overlying skull and brain parenchyma. Interestingly, the WHO grading system does not classify skull and bony invasion as an aggressive histologic criterion, while invasion into the brain parenchyma is considered the WHO grade II biologic behavior.[4]

Microscopic Features

Histologically, meningioma cells exhibit abundant cytoplasm without a distinct cytoplasmic border. Thus, meningioma tissues are frequently characterized as "syncytium-like" (Figure 11-2A). Tumor cell nuclei display delicate, vesicular chromatin with occasional central clearing (Figure 11-2A), or intranuclear pseudoinclusions. These cellular features are useful for "touch" or "squash" smear cytologic diagnoses.

Histologic Subtypes

Among several histologic subtypes of meningiomas, meningothelial, transitional, and fibrous subtypes are the most common. The histologic variants currently recognized by WHO are listed in Table 11-1. Meningiomas composed purely of one subtype are very rare, and most tumors show a mixture of several subtypes. Below is a brief description of meningioma subtypes, from more to less common. There were no significant differences in the recurrence rate among common WHO grade I meningioma variants.[17]

Meningothelial meningioma is one of the most common meningioma variants. It is characterized histologically by lobules of cells with abundant, indistinct cytoplasm (syncytium), delicate chromatin, occasional central nuclear clearing, and intranuclear pseudoinclusions (Figure 11-2A). Whorl and psammoma bodies are not common in this variant. Larger lobules of tumor cells should not be interpreted as sheeting or patternless pattern seen in atypical meningiomas.

Fibrous (fibroblastic) meningioma consists of spindle-shaped tumor cells intertwined with abundant collagen fibers arranged in parallel or storiform patterns (Figure 11-2B). Whorl and psammoma bodies are rare. This meningioma variant must be clinically distinguished from schwannomas, particularly in the cerebellopontine angle. If a clear diagnosis is not possible, an immunohistochemical staining for epithelial membrane antigen (EMA), vimentin, S100 protein, and claudin-1 should be utilized (Figure 11-2C and D).[18]

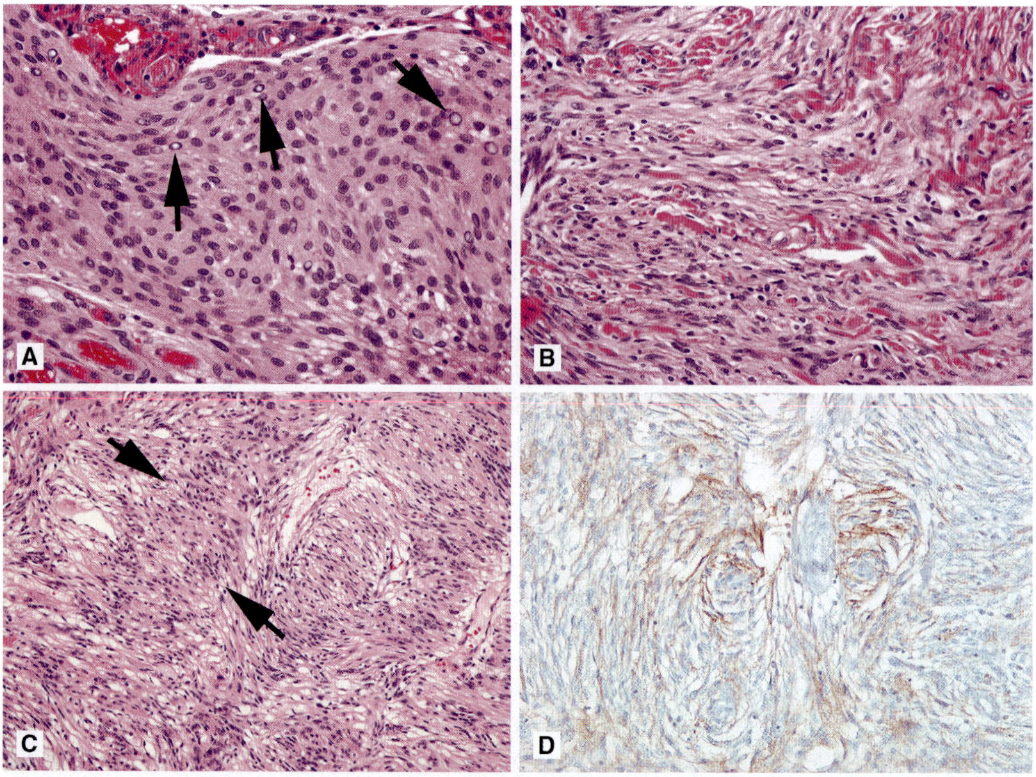

FIGURE 11-2: Prominent syncytia are characteristic of meningothelial meningiomas (**A**, H&E ×200). Extensive nuclear clearing (**A**, *arrows*) and intranuclear pseudoinclusions can be noted. Proliferating, spindle-shaped cells characteristic of fibrous meningioma are arranged in parallel or storiform patterns and exhibit no whorls or psammoma bodies; marked interstitial collagen deposition is noted (**B**, H&E ×400). Histologically, fibrous meningioma is similar to schwannoma: spindle-shaped tumor cells and Verocay body–like structures are noted (**C**, *arrows*, H&E ×200). Immunohistochemical analysis reveals claudin-1 (**D**, claudin-1 ×200) expression and lack of S100 protein staining (**D**, Courtesy by Dr. Mi Jung Kwon, Hallym, University Sacred Heart Hospital, Anyang, Korea.).

Table 11-1 Tumors of Meningothelial Cells (Modified According to the WHO Classifications)

Meningioma		9530/0[a]
WHO grade I	Meningothelial	9531/0
	Fibrous (fibroblastic)	9532/0
	Transitional (mixed)	9537/0
	Psammomatous	9533/0
	Angiomatous	9534/0
	Microcytic	9530/0
	Secretory	9530/0
	Lymphoplasmacyte rich	9530/0
	Metaplastic	9530/0
WHO grade II	Atypical	9539/1
	Chordoid	9538/1
	Clear cell	9538/1
WHO grade III	Anaplastic (malignant)	9530/3
	Papillary	9538/3
	Rhabdoid	9538/3

[a]Morphology code of the International Classification of Diseases for Oncology (ICD-O) and the Systematized Nomenclature of Medicine Behavior is coded: /0 for benign tumors; /1 for borderline tumors of uncertain behavior; and /3 for malignant tumors.

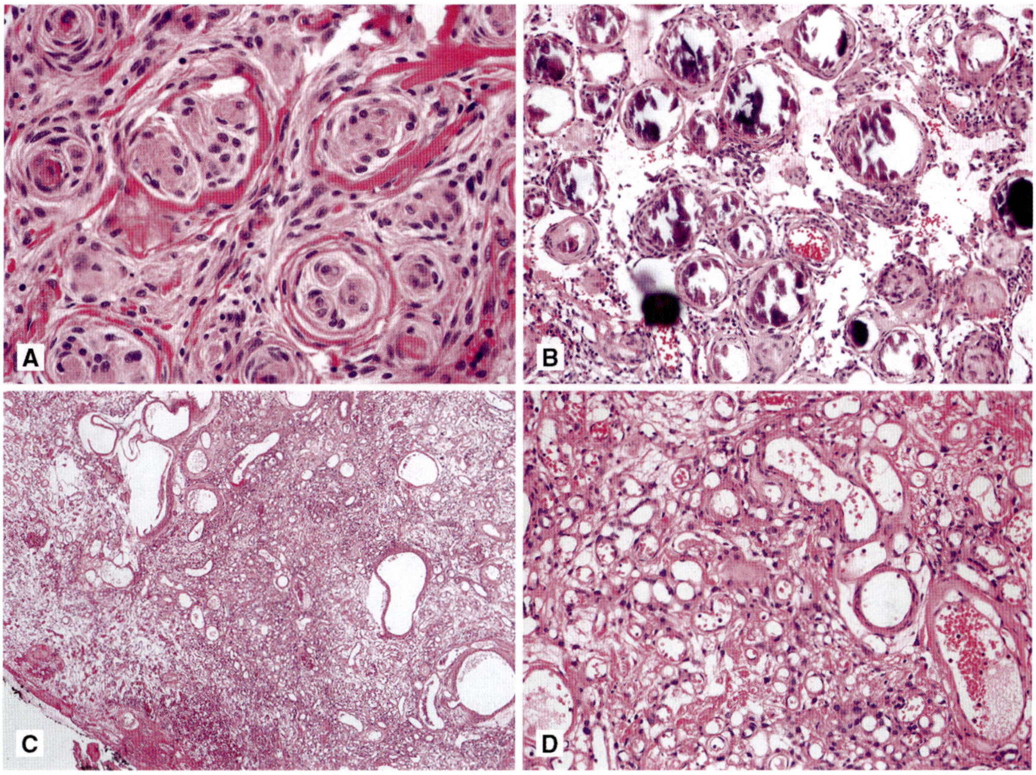

FIGURE 11-3: Prominent whorl pattern, characteristic of transitional meningioma is shown (**A**, H&E ×200). Psammomatous meningioma exhibits many calcified psammoma bodies (**B**, H&E ×200). An angiomatous meningioma displays many small- to medium-sized vessels (**C**, H&E ×40; **D**, H&E ×200).

Transitional meningioma is a transitional variant that exhibits characteristics of both, meningothelial and fibrous variants. Transitional meningiomas display vague lobular and fascicular cell patterns and are characterized by the presence of whorls and psammoma bodies (Figure 11-3A).

Psammomatous meningiomas are tumors with a distinct predominance of psammoma bodies throughout the tumor (Figure 11-3B). Subsequently, conventional meningothelial tumor cells are difficult to identify in these tumors. Psammomatous meningiomas typically occur in the spinal thoracic region of middle-aged women.

Angiomatous meningiomas are defined as meningiomas with high blood vessel density and vascular channels varying in size from small capillary-type vessels to large hyalinized vessels (Figure 11-3C and D). Histologically, this meningioma variant can be confused with vacuolated stromal cells in hemangioblastomas. A definitive diagnosis could be made on the bases of inhibin-α immunohistochemical analysis.[19] Clinically, although angiomatous meningiomas are frequently accompanied by the cerebral edema adjacent to the main mass, most of them exhibit a benign biologic behavior.

Microcystic meningioma is characterized by the formation of large, abundant, extracellular microcystic spaces that contain edematous fluid, and by tumor cells that appear stellate and vacuolated. Sometimes, numerous pleomorphic cells can also be seen (Figure 11-4A). Similar to angiomatous meningioma, this variant can be associated with a significant peritumoral cerebral edema, although it generally behaves in a benign fashion.

Secretory meningioma is characterized by numerous intracellular lumina that contain periodic acid Schiff (PAS)–positive eosinophilic secretions, also known as pseudopsammoma bodies (Figure 11-4B). These structures express carcinoembryonic antigen (CEA) (Figure 11-4C). In addition, the surrounding tumor cells express both cytokeratin (Figure 11-4D) and CEA.

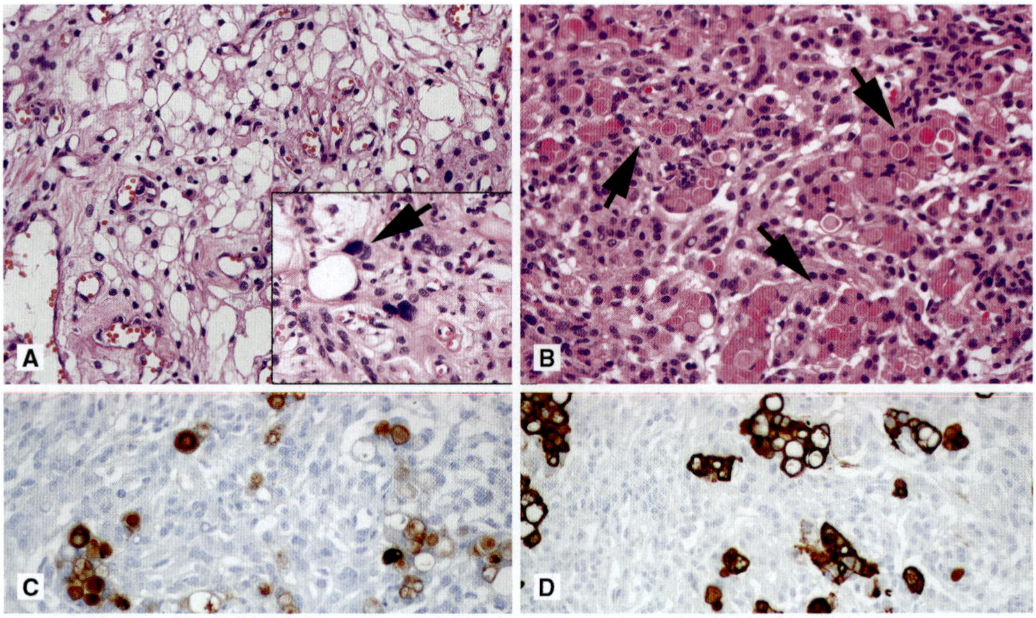

FIGURE 11-4: Microcystic meningioma is characterized by microcysts that exhibit nuclei at the periphery of tumor cells (**A**, H&E ×200). Occasionally, prominent nuclear atypia (**A**, **inset**, *arrow*, H&E ×400) is observed. Secretory meningioma is characterized by numerous intracellular lumina-containing eosinophilic secretory material, also known as pseudopsammoma bodies (**B**, *arrows*, H&E ×200). Carcinoembryonic antigen (CEA) can be detected in eosinophilic secretions and luminal cells (**C**, CEA immunostain ×400), while cytokeratin (CK) is expressed by the luminal cells (**D**, CK immunostain ×400).

Similar to angiomatous and microcystic meningiomas, secretory meningiomas are frequently accompanied by a significant peritumoral edema.

Lymphoplasmacyte-rich meningioma is a very rare variant that is characterized by the prominent infiltration of inflammatory cells, including lymphocytes and plasma cells (Figure 11-5A and B). This subtype should be differentiated from other disease entities that are associated with dense inflammatory infiltrates, such as idiopathic hypertrophic pachymeningitis, lymphoproliferative disease, Rosai-Dorfman disease,[20] and IgG4-related sclerosing disease, also known as IgG4-related pachymeningitis, which had recently been reported.[21,22] Although rare, a small number of this type of meningiomas showed increased numbers of IgG4 plasma cells,[23] differential diagnosis from IgG4-related pachymeningitis is often problematic. Systemic hematologic abnormalities associated with this variant, including hyperglobulinemia and iron refractory anemia, had been reported in some cases.[24]

Metaplastic meningioma is a rare variant characterized by the presence of metaplastic mesenchymal component(s), including osseous, cartilaginous, and lipomatous (Figure 11-5C), as well as pure or combined myxoid or xanthomatous tissues. Importantly, a metaplastic meningioma with prominent myxoid change should be differentiated from a high-grade chordoid meningioma. Absence of chordoma-like nesting tumor cells is important for a definitive histologic diagnosis.

Clear cell meningioma is predominantly composed of characteristic polygonal tumor cells with clear, glycogen-rich cytoplasm that is PAS positive and diastase sensitive (Figure 11-5D, inset). Perivascular and interstitial collagens are also prominent in these tumors (Figure 11-5D). However, based on our experience, not all tumor cells display PAS-positive glycogens in the cytoplasm. Since this meningioma variant should be differentiated from microcytic meningiomas, it is important to note that unlike the peripheral nuclei localization observed in microcytic meningiomas, nuclei of clear cell meningioma cells are located more centrally. In addition, clear cell meningiomas exhibit rare nuclear clearings and pseudoinclusions. Clinically, this meningioma variant is associated with an aggressive clinical behavior, frequent recurrences, and occasional cerebrospinal fluid seeding. Therefore, clear cell meningiomas are classified as WHO grade II tumors.

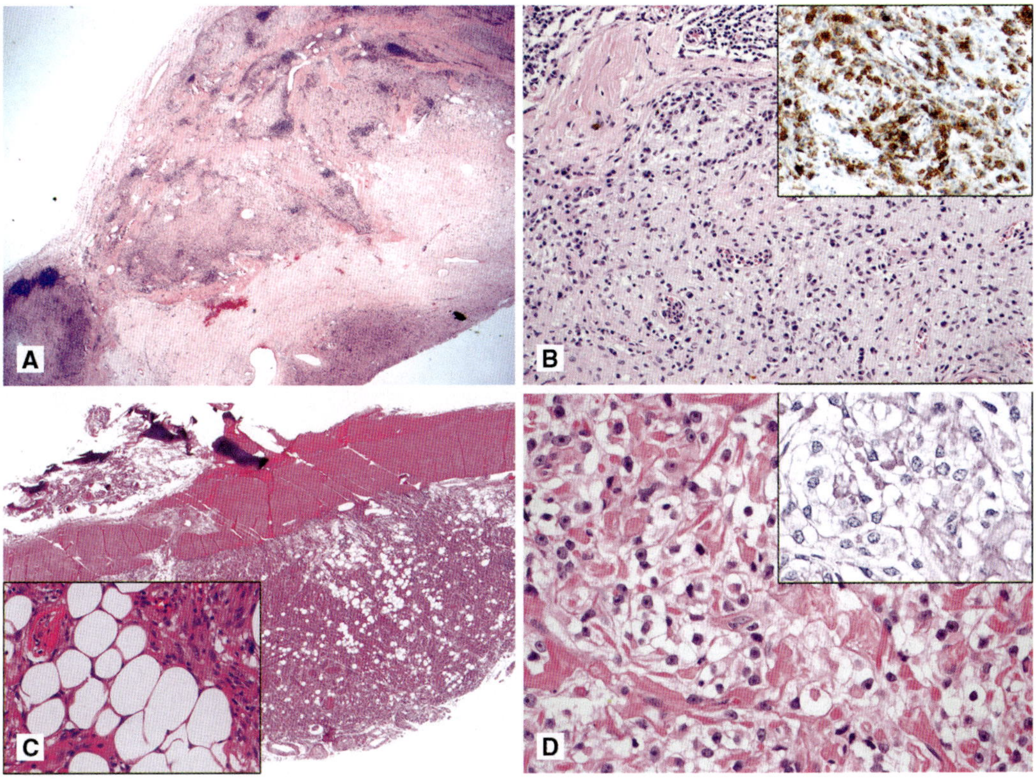

FIGURE 11-5: A lymphoplasmacyte-rich meningioma is shown as a dome-shaped mass with extensive inflammatory cell infiltrates (**A**, H&E ×12). A high-resolution image reveals marked syncytial meningothelial proliferation (**B**, **inset**, EMA immunostain ×100) associated with prominent plasma cell infiltration (**B**, H&E ×200). The lipomatous metaplastic meningioma shown is a dome-shaped mass with multifocal aggregates of lipid vacuoles (**C**, H&E ×12, and **inset** ×200). The clear cell meningioma shows diffuse proliferation of tumor cells characterized by clear cytoplasm, distinct nuclei, prominent nucleoli, and interstitial collagens (**D**, H&E ×400). Some clear cell tumor cells also display PAS-positive materials (**D**, **inset**, ×400).

Chordoid meningioma is similar histologically to a chordoma, and is characterized by cords and trabeculae of eosinophilic vacuolated cells in an abundant mucoid background (Figure 11-6A). Since chordoid areas are often focal, a pure form of this variant is very rare. In some cases, chordoid meningiomas may be accompanied by a hematologic disease, such as Castleman disease.[25] Chordoid meningiomas typically manifest as large masses associated with a high recurrence rate. Hence, they are classified as WHO grade II tumors.

Papillary meningioma is a rare disease variant characterized by the predominance of perivascular tumor cells arranged in a pseudopapillary pattern (Figure 11-6B). Papillary meningiomas are known to occur in younger patients, including children. Because this variant exhibits many overt malignant behaviors, such as brain invasion (75%), high rate of recurrence (55%), and metastases (25%), it is classified as WHO grade III. To ensure correct diagnosis, strict criteria defining the perivascular pseudopapillary pattern should be applied.

Rhabdoid meningioma is a rare variant, characterized by sheets of rhabdoid cells with plump, eosinophilic cytoplasm, eccentrically located nuclei, and prominent nucleoli (Figure 11-6C). In addition, the eosinophilic cytoplasm can contain whorled or compact waxy fibrils. Meningothelial meningioma with prominent eosinophilic cytoplasm due to degeneration may be confused with this variant. Practically, the morphologic mimickers such as metastatic rhabdoid tumors of the kidney and atypical teratoid/rhabdoid tumors should be excluded. Most rhabdoid meningiomas show high proliferation indices (Figure 11-6D) and other histologic features associated with atypical meningiomas. Moreover, these tumors often exhibit an aggressive biologic behavior and

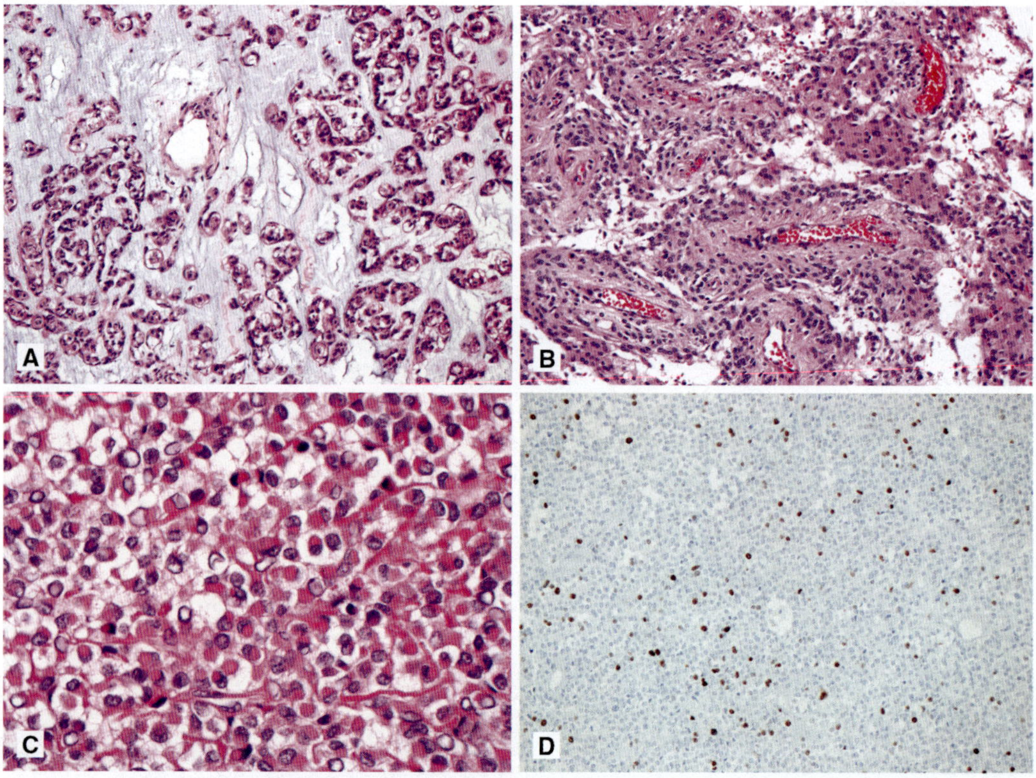

FIGURE 11-6: Chordoid meningiomas exhibit proliferation of meningothelial cells with trabeculae or cord-like appearance and a mucoid background staining pale blue (**A**, H&E ×200). Papillary meningiomas show meningothelial proliferation with prominent perivascular pseudopapillary arrangement and cellular atypia (**B**, H&E ×200). Rhabdoid meningiomas are characterized by the eosinophilic cytoplasm with prominent nucleoli (**C**, H&E ×600) and increased proliferation index (**D**, Ki-67 immunostain ×200).

thus correspond to WHO grade III. Biologic significance of focal rhabdoid cells present in other meningioma variants remains undetermined.

Cytologic Preparations (Squash and Touch Imprint)

Squash and touch smear preparations are very useful ancillary tools for intraoperative diagnosis. In such preparations, meningiomas usually exhibit cohesive syncytial clusters of meningothelial cells (Figure 11-7A and B). While the whorl formation varies, it could be diagnostic, if present. Smears often show oval nuclei with evenly dispersed, fine-to-coarse chromatin, and a small indistinct nucleolus. Intranuclear pseudoinclusions (Figure 11-7B) are also diagnostically useful. In addition, smear preparations can identify a variety of cytologic features common to specific histologic variants: bright eosinophilic pseudopsammoma bodies characteristic of secretory meningiomas, as well as cell mitoses and necrosis present in high-grade meningiomas (i.e., atypical and anaplastic meningiomas).

Immunohistochemistry

Previous reports had shown that meningioma cells commonly express the same dual antigen pattern, namely EMA and vimentin, as the normal arachnoid cap cells. In reality, the intensity of EMA expression could vary based on antibodies used, staining methods, and the tumor grade. CEA is expressed in pseudopsammoma bodies of secretory meningiomas (Figure 11-4C), while cytokeratin is expressed in cells surrounding pseudopsammoma bodies (Figure 11-4D). In addition to CEA, EMA, and vimentin, claudin-1 could also serve as a useful marker utilized in differential immunohistochemical diagnosis (Figure 11-2D).[18]

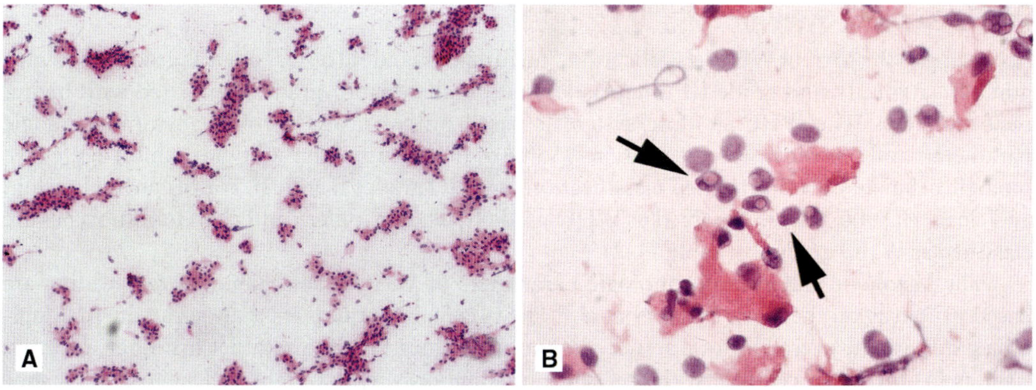

FIGURE 11-7: Typical squash smear findings of meningioma: a low-power image shows multiple cohesive meningothelial cell clusters (**A**, H&E ×100), while a high-power image reveals cells with plump cytoplasm, vesicular nuclei, syncytial pattern, and occasional intranuclear pseudoinclusions (**B**, *arrows*, H&E ×600).

Proliferation

Meningioma tumor grade directly correlates with the tumor cell proliferation rate, meaning that higher tumor grades have higher numbers of proliferating tumor cells. Hence, to assess the tumor cell proliferation rate, immunohistochemical test based on MIB-1/Ki-67 expression is very useful. A study by Maier et al.[26] reported that 4 or more mitoses and 20 or more mitoses in 10 high-power fields (HPFs) represent the cutoff values that separate the benign/atypical and atypical/anaplastic meningiomas, respectively. Consequently, the existing WHO grading system is based on these mitotic criteria. In the case of MIB-1/Ki-67 indices, benign tumors are characterized by the presence of 3.8% or fewer dividing cells, atypical meningiomas—by 7.2%, and anaplastic meningiomas—by 14.7%.[26] However, given that the immunohistochemical techniques vary considerably among different laboratories, generalization of the Ki-67 criteria is very difficult. Therefore, MIB-1/Ki-67 immunohistochemistry standardization is required for all clinical meningioma applications.

Phosphohistone-H3 (PHH3) is a histone protein that is involved in chromatin regulation and is known to be closely related to mitoses (Figure 11-8).[27] Recent evidence indicated that an anti-PHH3 antibody could be used as a sensitive and mitosis-specific marker in meningioma grading.[28,29] Levels of PHH3 reach their maximum during mitosis and are strongly correlated with the G2 to M transition. This is in direct contrast to MIB-1/Ki-67 expression, which identifies cells present in all cell cycle phases, except for G0.[29]

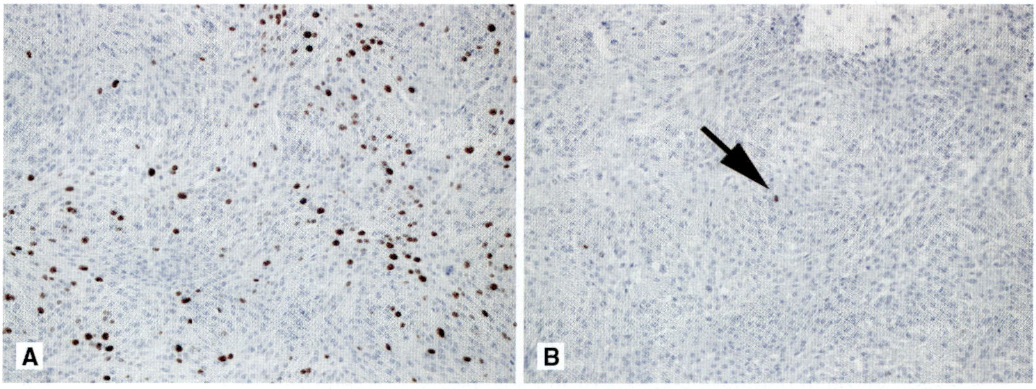

FIGURE 11-8: Immunohistochemical staining for MIB-1 (Ki-67) and PHH3 reveals that PHH3 expression (**B**, *arrow*, PHH3 ×100) is more specific for mitoses than is MIB-1 (Ki-67) (**A**, Ki-67 ×100).

WHO Grading System

According to the current WHO classification,[4] meningiomas could be classified as grade I (benign), grade II (atypical), and grade III (anaplastic), with higher tumor grades associated with higher recurrent rates. The WHO grading system is based on two axes: histologic/cytomorphologic parameters and specific histologic subtypes. Some of the meningioma subtypes exhibit aggressive biologic behaviors, leading to their classification as WHO grades II and III. For instance, chordoid and clear cell subtypes are classified as WHO grade II, while papillary and rhabdoid subtypes are classified as WHO grade III (Table 11-2).

The histologic and cytomorphologic parameters of WHO-based meningioma grading are based primarily on the work by Perry et al.[30] The two main parameters that define the meningioma grade are the overall mitotic activity in tumors (Figure 11-9B) and other histologic features, such as (a) increased cellularity, (b) presence of small cells with a high nuclear-to-cytoplasmic ratio (Figure 11-9A), (c) prominent nucleoli, (d) uninterrupted patternless or sheet-like growth (Figure 11-9A), and (e) foci of spontaneous or geographic necrosis (Figure 11-9C and D). If a meningioma shows an increased mitotic activity (4 or more mitoses per 10 HPFs) or three or more of the five histologic parameters listed above, the lesion can be diagnosed as an atypical meningioma (WHO grade II, Table 11-2). Conversely, meningioma masses that exhibit either the markedly increased mitotic indices (20 or more mitoses per 10 HPFs) or the apparent malignant cytologic features resembling carcinomas, sarcomas, or melanomas, can be diagnosed as anaplastic meningiomas (WHO grade III). Importantly, grade III meningiomas display an aggressive clinical behavior and are often fatal, with the median survival of less than 2 years.[30]

Besides mitotic indices, invasion into the brain parenchyma (Figure 11-10A) is also an important histologic parameter predictive of recurrence.[30] Therefore, strict histologic criteria that include irregular, tongue-like, or finger-like protrusions into the brain parenchyma without intervening leptomeninges, should be applied. However, care should be taken to not include a simple pushing tumor margin as evidence of the parenchymal invasion (Figure 11-10B). Work by Perry et al.[30] suggested that meningiomas that exhibit the invasion into the brain parenchyma should be considered WHO grade II, and should not be diagnosed as anaplastic meningiomas based solely on this finding.

Table 11-2 WHO Grading System for Meningiomas

WHO Grade I

- Histologic variant other than clear cell, chordoid, papillary, or rhabdoid
- Lack criteria of atypical and anaplastic meningiomas

WHO Grade II

- Clear cell or chordoid variant
- Mitotic index ≥4/10 high-power fields (HPF, defined as 0.16 mm^2)
- At least *three of five* following parameters:
  - Increased cellularity
  - Small cells with high nuclear-to-cytoplasmic ratio
  - Prominent nucleoli
  - Uninterrupted patternless or sheet-like growth
  - Foci of "spontaneous" or "geographic" necrosis

WHO Grade III

- Papillary or rhabdoid variant
- Cytology resembling that of carcinoma, melanoma, or high-grade sarcoma
- Markedly elevated mitotic index ≥20/10 HPF (defined as 0.16 mm^2)

Brain invasion (irregular, tongue-like protrusion) is prognostically considered WHO grade II.[4]

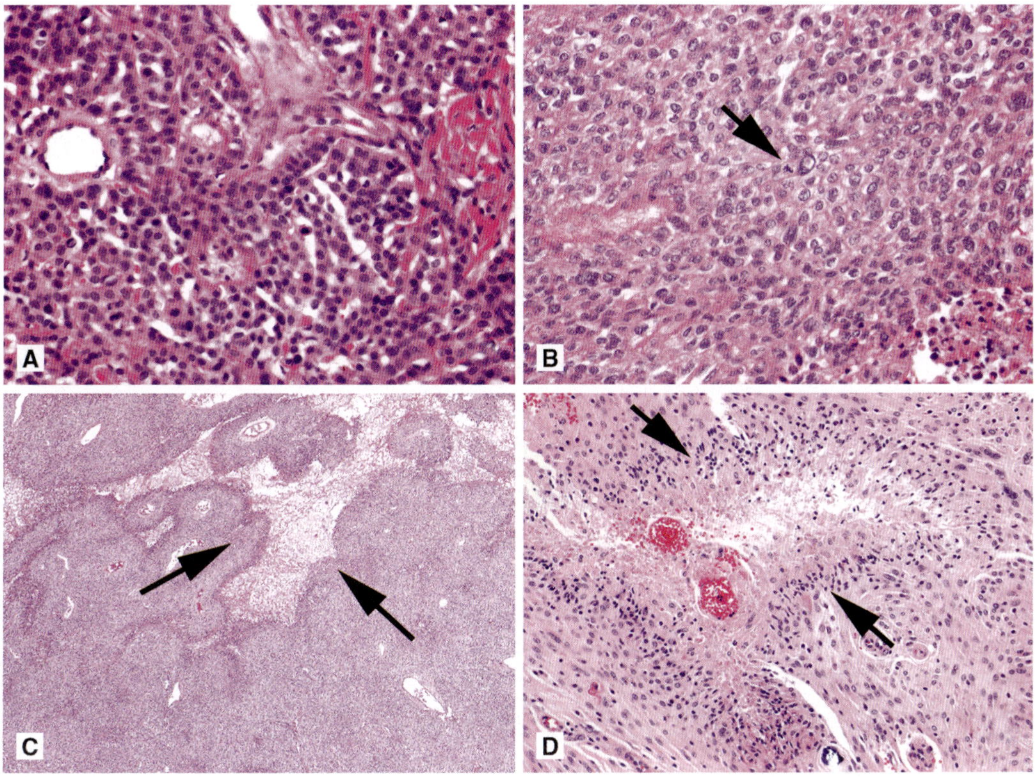

FIGURE 11-9: Histologic features of atypical meningiomas are shown in (**A**) and (**B**): increased cellularity, small cells with a high nuclear-to-cytoplasmic ratio, prominent nucleoli, and uninterrupted patternless or sheet-like growth (**A**, H&E ×400; **B**, H&E ×400). A mitotic figure (**B**, *arrow*) and spontaneous necrotic foci (**C** and **D**, *arrows*) are also shown (**B**, H&E ×400; **C**, H&E ×40; **D**, H&E ×200).

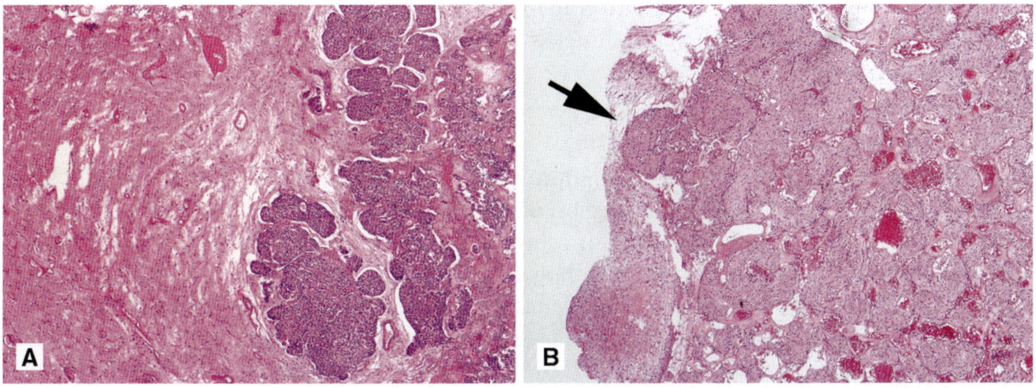

FIGURE 11-10: Histologic features of meningioma brain invasion are shown (**A**, H&E ×40). A simple tumor leading edge or margin (**B**, *arrow*, H&E ×40) should not be confused with brain invasion.

Embolized Meningioma

Surgical excision of hypervascular meningiomas could be catastrophic due to excessive blood loss. Hence, preoperative embolization may minimize the intraoperative tumor hemorrhage, thereby reducing the associated morbidity and mortality.[31] However, since this procedure results in histologic changes,[32] pathologists should be informed whether preoperative embolization had taken place prior to performing histologic evaluation of the tumor. Specifically, tumor necrosis (Figure 11-11) is frequently observed in embolized meningiomas and should not be

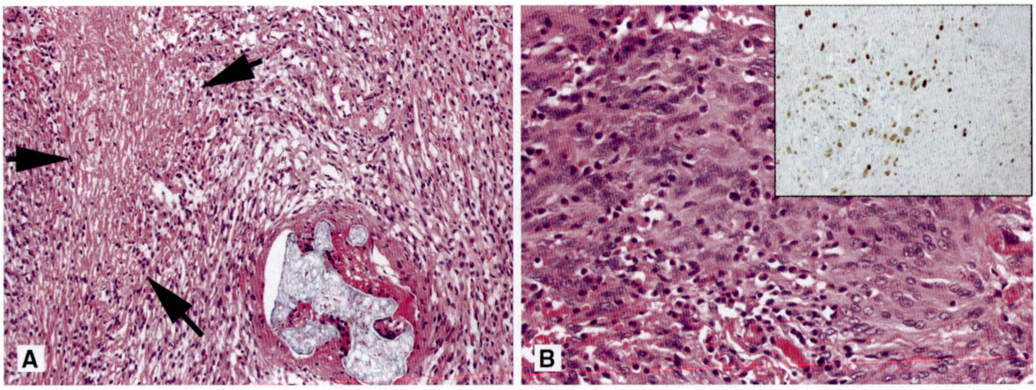

FIGURE 11-11: Necrosis due to embolization (**A**, *arrows*, H&E ×100) is shown. Meningioma tissue adjacent to the necrotic area exhibits prominent infiltration of acute inflammatory cells (**B**, H&E ×400), which can be identified immunohistochemically by MIB-1/Ki-67 staining (**B**, **inset**, Ki-67 ×100).

considered diagnostically in tumor grading. Additionally, embolization may lead to the influx of inflammatory cells into tumor areas surrounding necrosis. These inflammatory cells can stain positive for MIB-1/Ki-67 (Figure 11-11B), leading to overestimation of the proliferation index of the embolized tumor. Consequently, PHH3 immunohistochemical analysis of tumor tissues aimed at identifying the G2 to M mitoses phase could serve as an alternative ancillary diagnostic tool.

Prognostic Factors

The most important question regarding meningioma prognosis is related to its propensity for tumor recurrence, particularly in patients diagnosed with atypical meningiomas. Prognostic factors that define patient survival include proliferation indices, young age at diagnosis (<60 years of age), Simpson grade, and WHO histologic grade.[33–35] Simpson grade[35] is a grading system for surgically removed meningiomas, where grade 1 defines a complete macroscopic tumor removal complete with excision of its dural attachments and grade 5 defines a simple decompression with or without tumor biopsy.

Molecular Genetics of Meningiomas

Allelic loss of chromosome 22q is a common molecular genetic change seen in up to 60% of sporadic meningiomas.[36] Specifically, a region on chromosome 22q12.2, encoding the *NF2* tumor suppressor gene, which encodes merlin or schwannomin protein, is the most common genetic abnormality associated with early tumor pathogenesis.[37] In addition, other genetic changes, including the loss of protein 4.1 family or TSLC1, are associated with early benign meningiomas.[38] In an atypical meningioma, several chromosomal losses (1p, 6q, 10q, 14q, and 18q) or gains (1q, 9q, 12q, 15q, 17q, and 20q); activation of NOTCH, WNT, and IGF signaling; loss of the progesterone receptor; and activation of telomerase/hTERT are known to occur. Anaplastic meningiomas share the same chromosomal aberrations, with added frequent losses on 6q, 10q, 9p, and 12q, and gains or amplifications of 17q23.[38] In summary, meningioma tumorigenesis begins with the loss of 22q or *NF* gene mutation, and is compounded by the accumulation of additional chromosomal losses or gains, and activation or deactivation of various signaling pathways (Figure 11-12). Advances in cancer technology had led to recent genetic profiling of meningiomas. A study by Carvalho et al.[39] stratified meningiomas into low-proliferative and high-proliferative groups based on the gene expression microarray and array comparative genomic hybridization. The two tumor groups exhibit different proliferation indices, copy number aberrations, and other genetic changes.

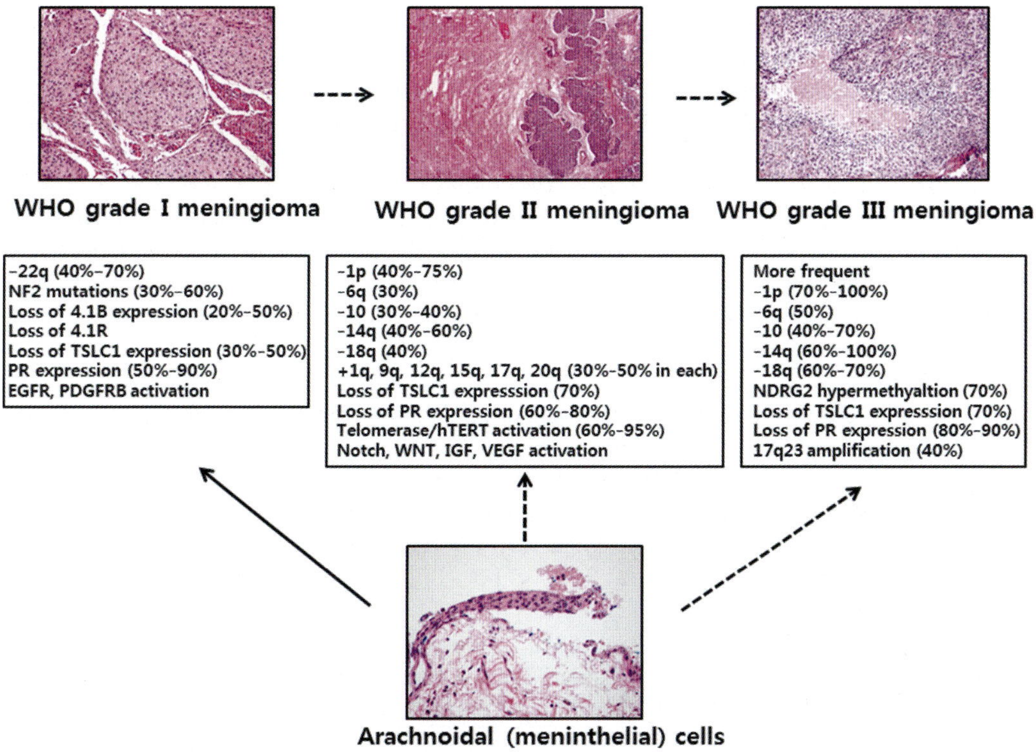

FIGURE 11-12: Summary of molecular tumorigenesis and malignant progression in meningioma.

HEMANGIOPERICYTOMA/SOLITARY FIBROUS TUMOR

Introduction

Hemangiopericytoma (HPC) is a highly cellular and vascularized mesenchymal tumor that exhibits characteristic thick-walled, branching "staghorn" vessels, also known as the hemangiopericytoma-like vasculature.[40] HPC tumors, typically WHO grade II or III, are classified as tumors of the CNS that present as dura-based masses and exhibit a high tendency to recur and metastasize outside the CNS.[40] The first HPC case was described in 1942 by Stout and Murray as a soft tissue tumor of pericytic origin.[41] In a previous report, Cushing and Eisenhardt described three variants of angioblastic meningioma, one of which could fall under the modern HPC classification. This tumor type was reclassified as a meningioma of hemangiopericytic type based on the 1979 WHO classification,[42] and then reclassified again as a mesenchymal, nonmeningothelial tumor based on the 1993 WHO classification.[43] This multistep reclassification reflects uncertainty of cell(s) of origin for this particular tumor.

The solitary fibrous tumor (SFT) of the CNS is a rare mesenchymal tumor that involves cranial and spinal meninges. Histologically, these tumors are characterized by the proliferating, spindle-shaped cells located in fascicles between prominent, eosinophilic bands of collagen. SFT was first described in 1931 by Klemperer and Coleman as a tumor containing spindle-shaped mesenchymal cells that arose from pleura.[44] Since then, SFTs had been found in other organs, including the CNS.[45] These tumors display characteristic immunoreactivity for CD34, Bcl-2, and CD99. Interestingly, histologic features of SFT do not correlate with their prognosis. Specifically, some of SFT are known to have high proliferation indices and had been reported to behave very aggressively.[46,47]

HPC and SFT—Two Variants of a Single Entity?

In contrast to soft tissue tumors, HPCs found in the CNS had been considered distinct from SFTs until recently, with evidence indicating that SFTs possess a more benign biologic behavior.[40,48] Morphologically, HPC and SFT can be distinguished based on the differences in collagen deposition, mitotic activity, and different levels of CD34 expression.[49,50] Clinically, it is important to differentiate between the meningeal HPC and SFT because a significantly higher proportion of HPCs recur, metastasize, and are associated with a diminished overall patient survival.[49] Interestingly, a recent whole-exome sequencing identified a fusion transcript common to both HPC and SFT. This new evidence indicates a common origin of these tumors, but further study is required in order to establish its biological significance.[51]

Incidence

Meningeal HPCs occur in approximately 0.4% of all primary CNS tumors.[40] Incidence of SFTs has not been reported, except for a study by Bisceglia et al.[51] that described 220 SFT cases in the CNS identified from a 15-year (1996 to 2011) literature search. A subsequent study[52] reported an additional five SFT cases, as well as 15 HPC and 786 meningioma cases among 806 primary meningeal-bases tumors diagnosed at a single institution between 1992 and 2009.

Macroscopic Findings

Macroscopic HPC and SFT findings are similar to those of meningiomas. These tumors present as dura-based tumors with a firm consistency. During surgery, meningeal HPCs appear as solid, well-demarcated tumors that tend to bleed during removal.[40]

Histology

HPC is composed of monotonous, closely packed, slightly spindled cells with little intervening stroma (Figure 11-13A and B). The cytoplasmic border of each tumor cell is indistinct, nuclei are round to oval with inconspicuous nucleoli, and rich reticulin fibers surround each tumor cell. A typical HPC is highly vascular and shows slit-like vascular channels lined by flat endothelial cells in a so-called staghorn pattern (Figure 11-13A). HPC can invade and destroy the adjacent bone or brain parenchyma. SFTs are composed of bland, spindled cells surrounded by dense collagenous matrix and prominent, branching blood vessels (Figure 11-13C and D). As mentioned above, HPC and SFT can be distinguished morphologically based on the differences in collagen deposition, mitotic activity, and levels of CD34 expression.[49,53]

Molecular Genetic Characteristics and Immunohistochemistry

Karyotypes of meningeal HPC and SFT show frequent abnormalities of chromosome 12, particularly in the 12q13-15 region, and of chromosome 3.[54] Contrary to meningiomas, the allelic loss of chromosome 22q, a chromosomal region harboring the *NF2* gene, has not been reported.[55] Recently, an integrative sequencing analysis identified a novel gene fusion between the NGFIA-binding protein 2 (*NAB2)* and the signal transducer and activator of transcription 6 (*STAT6*) in the majority of HPCs and SFTs.[56,57] Study authors suggested that this fusion was likely due to an intrachromosomal inversion that juxtaposed *NAB2* and *STAT6*.[56] *NAB2* is a transcriptional modulator of the zinc finger transcription factors *EGR1*, *EGR2*, and *EGR3*. NAB2 protein is highly expressed in a variety of tissues and is always localized in the nucleus. *STAT6* has a dual function as signal transducer and activator of transcription and is involved in interleukin-4 signaling. Normally, the STAT6 protein is predominantly expressed in the cytoplasm of various cell types. Limited experimental evidence indicated that the NAB2–STAT6 fusion protein promotes tumorigenesis by converting NAB2 from functioning as a transcriptional repressor to a transcriptional activator that acquires its activation domain from STAT6.[50] Moreover, the fusion protein localizes to the nucleus because the NAB2 break point is usually located in the C-terminal direction to its nuclear localization signal.[50] Therefore, an immunohistochemical analysis using the STAT6

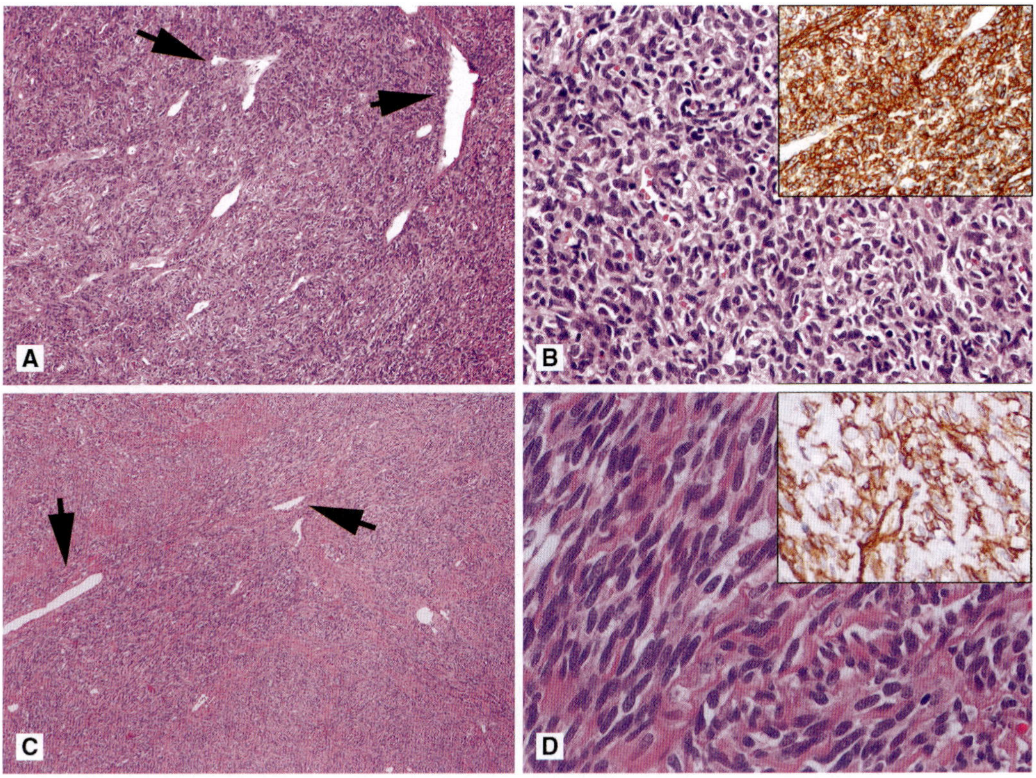

FIGURE 11-13: Typical histologic patterns of HPC and SFT. HPC is a hypercellular mass with a slit-like vascular pattern, also known as "staghorn" pattern (**A**, *arrows*, H&E ×40). Higher-power images exhibit short, proliferating, spindle-shaped tumor cells with little surrounding stroma (**B**, H&E ×400). CD34 expression is also observed (**B**, **inset**, CD34 immunostain ×200). SFT also displays slit-like vessels (**C**, *arrows*, H&E ×40), and a higher-power image reveals proliferating spindle-shaped cells with abundant intervening collagen fibers (**D**, H&E ×400). The SFT tumor also expresses CD34 (**D**, **inset**, CD34 immunostain ×400).

epitope may differentiate HPCs and/or SFTs from other mesenchymal tumors, as these tumors will be characterized by the nuclear STAT6 localization (Figure 11-14).[50] In addition, HPCs and SFTs are diffusely immunoreactive to vimentin in 85% of cases, and 80% to 100% of all cases display individual cells positive for factor XIIIa. Moreover, HPC exhibit a patchy CD34 immunopositivity in 33% to 100% of cases (Figure 11-13B, inset),[40,58] whereas all SFT cases showed diffuse CD34 positivity (Figure 11-13D, inset).[51] Lastly, both tumor types exhibit variable CD99 and Bcl2 expression, and almost all cases are negative for the expression of S100 protein, EMA, and claudin-1.[51]

Grading

WHO grade III (anaplastic) tumors show a high degree of mitotic activity (at least 5 mitoses per 10 HPFs) and/or necrosis, in addition to at least two of the following: hemorrhage, moderate-to-high nuclear atypia, and cellularity.[59] In SFT cases, hypercellularity and increased mitoses[46,47] had been suggested as histologic parameters of aggressive biology. Despite these suggestions, a strict grading guideline for SFT in the CNS has not been established (Table 11-3).

Prognostic Factors

Expression of proliferation markers carries prognostic implications in both, HPCs and SFTs.[40,51] Specifically, the MIB-1/Ki-67 labeling index cutoff values for HPC cases were suggested to be 10%[59] and 5%.[60] In SFT cases, a MIB-1/Ki-67 labeling index of greater than 5% had been suggested to serve as an adverse prognostic marker.[51]

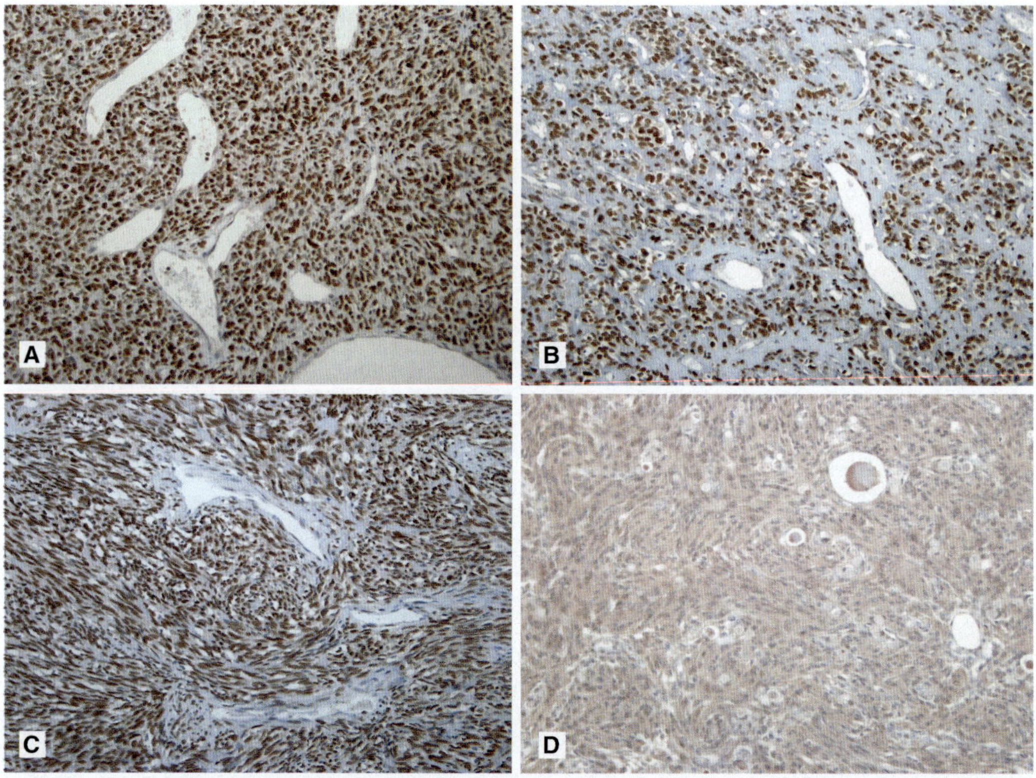

FIGURE 11-14: Immunohistochemical staining for STAT6. HPC and SFT tumor cells display a prominent nuclear STAT6 expression (**A**, **B**, **C**, STAT6 ×200). A vague, diffuse cytoplasmic STAT6 staining is deemed negative for STAT6 expression (a case of meningioma) (**D**, STAT6 ×200).

Table 11-3 WHO Grading System for Hemangiopericytoma/Solitary Fibrous Tumor

WHO Grade I

- (Solitary fibrous tumor[a])

WHO Grade II

- Hemangiopericytoma

WHO Grade III

- High degree of mitotic activity ≥5/10 high-power fields (HPF, defined as 0.16 mm^2) and/or
- Necrosis
  and
- At least two of the following:
  - Hemorrhage
  - Moderate-to-high nuclear atypia
  - Moderate-to-high cellularity

[a]Although the grading system of solitary fibrous tumor (SFT) is not described in the 2007 WHO bluebook, SFT is coded as a benign tumor in ICD-O (8815/0). To facilitate understanding, the authors provisionally categorized SFT as WHO grade I. In case of the SFT, hypercellularity and MIB-1/Ki-67 labeling indices ≥5% may serve as histologic parameters of aggressive biology.

ACKNOWLEDGMENTS

The authors express their gratitude to their mentor, Dr. Tai Seung Kim, for his inspiring and passionate teaching of neuropathology. Dr. S.H. Kim wishes to thank Dr. M. Joe Ma (Florida Hospital Center for Diagnostic Pathology), Dr. Jae Y. Ro (Weill Cornell Medical College), and Dr. Yeon-Lim Suh (Sungkyunkwan University, Samsung Seoul Hospital) for their excellent advice over the years.

References

1. Ng HK, Tse CC, Lo ST. Meningiomas and arachnoid cells: an immunohistochemical study of epithelial markers. *Pathology* 1987;19:253–257.
2. Ostrom QT, Gittleman H, Farah P, et al. CBTRUS statistical report: primary brain and central nervous system tumors diagnosed in the United States in 2006–2010. *Neuro Oncol* 2013;15(suppl 2):ii1–ii56.
3. Lee CH, Jung KW, Yoo H, et al. Epidemiology of primary brain and central nervous system tumors in Korea. *J Korean Neurosurg Soc* 2010;48:145–152.
4. Perry A, Louis DN, Scheithauer BW, et al. Meningiomas. In: Louis DN, Ohgaki H, Wiestler OD, et al., eds. *WHO Classification of Tumours of the Central Nervous System*. 4th ed. Lyon, France: International Agency for Research on Cancer; 2007:163–172.
5. Stemmer-Rachamimiv AO, Wiestler OD, Louis DN. Neurofibromatosis type 2. In: Louis DN, Ohgaki H, Wiestler OD, et al., eds. *WHO Classification of Tumours of the Central Nervous System*. 4th ed. Lyon, France: International Agency for Research on Cancer; 2007:210–214.
6. Scoles DR, Huynh DP, Morcos PA, et al. Neurofibromatosis 2 tumour suppressor schwannomin interacts with betaII-spectrin. *Nat Genet* 1998;18:354–359.
7. Louis DN, Ramesh V, Gusella JF. Neuropathology and molecular genetics of neurofibromatosis 2 and related tumors. *Brain Pathol* 1995;5:163–172.
8. Perry A, Giannini C, Raghavan R, et al. Aggressive phenotypic and genotypic features in pediatric and NF2-associated meningiomas: a clinicopathologic study of 53 cases. *J Neuropathol Exp Neurol* 2001;60:994–1003.
9. Ruttledge MH, Sarrazin J, Rangaratnam S, et al. Evidence for the complete inactivation of the NF2 gene in the majority of sporadic meningiomas. *Nat Genet* 1994;6:180–184.
10. Wiemels J, Wrensch M, Claus EB. Epidemiology and etiology of meningioma. *J Neurooncol* 2010;99:307–314.
11. Hijiya N, Hudson MM, Lensing S, et al. Cumulative incidence of secondary neoplasms as a first event after childhood acute lymphoblastic leukemia. *JAMA* 2007;297:1207–1215.
12. Friedman DL, Whitton J, Leisenring W, et al. Subsequent neoplasms in 5-year survivors of childhood cancer: the Childhood Cancer Survivor Study. *J Natl Cancer Inst* 2010;102:1083–1095.
13. Preston DL, Ron E, Yonehara S, et al. Tumors of the nervous system and pituitary gland associated with atomic bomb radiation exposure. *J Natl Cancer Inst* 2002;94:1555–1563.
14. Chang AS, Ross JS. Diagnostic neuroradiology: CT, MRI, fMRI, MRS, PET, and octreotide SPECT. In: Lee JH, ed. *Meningiomas*. London, UK: Springer; 2008:55–65.
15. Osawa T, Tosaka M, Nagaishi M, et al. Factors affecting peritumoral brain edema in meningioma: special histological subtypes with prominently extensive edema. *J Neurooncol* 2013;111:49–57.
16. Regelsberger J, Hagel C, Emami P, et al. Secretory meningiomas: a benign subgroup causing life-threatening complications. *Neuro Oncol* 2009;11:819–824.
17. Jellinger K, Slowik F. Histological subtypes and prognostic problems in meningiomas. *J Neurol* 1975;208:279–298.
18. Hahn HP, Bundock EA, Hornick JL. Immunohistochemical staining for claudin-1 can help distinguish meningiomas from histologic mimics. *Am J Clin Pathol* 2006;125:203–208.
19. Hoang MP, Amirkhan RH. Inhibin alpha distinguishes hemangioblastoma from clear cell renal cell carcinoma. *Am J Surg Pathol* 2003;27:1152–1156.
20. Forest F, N'Guyen AT, Fesselet J, et al. Meningeal Rosai-Dorfman disease mimicking meningioma. *Ann Hematol* 2014;93:937–940.

21. Tanboon J, Felicella MM, Bilbao J, et al. Probable IgG4-related pachymeningitis: a case with transverse sinus obliteration. *Clin Neuropathol* 2013;32:291–297.
22. Kim EH, Kim SH, Cho JM, et al. Immunoglobulin G4-related hypertrophic pachymeningitis involving cerebral parenchyma. *J Neurosurg* 2011;115:1242–1247.
23. Lal A, Dahiya S, Gonzales M, et al. IgG4 overexpression is rare in meningiomas with a prominent inflammatory component: a review of 16 cases. *Brain Pathol* 2014;24:352–359.
24. Gi H, Nagao S, Yoshizumi H, et al. Meningioma with hypergammaglobulinemia. Case report. *J Neurosurg* 1990;73:628–629.
25. Kepes JJ, Chen WY, Connors MH, et al. "Chordoid" meningeal tumors in young individuals with peritumoral lymphoplasmacellular infiltrates causing systemic manifestations of the Castleman syndrome. A report of seven cases. *Cancer* 1988;62:391–406.
26. Maier H, Wanschitz J, Sedivy R, et al. Proliferation and DNA fragmentation in meningioma subtypes. *Neuropathol Appl Neurobiol* 1997;23:496–506.
27. Hendzel MJ, Wei Y, Mancini MA, et al. Mitosis-specific phosphorylation of histone H3 initiates primarily within pericentromeric heterochromatin during G2 and spreads in an ordered fashion coincident with mitotic chromosome condensation. *Chromosoma* 1997;106:348–360.
28. Ribalta T, McCutcheon IE, Aldape KD, et al. The mitosis-specific antibody anti-phosphohistone-H3 (PHH3) facilitates rapid reliable grading of meningiomas according to WHO 2000 criteria. *Am J Surg Pathol* 2004;28:1532–1536.
29. Fukushima S, Terasaki M, Sakata K, et al. Sensitivity and usefulness of anti-phosphohistone-H3 antibody immunostaining for counting mitotic figures in meningioma cases. *Brain Tumor Pathol* 2009;26:51–57.
30. Perry A, Stafford SL, Scheithauer BW, et al. Meningioma grading: an analysis of histologic parameters. *Am J Surg Pathol* 1997;21:1455–1465.
31. Fiorella DJ, Deshmukh VR, McDougall CG, et al. Preoperative embolization of meningiomas. In: Lee JH, ed. *Meningiomas*. London, UK: Springer; 2008:89–99.
32. Perry A, Chicoine MR, Filiput E, et al. Clinicopathologic assessment and grading of embolized meningiomas: a correlative study of 64 patients. *Cancer* 2001;92:701–711.
33. Durand A, Labrousse F, Jouvet A, et al. WHO grade II and III meningiomas: a study of prognostic factors. *J Neurooncol* 2009;95:367–375.
34. Oya S, Kawai K, Nakatomi H, et al. Significance of Simpson grading system in modern meningioma surgery: integration of the grade with MIB-1 labeling index as a key to predict the recurrence of WHO grade I meningiomas. *J Neurosurg* 2012;117:121–128.
35. Simpson D. The recurrence of intracranial meningiomas after surgical treatment. *J Neurol Neurosurg Psychiatry* 1957;20:22–39.
36. Elder JB, Chiocca EA. Molecular and genetic characterization of meningiomas: future predictive assays and "personalized" treatment. *World Neurosurg* 2013;79:247–248.
37. Choy W, Kim W, Nagasawa D, et al. The molecular genetics and tumor pathogenesis of meningiomas and the future directions of meningioma treatments. *Neurosurg Focus* 2011;30:E6.
38. Riemenschneider MJ, Perry A, Reifenberger G. Histological classification and molecular genetics of meningiomas. *Lancet Neurol* 2006;5:1045–1054.
39. Carvalho LH, Smirnov I, Baia GS, et al. Molecular signatures define two main classes of meningiomas. *Mol Cancer* 2007;6:64.
40. Giannini C, Rushing EJ, Hainfellner JA. Haemangiopericytoma. In: Louis DN, Ohgaki H, Wiestler OD, et al., eds. *WHO Classification of Tumours of the Central Nervous System*. 4th ed. Lyon, France: International Agency for Research on Cancer; 2007:178–180.
41. Stout AP, Murray MR. Hemangiopericytoma: a vascular tumor featuring Zimmermann's pericytes. *Ann Surg* 1942;116:26–33.
42. Zulch KJ, ed. *Histological Typing of Tumours of the Central Nervous System*. Geneva, Switzerland: World Health Organization; 1979.
43. Kleihues P, Burger PC, Scheithauer BW, et al. *Histological Typing of Tumours of the Central Nervous System*. 2nd ed. Berlin; New York, NY: Springer-Verlag; 1993:xii, 112 p.
44. Klemperer P, Coleman BR. Primary neoplasms of the pleura. *Arch Pathol* 1931;11:385–412.
45. Carneiro SS, Scheithauer BW, Nascimento AG, et al. Solitary fibrous tumor of the meninges: a lesion distinct from fibrous meningioma. A clinicopathologic and immunohistochemical study. *Am J Clin Pathol* 1996;106:217–224.

46. Vassal F, Manet R, Forest F, et al. Solitary fibrous tumors of the central nervous system: report of five cases with unusual clinicopathological and outcome patterns. *Acta Neurochir* 2011;153:377–384.
47. Pakasa NM, Pasquier B, Chambonniere ML, et al. Atypical presentations of solitary fibrous tumors of the central nervous system: an analysis of unusual clinicopathological and outcome patterns in three new cases with a review of the literature. *Virchows Archiv* 2005;447:81–86.
48. Ng HK, Choi PC, Wong CW, et al. Metastatic solitary fibrous tumor of the meninges. Case report. *J Neurosurg* 2000;93:490–493.
49. Tihan T, Viglione M, Rosenblum MK, et al. Solitary fibrous tumors in the central nervous system. A clinicopathologic review of 18 cases and comparison to meningeal hemangiopericytomas. *Arch Pathol Lab Med* 2003;127:432–439.
50. Schweizer L, Koelsche C, Sahm F, et al. Meningeal hemangiopericytoma and solitary fibrous tumors carry the NAB2–STAT6 fusion and can be diagnosed by nuclear expression of STAT6 protein. *Acta Neuropathol* 2013;125:651–658.
51. Bisceglia M, Galliani C, Giannatempo G, et al. Solitary fibrous tumor of the central nervous system: a 15-year literature survey of 220 cases (August 1996–July 2011). *Adv Anat Pathol* 2011;18:356–392.
52. Mena H, Ribas JL, Pezeshkpour GH, et al. Hemangiopericytoma of the central nervous system: a review of 94 cases. *Hum Pathol* 1991;22:84–91.
53. Scheithauer BW, Fuller GN, VandenBerg SR. The 2007 WHO classification of tumors of the nervous system: controversies in surgical neuropathology. *Brain Pathol* 2008;18:307–316.
54. Martin AJ, Summersgill BM, Fisher C, et al. Chromosomal imbalances in meningeal solitary fibrous tumors. *Cancer Genet Cytogenet* 2002;135:160–164.
55. Joseph JT, Lisle DK, Jacoby LB, et al. NF2 gene analysis distinguishes hemangiopericytoma from meningioma. *Am J Pathol* 1995;147:1450–1455.
56. Chmielecki J, Crago AM, Rosenberg M, et al. Whole-exome sequencing identifies a recurrent NAB2–STAT6 fusion in solitary fibrous tumors. *Nat Genet* 2013;45:131–132.
57. Robinson DR, Wu YM, Kalyana-Sundaram S, et al. Identification of recurrent NAB2–STAT6 gene fusions in solitary fibrous tumor by integrative sequencing. *Nat Genet* 2013;45:180–185.
58. Perry A, Scheithauer BW, Nascimento AG. The immunophenotypic spectrum of meningeal hemangiopericytoma: a comparison with fibrous meningioma and solitary fibrous tumor of meninges. *Am J Surg Pathol* 1997;21:1354–1360.
59. Vuorinen V, Sallinen P, Haapasalo H, et al. Outcome of 31 intracranial haemangiopericytomas: poor predictive value of cell proliferation indices. *Acta Neurochir* 1996;138:1399–1408.
60. Probst-Cousin S, Bergmann M, Schroder R, et al. Ki-67 and biological behaviour in meningeal haemangiopericytomas. *Histopathology* 1996;29:57–61.

12 Hereditary Syndromes

▶ Nishant Tiwari
▶ Hidehiro Takei

NEUROFIBROMATOSIS TYPE 1

Neurofibromatosis type 1 (NF1; OMIM #162200), formerly known as "von Recklinghausen disease," is an autosomal dominant, multisystem genetic disorder with high penetrance and widely variable expressivity. NF1 is one of the most common single-gene disorders affecting neurologic functions. The mutation involves the *NF1* gene on chromosome 17q11.2, which encodes a GTPase activating protein, neurofibromin, which acts as K-ras suppressor.[1–3] Since neurofibromin regulates many pathways responsible for overactive cell proliferation, learning impairments, and skeletal defects, and plays a role in neuronal development, it is understandable that altered neurofibromin gene/protein can cause a variety of clinical manifestations of NF1.[4] The incidence of NF1 is 1:3,500 live births worldwide with a uniform distribution between males and females. Family history of NF1 in the first-degree relatives is seen in about 50% of cases,[1] and spontaneous mutation is seen in up to 50% of cases.

NF1 is caused by a germline inactivating mutation of neurofibromin gene, which is associated with loss of its inhibitory effect on the Ras-MAPK signaling pathway leading to increased transcription in response to growth factors. In addition, NF1 is now considered a part of larger disease spectrum called RASopathies, including Noonan syndrome, Costello syndrome, LEOPARD syndrome, and Legius syndrome.[5,6]

Clinical and Radiologic Findings

Clinical diagnosis is based on the presence of characteristic physical findings where the individual lesions appear at various ages. Multiple café au lait spots, plexiform neurofibroma, and pseudoarthrosis are often present by 1 year of age. Axillary/inguinal freckling, optic glioma, and scoliosis develop by the age of 7 years. Nonplexiform neurofibromas and iris hamartomas or Lisch nodules develop by adolescence. Other central nervous system (CNS) and peripheral malignancies arise in adults. One of the most common complications in patients with NF1 is cognitive and learning disability, and recently, a high prevalence of autism spectrum disorder has been reported in NF1 patients.[7] Three to seven percent of NF1 patients show some degree of cognitive impairment along with short stature and macrocephaly.[1,2] These features might represent the overlapping features with Noonan syndrome. Many have thus suggested neurofibromatosis–Noonan syndrome as a single entity that would encompass all such patients.[5,6]

Radiologically, T2-weighted MRI scans show focal areas of increased signal intensity, which are referred to as "unidentified bright objects (UBOs)," in up to 60% of brains of NF1 patients. Pathologically, UBOs may represent increased fluid within myelin associated with hyperplastic or dysplastic glial proliferation.[8] The clinical implications and functional characteristics of UBOs are not well understood, and UBOs are known to disappear with age.[3]

NF1-Associated Peripheral and Central Nervous System Neoplasms

A variety of nervous system neoplasms occur in association with NF1, and all involve tumorigenesis of neural crest-derived cells. These tumors include cutaneous neurofibromas, plexiform neurofibromas, malignant peripheral nerve sheath tumors, spinal neurofibromas, and astrocytomas.[9]

Spinal neurofibromas are presented in approximately 40% of patients with NF1. This is especially marked in individuals affected with familial spinal neurofibromatosis, a variant form of NF1, characterized by bilateral tumors involving multiple spinal nerve roots, which are often the only manifestation of NF1.[9]

In addition to peripheral neurofibromas, NF1 predisposes to CNS tumors, and up to 15% of all NF1 patients develop a brain tumor within the first two decades of life.[10] The vast majority of them are pilocytic astrocytomas (WHO grade 1) predominantly along the optic pathway and less commonly in the brainstem. Other histologic types of gliomas (i.e., diffuse astrocytoma, anaplastic astrocytoma, and glioblastoma) can also been seen.[11] Optic pathway gliomas are apparent on MRI before 6 years of age, but most are asymptomatic and remain so throughout life.[2] Symptomatic optic pathway gliomas in NF1 are usually stable for many years or very slowly progressive. Complete loss of neurofibromin is noted in NF1-associated optic gliomas.[9] In one study, multiple CNS tumors were seen in 20% of NF1 patients.[11]

NEUROFIBROMATOSIS TYPE 2

NF2 (OMIM #101000) is an autosomal dominant inherited tumor predisposition syndrome characterized by the development of neoplasms of the nervous system, most notably bilateral vestibular schwannomas. The penetrance is close to 100% at 60 years of age. This syndrome is known to be caused by constitutional mutations in the *NF2* gene on chromosome 22q12.2 that encodes the FERM (4.1 protein/Ezrin/Radixin/Moesin) domain protein, merlin/schwannomin.[12] Merlin is a tumor suppressor protein involved in regulation of cell proliferation in response to adhesive signaling.[12] NF2 has 1:33,000 estimated incidence.[13] Since in excess of 50% of patients represent *de novo* mutations, family history may be negative, making the diagnosis more difficult.[13,14] As many as one-third of simplex cases (i.e., single occurrence in a family) are mosaic for an *NF2* mutation, which are usually milder diseases.[14] Almost all affected individuals develop bilateral vestibular schwannomas by the age of 30 years.

Clinical Features and Diagnosis

Unlike in NF1, NF2 patients have few pigmentary abnormalities (e.g., café au lait spots), and the vast majority of symptoms are associated with tumor formations in the nervous system. The hallmark of NF2 is the development of bilateral vestibular schwannomas, and the presenting symptoms include tinnitus, balance problems, and hearing loss. Schwannomas also occur on other cranial nerves, spinal nerve roots, and peripheral nerves. In addition, meningiomas (the second most common tumor type of NF2), ependymomas, and very rarely, astrocytomas are other brain tumors seen in NF2 patients. Diagnosis of NF2 is based on clinical criteria (Table 12-1).[15,16] Molecular diagnosis is also available, and identification of pathogenic *NF2* mutation in blood or in two separate tumors from the same individuals confirms the diagnosis.[14]

Variable expressivity of *NF2* among individuals results in varying size, location, and number of tumors. At least two clinical subtypes of NF2 have been described: The mild (Gardner) type has a late onset and a comparatively benign course with fewer tumors, whereas the severe (Wishart) type has an early onset and rapid aggressive clinical course with marked predisposition to meningiomas and ependymomas in addition to vestibular schwannomas.[17] The majority of clinical pictures of NF2 lie between these two extremes. Genotype–phenotype correlation has been reported: Truncating mutations (nonsense and frameshift mutations), leading to a smaller and probably nonfunctional NF2 protein product, are more often associated with severe (Wishart) type, while missense mutations cause predominantly mild (Gardner) type.[14]

Table 12-1 Diagnostic Criteria for Neurofibromatosis Type 2

1.	**Bilateral vestibular schwannomas**				
2.	**First-degree relative with NF2**	**AND**	Unilateral vestibular schwannoma	**OR**	Any two of the following: • Meningioma • Ependymoma • Neurofibroma • Nonvestibular schwannoma • Posterior subcapsular lens opacities
3.	**Unilateral vestibular schwannoma**	**AND**	Any two of the following • Meningioma • Ependymoma • Neurofibroma • Schwannoma • Posterior subcapsular lens opacities		
4.	**Multiple Meningiomas**	**AND**	Unilateral vestibular schwannoma	**OR**	Any two of the following: • Ependymoma • Neurofibroma • Nonvestibular schwannoma • Cataract

NF2-Associated Brain Tumors

1. In addition to vestibular nerves, schwannomas can also develop on other cranial nerves and peripheral nerves. In the spinal cord, schwannomas arise on the dorsal root and typically present as so-called dumbbell tumors, which occasionally cause diagnostic confusion between NF1 and NF2. NF2-associated schwannomas have a similar histology to sporadic tumors, but multifocal nerve involvement and whorl formation are more frequent.[18] Hybrid tumors (i.e., benign nerve sheath tumors with characteristic features of both neurofibromas and schwannomas) are reported in the setting of NF1, NF2, and schwannomatosis[19] (Figure 12-1). There may be a patchy loss of SMARCB1 (INI-1) immunoreactivity, which is also seen in schwannomatosis.
2. Meningiomas are seen in approximately half of individuals with NF2 in patient series.[14] High frequency of NF2 was reported in pediatric meningioma patients, and meningioma may be the initial manifestation of NF2 in this age group. It is suggested that NF2-associated meningiomas exhibit an aggressive histologic, genetic, and clinical phenotype.[20] Fibroblastic and transitional subtypes may be more associated with NF2-associated meningiomas.
3. Ependymomas are found in 33% to 55% of NF2 patients by imaging, with a predilection for the cervical cord and cervicomedullary junction, in contrast to sporadic tumors, which are more commonly located in the brain.[21] Multiple ependymomas are common and usually have low-grade histology. NF2-associated ependymomas show an indolent growth pattern.[21]

Differential Diagnosis from NF1

1. No cognitive problems (mental retardation and learning disability) are seen in individuals with NF2, while they are known to be present in some patients with NF1.

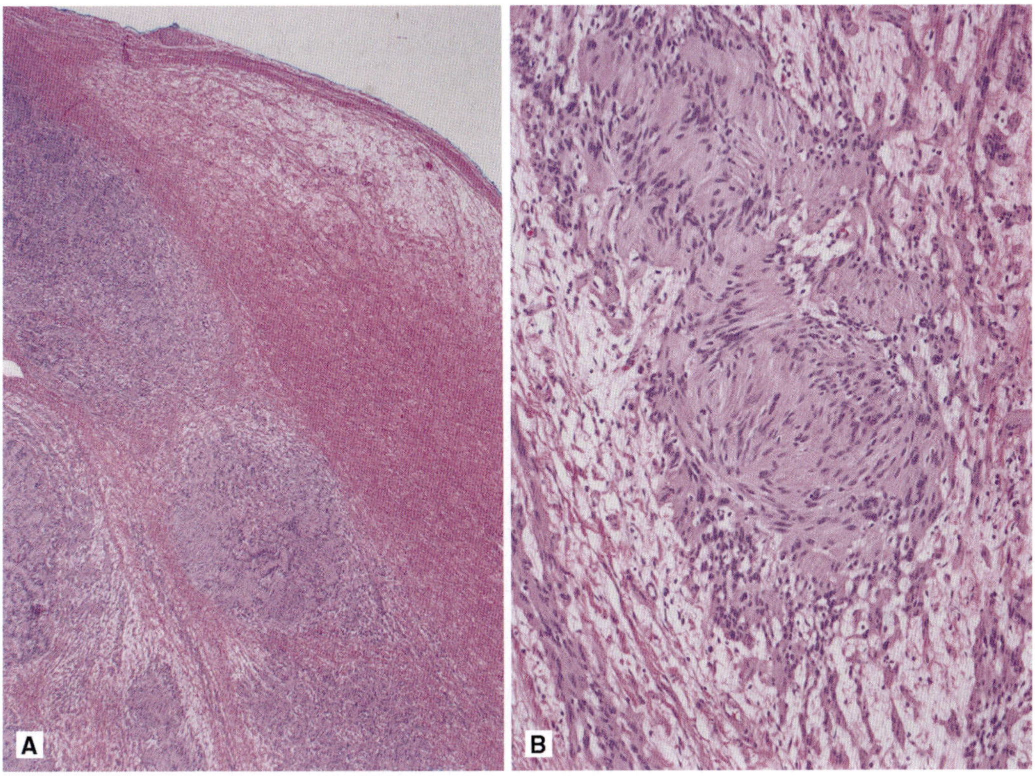

FIGURE 12-1: Hybrid neurofibroma/schwannoma. Low-power view showing an encapsulated tumor composed of schwannoma-like nodules surrounded by neurofibroma-like areas with abundant collagen and myxoid change (**A**). High-power view showing a schwannoma-like nodule with prominent Verocay bodies (Antoni A region) (**B**).

2. Malignant transformation is very rarely seen in schwannomas in NF2 patients, while there is some risk of malignant transformation of neurofibromas in NF1 patients.
3. Significant numbers of Lisch nodules (i.e., iris hamartomas) and café au lait macules are not features of NF2.[14]

SCHWANNOMATOSIS

Schwannomatosis (OMIM #162091), also called NF type 3, is the third major form of neurofibromatosis, clinically and genetically distinct from NF1 and NF2. It is characterized by the development of multiple schwannomas in the absence of bilateral vestibular schwannomas. Constitutional mutations of chromatin remodeling gene *SMARCB1* at 22q11.23 have been found in approximately 50% of familial and less than 10% of sporadic schwannomatosis cases.[22] The majority of cases of schwannomatosis are sporadic, and case series suggest that only 15% to 25% of cases are inherited from an affected parent (i.e., familial).[23] The tumorigenesis is thought to occur through a 4-hit, 3-step mechanism for *SMARCB1* and *NF2* inactivation, beginning with a germline mutation in *SMARCB1* (hit 1), which is followed by loss of a portion of chromosome 22 that contains the second *SMARCB1* allele and one *NF2* allele (hits 2 and 3), and by mutation of the remaining wild-type *NF2* allele (hit 4).[23] Recently, *LZTR1* gene (on chromosome 22q11) has been shown to be responsible for 22q-related schwannomatosis cases lacking mutations in *SMARCB1*.[24]

Clinical Features and Diagnosis

Multiple schwannomas arise from peripheral, spinal, and (rarely) cranial nerves, but spare the vestibular nerves. Disease onset is usually in the second and third decades, and the major first symptom is pain.[25] Chronic pain is the most common symptom, often exceeds neurologic

Table 12-2 Proposed Diagnostic Criteria for Schwannomatosis

Molecular Diagnosis		
1.	Two or more pathologically proved schwannomas or meningiomas **AND**	At least two tumors with LOH for chromosome 22 and two different *NF2* mutations
2.	One pathologically proved schwannoma or meningioma **AND**	Germline *SMARCB1* pathogenic mutation
Clinical Diagnosis		
1.	Two or more nonintradermal schwannomas (one with pathologic confirmation) **AND**	No bilateral vestibular schwannomas by high-quality MRI
2.	One pathologically confirmed schwannoma or intracranial meningioma **AND**	Affected first-degree relative

LOH, loss of heterozygosity.
Data from Plotkin SR, Blakeley JO, Evans DG, et al. Update from the 2011 International Schwannomatosis Workshop: from genetics to diagnostic criteria. *Am J Med Genet Part A* 2013;161A:405–416.

disability of tumors, and is difficult to treat, although the etiology of pain in schwannomatosis is unclear.[26] About a third of patients have a unique segmental presentation and only involve a single limb or side of body/spine (single nerve distribution).

In addition to schwannomas, the occurrence of multiple intracranial meningiomas was reported in some schwannomatosis families with *SMARCB1* germline mutations.[27] Taking account of the possibility of multiple meningiomas as a presenting feature as well as incorporating molecular testing as a diagnostic tool, the new diagnostic criteria were proposed in the 2011 International Schwannomatosis Workshop (Table 12-2).

Histologically, schwannomas in schwannomatosis is generally indistinguishable from sporadic schwannomas. One study reported a high percentage of hybrid neurofibromas/schwannomas[19] (Figure 12-1). A mosaic pattern of immunohistochemical stain for SMARCB1/INI1 is seen in schwannomatosis-associated schwannomas.

TUBEROUS SCLEROSIS COMPLEX

Tuberous sclerosis complex (TSC) is an autosomal dominant disorder of cellular differentiation and proliferation affecting virtually any or all organ systems in the body. Characteristically, the disease manifestations are highly diverse in both organ involvement and severity. The most common findings are benign tumors in the brain, skin, kidneys, lung, and heart. CNS tumors are the leading cause of morbidity and mortality. TSC is the second most common hereditary tumor syndrome with an incidence of 1 per 5,800 live births.[28]

TSC results from mutations in the *TSC1* gene on chromosome 9q34, encoding for hamartin (OMIM #191100), or *TSC2* gene on chromosome 16p13.3, encoding for tuberin (OMIM #613254). Two-thirds of TSC cases are caused by sporadic *TSC1* or *TSC2* mutations, while the remainder of affected patients have an inherited *TSC1* or *TSC2* mutation. No hotspots for mutations are found in these genes. *TSC2* mutations account for 60% of TSC patients, with 30% expressing *TSC1* mutations.[29] Patients with *TSC2* mutations tend to exhibit more severe phenotype than do those with *TSC1* mutations. In 2% to 3% of patients, large genomic deletion in *TSC2* also involves the adjacent gene, polycystic kidney disease type 1 (*PKD1*) (i.e., *TSC2/PKD1* contiguous gene deletion syndrome). Inactivation of both alleles of *TSC1* or *TSC2* is needed for tumor development.

Hamartin and tuberin bind to form a heterodimeric complex responsible for limiting the activity of an important intracellular regulator of cell growth and metabolism known as mammalian target of rapamycin complex (mTORC1) *via* inhibition of Ras homolog enriched in brain (Rheb), a small G protein of the Ras family, by the GTPase-activating protein activity of hamartin–tuberin complex.[29,30] The loss-of-function mutations of *TSC1* or *TSC2* gene lead to a defective cell size, migration, proliferation, and differentiation. Rapamycin and its derivatives (e.g., everolimus), mTOR inhibitors, have been shown to be effective in treating some of TSC manifestations.[31,32]

Clinical Features and Diagnosis

The diagnosis of TSC is largely based on clinical features that define major and minor diagnostic criteria. According to the most recently updated TSC diagnostic criteria in 2012 (Table 12-3), two diagnostic classes (i.e., possible and definite) are assigned based on the appearance of defined

Table 12-3 Diagnostic Criteria for Tuberous Sclerosis Complex 2012

A. Genetic diagnostic criteria			
Definite diagnosis	**Identification of either a *TSC1* or *TSC2* pathogenic mutation in DNA from normal tissue** (Pathogenic mutation is defined as a mutation that clearly inactivates the function of the TSC1 or TSC2 proteins, prevents protein synthesis, or is a missense mutation whose effect on protein function has been established by functional assessment.)		
B. Clinical diagnostic criteria			
	Definite diagnosis	2 major features **OR**	1 major with ≥2 minor features
	Possible diagnosis	1 major feature **OR**	≥2 minor features
Major features	Skin	• Hypomelanotic macules ("ash leaf spots") • Angiofibromas or fibrous cephalic plaque • Ungual fibromas • Shagreen patch	
	Central nervous system/eye	• Multiple retinal hamartomas • Cortical dysplasias (including tubers and cerebral white matter radial migration lines) • Subependymal nodules • Subependymal giant cell astrocytoma	
	Others	• Cardiac rhabdomyoma • Lymphangioleiomyomatosis • Angiomyolipoma	
Minor features		• "Confetti" skin lesions • Dental enamel pits • Intraoral fibromas • Retinal achromic patch • Multiple renal cysts • Nonrenal hamartomas	

The coexistence of major clinical features "Lymphangioleiomyomatosis" and "Angiomyolipomas" does not meet criteria for a definite diagnosis. One more major or two more minor features would be required.

Data from Northrup H, Krueger DA. Tuberous sclerosis complex diagnostic criteria update: recommendations of the 2012 International Tuberous Sclerosis Complex Consensus Conference. *Pediatr Neurol* 2013;49:243–254.

features in multiple organ systems.[33] In addition, molecular genetic testing is included for the first time in the criteria. Identification of either a *TSC1* or *TSC2* pathogenic mutation in DNA from normal tissue is sufficient to make a definite diagnosis. While the overall mutation detection rate in patients with TSC is around 85% to 90%, approximately 10% to 15% of clinically defined TSC patients have no mutations identified by conventional methods.[29,30]

Neuropathologic Manifestations and Pathologic Features

The classic neuropathologic manifestations of TSC include cortical dysplasias (including cortical tubers and cerebral white matter radial migration lines; CWMRMLs), subependymal nodules (SENs), and subependymal giant cell astrocytomas (SEGAs). SEGAs and cortical dysplasias are associated with neurologic features, while SENs are believed to be asymptomatic.

Cortical Dysplasias

Cortical dysplasias are focal developmental abnormalities and include cortical tubers and CWMRMLs. Both lesions represent a single "major feature" in the 2012 TSC diagnostic criteria since they overlap each other clinically and pathologically.[33] These lesions are commonly associated with intractable epilepsy and learning disabilities in TSC.

Cortical tubers constitute the hallmark of the disease and are observed in approximately 90% of TSC patients. Tubers are well circumscribed, mostly supratentorial lesions that can often be easily identified by gross examination of the brain as protuberant, tan-white, firm/rubbery gyral expansion. Tubers have a variable appearance with mushroom-shaped gyri and loss of the gray–white matter junction. Tubers are characterized histologically by the presence of cells with aberrant morphologies such as dysmorphic neurons (DNs), numerous large astrocytes, and a unique cell type known as giant cells (GCs).[29,34] DNs exhibit an enlarged cell body with conspicuous Nissl substance, aberrant axonal projections (loss of radial orientation with respect to the pial surface), and dendritic arbors. Immunohistochemically, DNs typically express neurofilament protein. GCs have very large cell soma and a laterally displaced nucleus, lacking clear polarization into axonal or dendritic segments, and absence of Nissl substance in contrast to DNs. GCs are periodic acid–Schiff positive. These cells are very similar to balloon cells seen in sporadic focal cortical dysplasia type 2B. Increased numbers of astrocytes of different size and shape, highlighted with GFAP immunohistochemistry, are also noted in tubers. Some enormous gemistocytic astrocytes with abundant eosinophilic cytoplasm may be found.[34] In older children and adults, tubers may be calcified or undergo cystic degeneration. The pathologic alteration may be confined within the cortical mantle or extend to the deep subcortical white matter. Interestingly, the cytoarchitecture of the cerebral cortex surrounding the tubers is typically normal.

CWMRMLs run from the ventricles through the cerebral mantle to the normal cortex or to the cortical tuber. Histologically, these lesions are almost identical to those seen in the cortical tubers.[35]

Subependymal Nodule and Subependymal Giant Cell Astrocytoma

SENs are nodular lesions located on the surfaces of lateral and third ventricles, detected by imaging in about 80% of TSC patients.[33] These lesions develop in fetal life and often degenerate or calcify during later life.[34] Grossly, SENs occur singly or in rows (candle guttering) and usually measure less than 1 cm.

In contrast, SEGAs occur in only 10% to 15% of TSC patients and generally appear within the first 20 years of life.[29,34] They correspond to WHO grade I and generally exceed 1 cm in diameter. SEGAs usually extend into lateral ventricle and can obstruct the foramen of Monro, causing hydrocephalus.

Microscopically, SENs are typically covered by ependymal lining and can have extensive vascularization. SEGA and SEN are histologically very similar (Please refer to Chapter 3 for detailed description).

VON HIPPEL-LINDAU DISEASE

von Hippel-Lindau disease (VHL; OMIM #193300) is a familial syndrome characterized by development of various hypervascular neoplasms and cysts. VHL disease is an autosomal dominant disease with marked phenotypic variability and age-dependent penetrance. The incidence is 1 in 30,000 to 50,000 live births. The most common age at clinical presentation is in the third and fourth decades. VHL disease is caused by germline mutations in the *VHL* tumor suppressor gene located on chromosome 3p25.3. Biallelic *VHL* inactivation is required for tumor formation (i.e., two hit model of tumorigenesis).

VHL protein (pVHL) is involved in a critical pathway for adaptation of cells to hypoxia by proteolytic degradation of the α subunits of hypoxia-inducible transcription factor (HIF)-1 and HIF-2. When pVHL expression is lost or is functionally inactivated, HIF-1 and -2 are stabilized and stimulate expression of genes involved in angiogenesis, anaerobic metabolism, and numerous other cellular functions (e.g., *VEGF*, *PDGFβ*, *TGFα*, *erythropoietin*, *Cyclin D1*).[36]

Clinical Features and Diagnosis

The most common tumors seen in VHL disease include retinal and CNS hemangioblastomas (HBs), clear cell renal cell carcinoma (CCRCC), pheochromocytoma (Pheo), endolymphatic sac tumor (ELST), and pancreatic islet cell tumors. Diagnosis of VHL disease is often based on clinical criteria: (a) patients with a positive family history: a CNS HB, CCRCC, or Pheo; and (b) patients with no family history of VHL disease: two or more CNS HBs AND a visceral tumor (excluding epididymal and renal cysts). As many as 20% of patients with VHL disease are caused by *de novo* mutations. The initial mutation of a *de novo* cases might result in disease mosaicism, which can cause a diagnostic challenge.[37] Familial VHL disease is classified phenotypically into types 1 and 2 based on absence or presence of Pheo, respectively.[37] Genetic testing detects mutations in greater than 95% of nonmosaic patients with classical VHL disease.[36,37] Surveillance of affected and asymptomatic gene carriers can reduce morbidity and mortality.

Hemangioblastoma

CNS HBs are a cardinal feature of VHL disease, affecting 60% to 80% of patients, and are associated with major morbidity although they are benign (WHO grade I tumor). They usually seen in cerebellum (around the fourth ventricle and less commonly in the cerebellar hemispheres), followed by the spinal cord, brainstem, lumbosacral nerve roots, and (very rarely) supratentorial regions.[38] HBs are the presenting feature in about 40% of VHL cases, and the average age of presentation is 33 years.[37] Conversely, about 30% of all patients with cerebellar HBs have VHL disease, while about 80% of those with spinal HBs have this disease.[39] Of interest, HBs are the only brain tumors associated with polycythemia, caused by the unregulated secretion of erythropoietin, which is encountered in 9% to 20% of intracranial tumors, but not in spinal tumors.[38] The histogenesis of HB is uncertain. Radiologically, the classic appearance of cerebellar HBs on MRI is a well-demarcated cystic lesion with a contrast enhancing mural nodule.

Grossly, HB is usually a well-circumscribed lesion but without true capsules. The solid area/mural nodule presents as an orange-red, firm mass.

Histologically, HB is highly cellular and vascularized, and is composed of haphazardly oriented small capillaries and sinusoidal channels lined by plump endothelial cells that are separated by larger, vacuolated, lipid-containing cells ("stromal cells"). Stromal cells, representing the neoplastic component of HB, commonly show degenerative nuclear atypia. Mast cells are commonly present within the tumor, and foci of extramedullary hematopoiesis may be seen. HBs are subdivided into two variants: a reticular variant, where stromal cells are evenly distributed among the capillary network; and a cellular variant, in which stromal cells are arranged in larger sheets or nests[38] (Figure 12-2B and C). The tumor is usually separated from the adjacent brain tissue by a rim of gliosis with Rosenthal fibers that are often abundant.

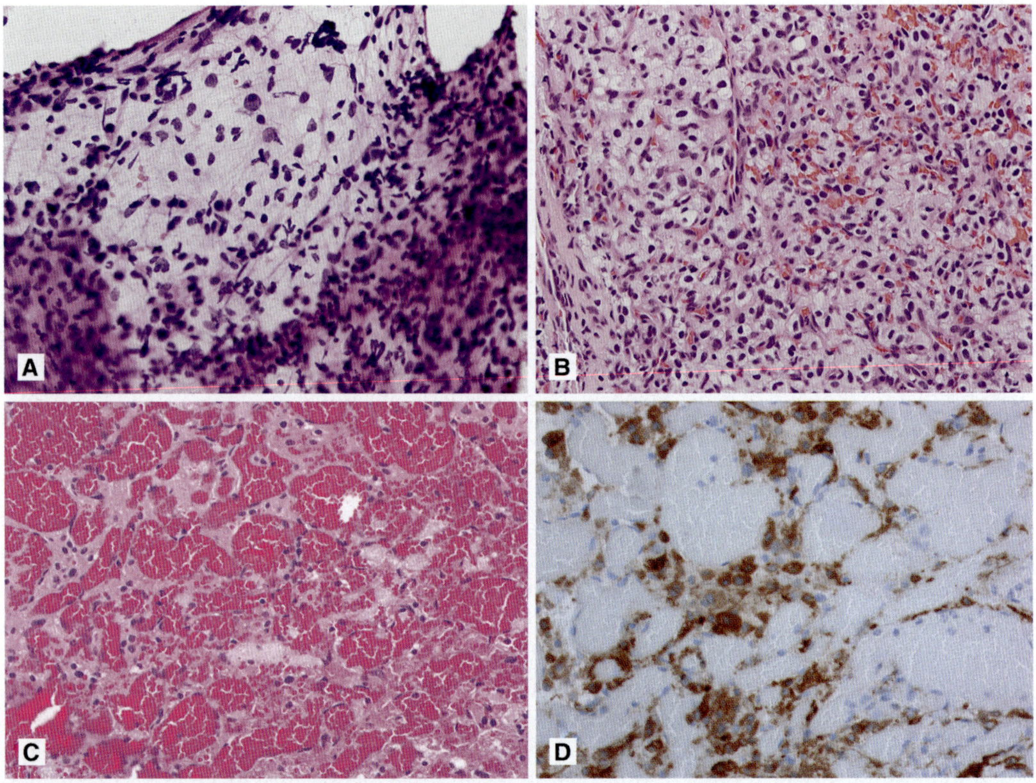

FIGURE 12-2: Hemangioblastoma. Cytologic squash preparation: sheet of stromal cells with nuclear pleomorphism and clear cytoplasm is noted. Perivascular neutrophils are commonly seen (**A**). Histologic section of cellular variant: sheets and nests of stromal cells separated by thin capillaries are seen (**B**). Histologic section of reticular variant: abundant congested capillaries with scattered stromal cells among them are identified (**C**). Inhibin-A immunohistochemistry: stromal cells among dilated capillaries are highlighted (**D**).

Immunohistochemically, inhibin-A (Figure 12-2D) and aquaporin-1 (a widely expressed water channel protein), respectively, show strong cytoplasmic positivity and plasma membrane positivity of stromal cells in the majority of HB cases.[40]

Histologic differential diagnosis of HB includes metastatic CCRCC (especially in VHL patients) and angiomatous/microcystic meningioma. A panel of immunohistochemistry is of great help in this distinction (Table 12-4). Carney et al. proposed the combined use of PAX2, PAX8, and inhibin-A to resolve the differential diagnosis of HB (PAX2−, PAX8−, inhibin-A+) versus metastatic CCRCC (PAX2+, PAX8+, inhibin-A−).[41] Of note, inhibin-A and epithelial membrane antigen (EMA) immunoreactivity is seen in a significant percentage of RCC and HB cases, respectively.

Table 12-4 Immunohistochemistry for Differential Diagnosis: Hemangioblastoma versus Metastatic Renal Clear Cell Carcinoma

	Inhibin-A	Aquaporin-1	D2-40	RCC	CD10	PAX2	PAX8	EMA	AE1/AE3
CNS hemangioblastoma	(++)	(++)	(+)	(−)	(−)	(−)	(−)	(+/−)	(−)
Renal clear cell carcinoma	(−/+)	(−/+)	(−/+)	(+/++)	(++)	(++)	(++)	(++)	(++)

RCC, renal cell carcinoma marker.

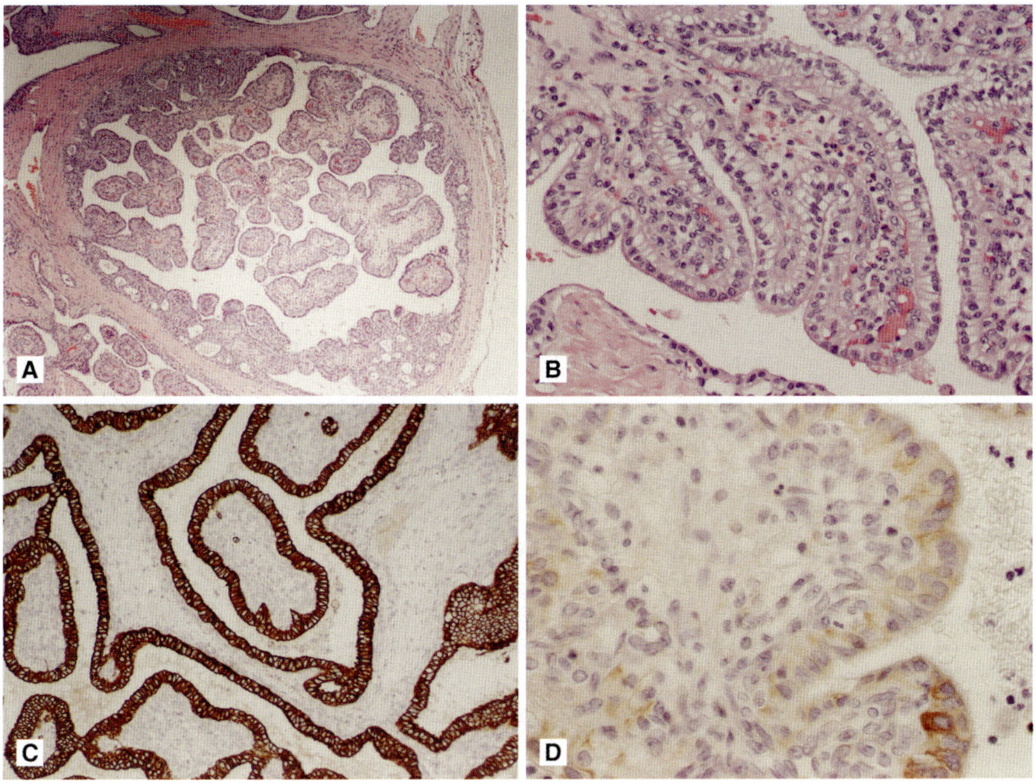

FIGURE 12-3: Endolymphatic sac tumor. Tubulopapillary arrangement of tumor cells is seen (**A**). Broad complex papillae lined by cuboidal to columnar epithelial cells with clear cytoplasm are seen (**B**). Cytokeratin-7 immunohistochemistry: tumor cells are diffusely and strongly labeled (**C**). GFAP immunohistochemistry: some tumor cells are weakly positive (**D**).

Endolymphatic Sac Tumor

ELST is a primary low-grade, locally invasive neuroectodermal neoplasm originating from the intraosseous portion of the endolymphatic sac epithelium. It is rare in the general population and is frequently associated with VHL disease. Bilateral ELSTs are considered pathognomonic for VHL disease. ELST can be detected radiologically in up to 11% of patients with VHL disease.[36,37] The most frequent clinical presentation is progressive hearing loss (mean age 22 years).

Histologically, HB is characterized by papillotubular structures lined by a single layer of bland cuboidal or columnar epithelium with clear to eosinophilic cytoplasm (Figure 12-3A and B). Cystic spaces, sclerotic collagenous bands, thyroid-like follicles, hemorrhage, and siderophages are often seen. Mitotic figures are rarely seen.

Immunohistochemically, the tumor cells are positive for pancytokeratin, cytokeratin-7 (Figure 12-3C), and EMA. They are variably immunoreactive with GFAP (Figure 12-3D).

Differential diagnosis includes choroid plexus papilloma, papillary ependymoma, metastatic CCRCC, adenoma of the middle ear, and paraganglioma. Radiologic evaluation is crucial for this differential diagnosis. Immunohistochemical stains for the differential diagnosis are shown in Table 12-5.

TURCOT SYNDROME

Turcot syndrome (TS) is a rare familial disorder clinically characterized by the combination of colorectal polyposis/adenomas/carcinomas and primary tumors of the CNS. At the molecular genetic level, TS represents two distinct inherited diseases: hereditary nonpolyposis colorectal cancer syndrome (or Lynch syndrome) due to germline mutations in the mismatch repair

Table 12-5 Immunohistochemistry for Differential Diagnosis of Endolymphatic Sac Tumor (ELST)

	Pancytokeratin	EMA	Synaptophysin/ Chromogranin A	GFAP	Transthyretin	Others
ELST	(+)	(+)	(−)	(+/−)	(−)	
Choroid plexus papilloma	(+)	(+)	(−)	(−/+)	(+)	EAAT-1[a] (91%); Kir7.1[b] (100%)
Papillary ependymoma	(−)	(−/+)	(−)	(+)	(−)	
Metastatic renal cell carcinoma	(+)	(+)	(−)	(−)	(−)	PAX-8 (+); PAX-2 (+)
Adenoma of the middle ear	(+)	(+)	(+)		(−)	
Paraganglioma	(−)	(−)	(+)	(−)	(−)	

[a]Excitatory amino acid transporter-1.
[b]Inwardly rectifying potassium channel 7.1.

genes (*MLH1*, *MSH2*, *MSH6*, and *PMS2*),[42] and familial adenomatous polyposis syndrome caused by germline mutations in *adenomatous polyposis coli* (*APC*) gene. The brain tumor that is most frequently associated with the former disease is glioblastoma, while the latter is medulloblastoma (MB). In the former disease, the microsatellite instability is less pronounced in glioblastomas than in colorectal neoplasms.[43] Brain tumors are the major cause of death in patients with TS.

GORLIN SYNDROME (NEVOID BASAL CELL CARCINOMA SYNDROME)

Nevoid basal cell carcinoma syndrome (NBCCS; OMIM #109400), also known as Gorlin syndrome and basal cell nevus syndrome, is an autosomal dominant familial syndrome that predisposes to a cluster of malformative and neoplastic growths involving the CNS, skin, and bone. The characteristic lesions include (multiple or pediatric) basal cell carcinomas (BCCs), odontogenic keratocysts of the jaw, MBs, and skeletal abnormalities. The incidence is reportedly as high as 1 in 19,000 births.[44] NBCCS is caused by germline mutations in genes involving the hedgehog signaling pathway, including *PTCH1* (most common) on chromosome 9q22, *PTCH2* on 1p32, and *SUFU* on 10q24-q25. Germline (loss-of-function) mutations in *PTCH1* gene are found in approximately 75% of patients meeting clinical criteria of NBCCS.[44] Genotype–phenotype correlations are not evident.

In the CNS, MBs and lamellar calcification of the falx cerebri (LCFC) are listed as major diagnostic criteria of NBCCS. Up to 5% of patients with NBCCS develop MB. The average age of onset of MB in NBCCS patients is much earlier than in sporadic MBs (2 and 7 years, respectively).[44,45] Since the incidence of MBs is higher at younger ages, younger age of presentation with MB should raise suspicion for NBCCS.[46] Histologically, desmoplastic/nodular variant of MB is strongly associated with NBCCS. The management and prognosis is similar to that of sporadic disease with the exception of the increased sensitivity to radiation, leading to development of secondary radiation-induced neoplasms (most commonly, multiple meningiomas and BCCs in the radiation field).[44–47] Identification of the patients with NBCCS is important for selection of appropriate adjuvant treatment.

Ectopic calcifications are frequent findings in NBCCS. LCFC is common in NBCCS patients with the incidence ranging from 65% to 92%.[46] Other sites of ectopic calcifications include tentorium cerebelli, petroclinoid ligament, and diaphragm sellae.[46]

COWDEN SYNDROME

Cowden syndrome (CS; OMIM #15835), also known as multiple hamartoma syndrome, is characterized by a wide variety of hamartomas (most commonly of the skin and mucosa), with increased risk of various malignancies (breast, thyroid, and endometrial carcinomas). Most patients with autosomal dominant CS are caused by germline mutations of *PTEN*, encoding phosphatase and TENsin homolog deleted on chromosome 10. *PTEN* is a well-characterized tumor suppressor phosphatase involved in cellular regulation *via* G1 cell cycle arrest and apoptosis.[48] CS has an incidence of 1 in 200,000 live births with female predominance.[48] CS along with Proteus syndrome, Proteus-like syndrome and Bannayan-Riley-Ruvalcaba syndrome are associated with *PTEN* germline mutations and collectively classified as PTEN hamartoma tumor syndrome (PTHS).[48,49]

In the CNS, adult-onset, Lhermitte-Duclos disease (LDD), also known as "dysplastic gangliocytoma of cerebellum," and macrocephaly are listed in the major criteria of most recently published, revised PTHS clinical diagnostic criteria proposed by Pilarski et al.[50] On the other hand, adult-onset LDD is recognized as a pathognomonic criterion for CS according to the International Cowden Consortium for CS in 2004.[51] (Please refer to Chapter 6 for detailed clinical and pathologic features.)

LI-FRAUMENI SYNDROME

Li-Fraumeni syndrome (LFS; OMIM #151623) is a familial cancer predisposing syndrome caused by germline mutations of *TP53* located on chromosome 17p13.1. It is an autosomal dominant disease, and deleterious (disease causing) germline mutations in *TP53* are identified in approximately 70% of LFS.[52,53] The diagnosis is rendered based on a set of clinical classification criteria. Component or "core" LFS tumors include soft tissue and bone sarcomas, premenopausal breast cancers, brain tumors, adrenal cortical carcinomas, and leukemias.[54] These malignancies tend to occur at significantly earlier ages.

Brain tumors occur in 9% to 16% of individuals with *TP53* mutations.[55] Glioblastomas/astrocytomas are most common, but MB, supratentorial primitive neuroectodermal tumors, and choroid plexus carcinomas (CPCs) can be seen.[56] It is reported that 50% of patients with CPC were positive for germline *TP53* mutations.[55] Histologically there is no specific difference from sporadic cases; however, due to germline mutations in *TP53* these patients would be sensitive to radiation therapy and are likely to develop secondary neoplasms.[52]

RHABDOID TUMOR PREDISPOSITION SYNDROMES

Rhabdoid tumor predisposition syndromes (RTPSs) are autosomal dominant cancer syndromes predisposing to renal or extrarenal malignant rhabdoid tumors (MRTs) and to atypical teratoid rhabdoid tumor (ATRT) in the CNS. The diseases usually occur in infancy or childhood and characteristically have a dismal prognosis. At the molecular genetic level, there are two known types based on the gene involved: heterozygous germline mutations in *SMARCB1* (aliases *INI1*, *hSNF5*, *BAF47*) on chromosome 22q11.2 causing RTPS1 (OMIM #609322), and those in *SMARCA4/BRG1* on 19p13.2 causing (very rare) RTPS2 (OMIM #613325).[57,58] Both of these genes are tumor suppressors and encode for core subunits of the ATP-dependent SWI/SNF chromatin–remodeling complex, a master regulator of gene expression involved in caner. Biallelic somatic inactivation of *SMARCB1* underlie 95% of MRTs.[58]

RTPS1 (mutant *SMARCB1*) accounts for the vast majority of cases. The penetrance is not complete, and approximately 20% of MRTs are due to presumed sporadic germline mutations of *SMARCB1*.[59] Clinically, patients with RTPS1 have earlier-onset presentation compared to those with sporadic rhabdoid tumors. In the CNS, approximately one-third of ATRT patients have germline *SMARCB1* mutations.[59] Of note is that *SMARCB1* mutations are also associated with schwannomatosis.

CARNEY COMPLEX

Carney complex (CNC) is an autosomal dominant, multiple endocrine neoplasia syndrome that was originally described in 1985 by Carney et al. as "the complex of myxomas, spotty skin pigmentation and endocrine over activity."[60] Genetically, two gene loci associated with a predisposition to CNC have been reported: 17p22-24 locus (mutations identified in the protein kinase A regulatory subunit-1-alpha gene; *PRKAR1A*) for CNC type 1 (OMIM #160980) and the 2p16 locus for CNC type 2 (OMIM #605244). The gene responsible for CNC type 2 remains unknown. Inactivating heterozygous germline mutations of *PRKAR1A*, resulting in PRKAR1A haploinsufficiency, are present in up to 70% of the patients diagnosed with CNC.[61,62] The non-*PRKAR1A*-associated CNC (i.e., CNC type 2) is less severe, appears later in life, and mostly in a sporadic fashion.[61]

Pituitary adenomas, especially growth hormone (GH) and GH and prolactin (GH-PRL) secreting adenomas, are known to be seen in CNC patients.[61] Radiologically, the tumors are usually microadenomas (i.e., <1 cm).[63] Acromegaly due to GH-producing pituitary adenoma is one of the major diagnostic features for CNC and the incidence has been estimated at less than 15% in patients with this disease.[63]

Psammomatous melanotic schwannoma (PMS) is another major diagnostic feature for CNC. It can be found in up to 8% of the subjects and is most commonly seen in the gastrointestinal tract and spinal nerve roots (especially cervical and thoracic spine).[61,63] PMS is characterized by melanin-containing cells having ultrastructural characteristics of Schwann cells. It is potentially malignant with metastasis in contrast to classical schwannomas.

References

1. Tonsgard JH. Clinical manifestations and management of neurofibromatosis type 1. *Semin Pediatr Neurol* 2006;13:2–7.
2. Jett K, Friedman JM. Clinical and genetic aspects of neurofibromatosis 1. *Genet Med* 2010;12:1–11.
3. Arun D, Gutmann DH. Recent advances in neurofibromatosis type 1. *Curr Opin Neurol* 2004;17:101–105.
4. Le LQ, Parada LF. Tumor microenvironment and neurofibromatosis type 1: connecting the GAPs. *Oncogene* 2007;26:4609–4616.
5. Jorge AA, Malaquias AC, Arnhold IJ, et al. Noonan syndrome and related disorders: a review of clinical features and mutations in genes of the RAS/MAPK pathway. *Horm Res* 2009;71:185–193.
6. Tartaglia M, Gelb BD, Zenker M. Noonan syndrome and clinically related disorders. *Best Pract Res Clin Endocrinol Metab* 2011;25:161–179.
7. Garg S, Green J, Leadbitter K, et al. Neurofibromatosis type 1 and autism spectrum disorder. *Pediatrics* 2013;132:e1642–e1648.
8. DiPaolo DP, Zimmerman RA, Rorke LB, et al. Neurofibromatosis type 1: pathologic substrate of high-signal-intensity foci in the brain. *Radiology* 1995;195:721–724.
9. Laycock-van Spyk S, Thomas N, Cooper DN, et al. Neurofibromatosis type 1-associated tumours: their somatic mutational spectrum and pathogenesis. *Hum Genomics* 2011;5:623–690.
10. Hernáiz Driever P, von Hornstein S, Pietsch T, et al. Natural history and management of low-grade glioma in NF-1 children. *J Neurooncol* 2010;100:199–207.

11. Guillamo JS, Créange A, Kalifa C, et al.; Réseau NF France. Prognostic factors of CNS tumours in neurofibromatosis 1 (NF1): a retrospective study of 104 patients. *Brain* 2003;126:152–160.
12. Cooper J, Giancotti FG. Molecular insights into NF2/Merlin tumor suppressor function. *FEBS Lett* 2014;588:2743–2752.
13. Evans DG, Howard E, Giblin C, et al. Birth incidence and prevalence of tumour prone syndromes: estimates from a UK genetic family register service. *Am J Med Genet* 2010;152A:327–332.
14. Evans DG. Neurofibromatosis 2 (bilateral acoustic neurofibromatosis, central neurofibromatosis, NF2, neurofibromatosis type II). *Genet Med* 2009;11:599–610.
15. Evans DGR, Huson S, Donnai D, et al. Clinical study of type 2 neurofibromatosis. *Q J Med* 1992;84:603–618.
16. Baser ME, Friedman JM, Wallace AJ, et al. Evaluation of diagnostic criteria for neurofibromatosis 2. *Neurology* 2002;59:1759–1765.
17. Reed N, Gutmann DH. Tumorigenesis in neurofibromatosis: new insights and potential therapies. *Trends Mol Med* 2001;7:157–162.
18. Hilton DA, Hanemann CO. Schwannomas and their pathogenesis. *Brain Pathol* 2014;24:205–220.
19. Harder A, Wesemann M, Hagel C, et al. Hybrid neurofibroma/schwannoma is overrepresented among schwannomatosis and neurofibromatosis patients. *Am J Surg Pathol* 2012;36:702–709.
20. Perry A, Giannini C, Raghavan R, et al. Aggressive phenotypic and genotypic features in pediatric and NF2-associated meningiomas: a clinicopathologic study of 53 cases. *J Neuropathol Exp Neurol* 2001;60:994–1003.
21. Plotkin SR, O'Donnell CC, Curry WT, et al. Spinal ependymomas in neurofibromatosis type 2: a retrospective analysis of 55 patients. *J Neurosurg Spine* 2011;14:543–547.
22. Smith MJ, Wallace AJ, Bowers NL, et al. Frequency of SMARCB1 mutations in familial and sporadic schwannomatosis. *Neurogenetics* 2012;13:141–145.
23. Plotkin SR, Blakeley JO, Evans DG, et al. Update from the 2011 International Schwannomatosis Workshop: from genetics to diagnostic criteria. *Am J Med Genet A* 2013;161A:405–416.
24. Piotrowski A, Xie J, Liu YF, et al. Germline loo-of-function mutations in LZTR1 predispose to an inherited disorder of multiple schwannomas. *Nat Genet* 2014;46:182–187.
25. Gonzalvo A, Fowler A, Cook RJ, et al. Schwannomatosis, sporadic schwannomatosis, and familial schwannomatosis: a surgical series with long-term follow-up. *J Neurosurg* 2011;114:756–762.
26. Merker VL, Esparza S, Smith MJ, et al. Clinical features of schwannomatosis: a retrospective analysis of 87 patients. *Oncologist* 2012;17:1317–1332.
27. van den Munckhof P, Christiaans I, Kenter SB, et al. Germline SMARCB1 mutation predisposes to multiple meningiomas and schwannomas with preferential location of cranial meningiomas at the falx cerebri. *Neurogenetics* 2012;13:1–7.
28. O'Callaghan F, Shiell A, Osborne J, et al. Prevalence of tuberous sclerosis estimated by capture–recapture analysis. *Lancet* 1998;352:318–319.
29. Crino PB. Evolving neurobiology of tuberous sclerosis complex. *Acta Neuropathol* 2013;125:317–332.
30. Curatolo P, Bombardieri R, Jozwiak S. Tuberous sclerosis. *Lancet* 2008;372:657–668.
31. Hassakari J. Everolimus. *Recent Results Cancer Res* 2014;201:373–392.
32. Franz DN. Everolimus in the treatment of subependymal giant cell astrocytomas, angiomyolipomas, and pulmonary and skin lesions associated with tuberous sclerosis complex. *Biologics* 2013;7:211–221.
33. Northrup H, Krueger DA. Tuberous sclerosis complex diagnostic criteria update: recommendations of the 2012 International Tuberous Sclerosis Complex Consensus Conference. *Pediatr Neurol* 2013;49:243–254.
34. Grajkowska W, Kotulska K, Jurkiewicz E, et al. Brain lesions in tuberous sclerosis complex. *Rev Folia Neuropathol* 2010;48:139–149.
35. Curatolo P, Bombardieri R, Pinci M, et al. Recent advances in tuberous sclerosis. *World J Pediatr* 2006;3:177–186.
36. Maher ER, Neumann HPH, Richard S. von Hippel-Lindau disease: a clinical and scientific review. *Eur J Hum Genet* 2011;18:617–623.
37. Lonser RR, Glenn GM, Walther M, et al. von Hippel-Lindau disease. *Lancet* 2003;361: 2059–2067.
38. Hussein MR. Central nervous system capillary hemangioblastoma: the pathologist's view-point. *Int J Exp Pathol* 2007;88:311–324.
39. Leung RS, Biswas SV, Duncan M, et al. Imaging features of von Hippel-Lindau disease. *Radiographics* 2008;28:65–79.

40. Takei H, Powell SZ. Novel immunohistochemical markers in the diagnosis of nonglial tumors of nervous system. *Adv Anat Pathol* 2010;17:150–153.
41. Carney EM, Banerjee P, Ellis CL, et al. PAX2(−)/PAX8(−)/inhibin A(+) immunoprofile in hemangioblastoma: a helpful combination in the differential diagnosis with metastatic clear cell renal cell carcinoma to the central nervous system. *Am J Surg Pathol* 2011;35:362–367.
42. Hegde MR, Chong B, Blazo ME, et al. A homozygous mutation in MSH6 causes Turcot syndrome. *Clin Cancer Res* 2005;11:4689–4693.
43. Hamilton SR, Liu B, Parsons RE, et al. The molecular basis of Turcot's syndrome. *N Engl J Med* 1995;332:839–847.
44. Bree AF, Shah MR; for the BCNS Colloquium Group. Consensus statement from the first international colloquium on basal cell nevus syndrome (BCNS). *Am J Med Genet A* 2011;155:2091–2097.
45. Taylor SF, Cook AE, Leatherbarrow B. Review of patients with basal cell nevus syndrome. *Ophthal Plast Reconstr Surg* 2006;22:259–265.
46. Sartip K, Kaplan A, Obeid G, et al. Neuroimaging of nevoid basal cell carcinoma syndrome (NBCCS) in children. *Pediatr Radiol* 2013;43:620–627.
47. Amlashi SF, Riffaud L, Brassier G, et al. Nevoid basal cell carcinoma syndrome: relation with desmoplastic medulloblastoma in infancy. A population-based study and review of the literature. *Cancer* 2003;98:618–624.
48. Bennett KL, Mester J, Eng C. Germline epigenetic regulation of KILLIN in Cowden and Cowden-like syndromes. *JAMA* 2010;304:2724–2731.
49. Hobert JA, Eng C. PTEN hamartoma tumor syndrome: an overview. *Genet Med* 2009;11:687–694.
50. Pilarski R, Burt R, Swisher E, et al. Cowden syndrome and the PTEN hamartomatous tumor syndrome: systematic review and revised diagnostic criteria. *J Natl Cancer Inst* 2013;105:1607–1616.
51. Blumenthal GM, Dennis PA. PTEN hamartoma tumor syndromes. *Eur J Hum Genet* 2008;16:1289–1300.
52. McBride KA, Ballinger ML, Killick E, et al. Li-Fraumeni syndrome: cancer risk assessment and clinical management. *Nat Rev Clin Oncol* 2014;11:260–271.
53. Mai PL, Malkin D, Garber JE, et al. Li-Fraumeni syndrome: report of a clinical research workshop and creation of a research consortium. *Cancer Genet* 2012;205:479–487.
54. Kamihara J, Rana HQ, Garber JE. Germline TP53 mutations and the changing landscape of Li-Fraumeni syndrome. *Hum Mutat* 2014;35:654–662.
55. Tabori U, Shlien A, Baskin B, et al. TP53 alterations determine clinical subgroups and survival of patients with choroid plexus tumors. *J Clin Oncol* 2010;28:1995–2001.
56. Sorrell AD, Espenschied CR, Culver JO, et al. Tumor protein (9TP53) testing and Li-Fraumeni syndrome: current status of clinical applications and future directions. *Mol Diagn Ther* 2013;17:31–47.
57. Schneppenheim R, Frühwald MC, Gesk S, et al. Germline nonsense mutation and somatic inactivation of SMARCA4/BRG1 in a family with rhabdoid tumor predisposition syndrome. *Am J Hum Genet* 2010;86:279–284.
58. Witkowski L, Lalonde E, Zhang J, et al. Familial rhabdoid tumour 'avant la lettre'—from pathology review to exome sequencing and back again. *J Pathol* 2013;231:35–43.
59. Schiffman HD, Geller JI, Mundt E, et al. Meeting report. Update on pediatric cancer predisposition syndromes. *Pediatr Blood Cancer* 2013;60:1247–1252.
60. Carney JA, Gordon H, Carpenter PC, et al. The complex of myxomas, spotty pigmentation, and endocrine overactivity. *Medicine* 1985;64:270–283.
61. Salpea P, Stratakis CA. Carney complex and McCune Albright syndrome: an overview of clinical manifestations and human molecular genetics. *Mol Cell Endocrinol* 2014;386:85–91.
62. Espiard S, Bertherat J. Carney complex. *Front Horm Res* 2013;41:50–62.
63. Courcoutsakis NA, Tatsi C, Patronas NJ, et al. The complex of myxomas, spotty skin pigmentation and endocrine overactivity (Carney complex): imaging findings with clinical and pathological correlation. *Insights Imaging* 2013;4:119–133.

Tumors of Cranial and Peripheral Nerves and Other Tumors

13

Yeon-Lim Suh

INTRODUCTION

Peripheral nerve tumors are classified according to the specific features of their cellular differentiation. These tumors occur sporadically or as manifestations of genetic syndromes, such as neurofibromatosis type 1 (NF-1) and type 2 (NF-2) or schwannomatosis. Most peripheral nerve tumors are benign, but malignant transformation does occur.

SCHWANNOMA

Schwannomas are the most common benign tumors and have been referred to by various names in the literature, such as neuromas, neurinomas, and neurilemmomas.[1] This tumor is composed entirely of Schwann cells.

Clinical Findings

Schwannomas represent 8% to 9% of intracranial tumors.[2,3] Vestibular schwannoma is the most common and accounts for approximately 78% of cerebellopontine angle tumors.[4] Trigeminal nerve schwannoma is the second most common, but very rare, representing 0.8% to 8% of all intracranial schwannomas.[5] Schwannomas of the spinal cord constitute approximately 30% of primary spinal neoplasms, and have a predilection for sensory nerve root. Schwannomas may occur rarely in the parenchyma of the brain and spinal cord, and the ventricle.[6,7] Intracranial schwannomas occur most frequently in adults, with a female preponderance. Cerebral or spinal parenchymal schwannomas more frequently affect children with a male predominance.[7] Bilateral tumors are very rare (0.26%) and always associated with NF-2; they develop earlier, with a peak incidence around the third decade. Clinical and radiologic features of intracranial schwannomas may vary according to the parent nerve involvement. Generally, these tumors present as mass lesions producing neurologic dysfunction. Treatment options include observation, using serial MRIs, microsurgical resection, stereotactic radiosurgery, and fractionated radiotherapy.

Genetics

Extensive research has indicated the *NF2* gene as an integral part of schwannoma tumorigenesis even in sporadic tumors.[8] The underlying genetic events are predominantly small frameshift mutations,[9] and such mutations are accompanied by loss of the remaining wild-type allele on chromosome 22 in most cases. Loss of merlin (the growth inhibitory protein product of the *NF2* gene) is a universal finding in schwannomas, regardless of the underlying mutational or allelic status,[10] suggesting that loss of *NF2* protein function is a prerequisite for tumor formation. Mutations in the *SMARCB1* gene at 22q11.23 have been identified in approximately 50% of familial and less than 10% of sporadic schwannomatosis cases, and are considered to be implicated as an underlying cause of the schwannomatosis.[11] Recently, germline loss-of-function mutations in *LZTR1* were found in approximately 80% of schwannomatosis cases lacking mutations in *SMARCB1*.[12]

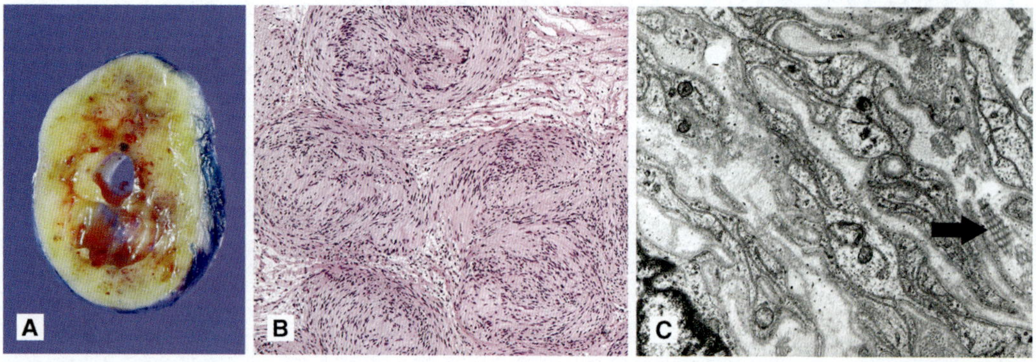

FIGURE 13-1: Schwannoma. Note a well-circumscribed, yellowish mass with hemorrhage and cystic change (**A**). Note alternating cellular Antoni A with Verocay bodies and loose, myxoid Antoni B areas (**B**). Electron micrograph illustrating long, thin intertwining processes covered by basal lamina and long spacing collagen (*arrow*) (**C**).

Pathologic Findings

Grossly, schwannomas are typically well encapsulated and tend to displace the parent nerve eccentrically. The cut surface is grayish tan or yellow with hemorrhage and cystic changes (Figure 13-1A). Microscopically, tumors consist of Antoni A and B areas (Figure 13-1B). Antoni A consists of compact spindle cells with buckled, cigar-shaped nuclei and indistinct cytoplasm. The nuclear palisading with intervening nuclear-free zones, referred to as Verocay bodies, is uncommon in intracranial schwannomas. Antoni B areas consist of less cellular, haphazardly arranged cells in the loosely textured matrix. Cystic changes, vascular hyalinization, hemosiderin deposits, and infiltrates of inflammatory cells are common. Bizarre and pleomorphic nuclei are found frequently in ancient schwannomas. Tumor cells diffusely and strongly express S100 protein, and often express Leu-7 and glial fibrillary acidic protein (GFAP). Most tumors show membranous staining for type IV collagen and laminin.[13] Ultrastructurally, tumor cells have long, thin intertwining processes that are covered by basal lamina (Figure 13-1C). Small junctions and long-spacing collagen are often present. These ultrastructural features are similar in various types of schwannomas. The cells of melanotic schwannoma (MS) are also similar, except for the presence of melanosomes. These features may be sparse or absent in malignant peripheral nerve sheath tumors (MPNST).[14]

Cellular Schwannoma

Cellular schwannomas accounted for 4.6% of benign peripheral nerve tumors in a large series of 70 cases.[15] Patient ages ranged from 15 to 80 (median, 47.7) years. The female:male ratio was 1.6:1. Paravertebral and intraspinal locations, including the sacrum (64%), extremities (25%), and the intracranial space (8%), were most common, and rare examples of cranial nerves have been described.[16] Tumors are surgically curable with complete excision. Grossly, the tumors are ovoid to lobulated; firm and rubbery, with complete or partial encapsulation; and occasionally multinodular or plexiform (Figure 13-2A). Histologically, tumors consist of predominantly Antoni A areas without nuclear palisading or Verocay bodies (Figure 13-2B). Hyperchromasia, nuclear atypia, thick hyalinized blood vessels, and lymphohistiocytic infiltrates, especially underneath tumor capsules, are common. Mitotic activity <1/10 high-power fields (HPF) is frequent, but not atypical. Necrosis is rarely observed. Recurrent tumors may express p53. Recurrence is significantly correlated with mitotic index in tumors with incomplete resection. Malignant transformation is very rare. Cellular schwannomas may present diagnostic problems due to their histologic similarity to MPNSTs. Immunoreactivity for S100 protein is helpful in the differential diagnosis: diffuse in cellular schwannoma versus patch pattern in MPNST.

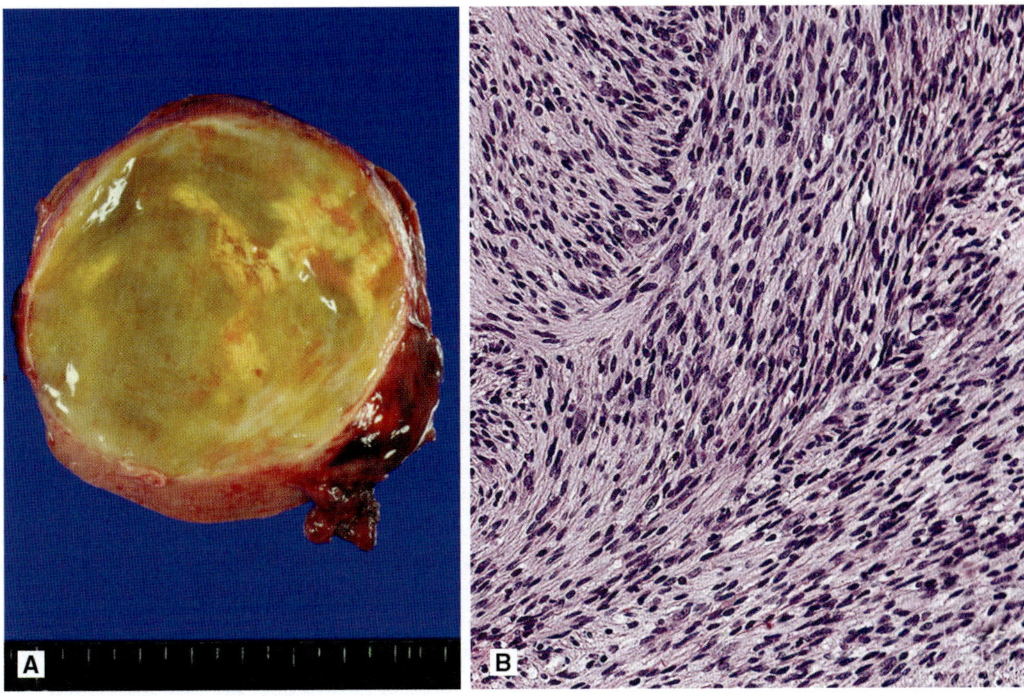

FIGURE 13-2: Cellular schwannoma. Note a well-circumscribed, yellow-tan mass (**A**) and highly cellular tumor without Verocay bodies (**B**).

Plexiform Schwannoma

Plexiform schwannoma (PS) is a rare variant of schwannoma, representing 5% of schwannomas.[17] PS represents 23% of head and neck examples, and 15% of cutaneous schwannomas.[18] This tumor occurs predominantly in children and young adults as a slowly growing, asymptomatic, nodular lesion in the dermis and subcutis. Deep-seated PSs are rare and mostly affect the extremities and pelvis, and viscera.[19] Rare cases involving the cervical spine and peripheral nerves have been reported.[20] PSs rarely occur in patients with NF-2 or schwannomatosis.[21] Tumors can recur locally due to the multinodular growth pattern, but no metastasis or malignant transformation has been reported. Tumors are curable with complete surgical excision. A recent cytogenetic study revealed trisomy of chromosomes 17 and 18 in a PS,[22] but the lack of involvement of chromosome 22. Histopathologic features of PS are similar to those of a conventional schwannoma, but more Antoni A than Antoni B is seen (Figure 13-3). PS often exhibits worrisome morphologic features, such as increased cellularity, mild-to-moderate nuclear pleomorphism, and mitosis. However, these tumors show a benign behavior.[23] PSs are uniformly positive for S100 protein, collagen type IV, and laminin. Conventional or cellular schwannomas may show intratumoral nodularity, simulating a plexiform or multinodular pattern of PS. However, they have tumor tissues in internodular areas.[18] Plexiform neurofibromas with cellular schwannian nodules may mimic PS. In such cases, the clinical setting of NF-1 and immunohistochemistry are helpful in differential diagnosis. Plexiform neurofibromas contain S100-positive and S100-negative cells, and neurofilament-positive residual axons within tumor nodules. For distinguishing MPNST, immunohistochemistry for S100 protein, laminin, and collagen type IV are useful: diffuse and strong positivity in PSs, while negative or weak, patchy reactivity in MPNSTs.

Melanotic Schwannoma

Melanotic schwannoma (MS) is a rare variant of pigmented peripheral nerve tumors, composed of melanin-containing spindle-to-epithelioid cells with immunohistochemical and ultrastructural schwannian differentiation.[24] MS is variably associated with the Carney complex. Tumors

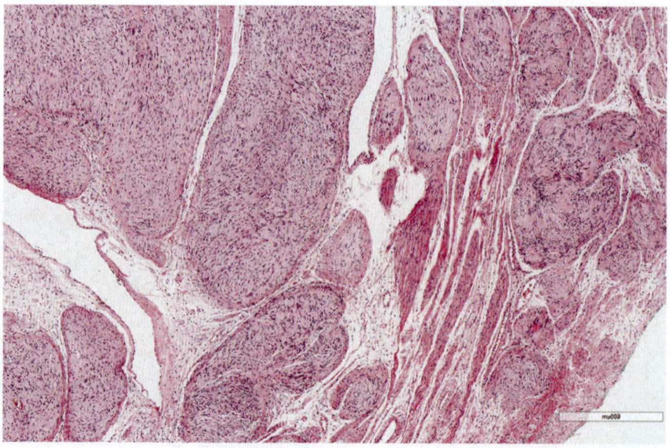

FIGURE 13-3: Plexiform schwannoma. Note a multinodular or plexiform growth of Schwann cells along nerve fascicles.

have a predilection for spinal nerve roots, but may occur in other locations, such as the mediastinum, sacrum, cauda equina, fifth cranial nerve, and cerebellum.[25] There are two varieties: psammomatous type and nonpsammomatous. The clinicopathologic features of both types are apparently identical. Local recurrences and metastasis have been reported. MSs differ significantly from conventional schwannoma or malignant melanoma at the genomic level. MSs show significant down-regulation of several genes important for Schwann cell function, including *PMP22*, *PMP2*, and *MPZ*.[25] Grossly, tumors are dark brown to black, and generally circumscribed but unencapsulated. Histologically, spindle and epithelioid cells containing melanin pigments are arranged in short fascicles and sheets. The nuclear morphology varies significantly. Vacuolated, adipocyte-like cells are found occasionally. Tumor cell necrosis or mitosis may be seen. The mitotic rate >2/10 HPF is significantly correlated with metastases. Tumor cells express both S100 protein and melanocytic markers, such as HMB45, tyrosinase, and Melan-A. The Ki-67-labeling index is less than 5% in most cases. The differential diagnosis includes malignant melanoma and meningeal melanocytoma.[1] Immunohistochemical staining for collagen type IV and laminin is helpful: Staining is completely negative in melanocytic tumors, in contrast to membranous staining in MSs.

Schwannomatosis

Schwannomatosis is a recently recognized, uncommon type of peripheral nerve sheath tumor, characterized by multiple noncutaneous, nonvestibular schwannomas. This disease is clinically and genetically distinct from NF-2. Patients with schwannomatosis tend to be younger than are those presenting with solitary schwannomas. Familial occurrence is uncommon.[26] The most common clinical symptom is chronic pain unassociated with a mass.[27] The pain is usually persistent, despite aggressive surgical and medical treatments. Definite diagnostic criteria include patient age greater than 30 years and two or more nonintradermal schwannomas, at least one with histologic confirmation or one pathologically confirmed schwannoma plus a first-degree relative who meet the above criteria.[28]

NEUROFIBROMA

Neurofibroma is defined by the World Health Organization (WHO) as a well-demarcated intraneural or diffuse infiltrative extraneural tumor consisting of a mixture of cell types, including Schwann cells, perineurial-like cells, and fibroblasts.[2] Neurofibroma has three growth patterns: localized, diffuse, or plexiform.[29] Approximately 10% of neurofibromas are associated with NF-1. Diffuse and plexiform neurofibromas are closely associated with NF-1. Multiple and plexiform neurofibromas are nearly pathognomonic of NF-1. Plexiform and localized intraneural neurofibroma are significant precursors of MPNST. Localized cutaneous neurofibroma is the most common, and plexiform neurofibroma is the rarest form.

Genetics

A monoclonal origin has been documented in tumors occurring sporadically as well as in tumors with NF-1.[30] Allelic loss of the *NF1* gene region of 17q has been confirmed in S100 protein immunoreactive Schwann cells, suggesting that the Schwann cell is the primary neoplastic component in this tumor.[31] Regarding tumorigenesis, all NF-1 patients have *NF1* germline mutations, and tumors are apparently initiated by loss of the second wild-type allele.[32] *NF1* alterations also appear to be involved in the genesis of sporadic neurofibromas.[33] Other chromosomal losses are not common, but have been reported on 19q and 22q in NF-1-associated and NF-1-unassociated tumors.[34]

Neurofibroma Variants

Localized neurofibromas present mostly as solitary, cutaneous nodules (localized cutaneous neurofibroma), and less often present as a circumscribed mass involving the peripheral nerve (localized intraneural neurofibroma). Diffuse neurofibroma is characterized by infiltrative growth involving the skin and subcutis (diffuse cutaneous neurofibroma) or extensive to massive involvement of the soft tissue (massive soft tissue neurofibroma). Plexiform neurofibroma is defined by the involvement of numerous adjacent nerve fascicles or multiple components of a nerve plexus.

Clinical and Pathologic Findings

All ages and both genders are affected. Localized cutaneous neurofibroma grows slowly as a painless nodule, and localized intraneural neurofibroma appears as a fusiform expansion of the affected nerve trunk. Diffuse neurofibroma presents as a plaque-like elevation of the skin in the head and neck regions. Plexiform neurofibroma always develops during early childhood. Plexiform neurofibroma involving the entire extremity is known as elephantiasis neuromatosa. Grossly, cutaneous neurofibromas are circumscribed (Figure 13-4A), or diffuse and involve skin and subcutaneous tissues (Figure 13-4B). Localized intraneural neurofibroma shows a nerve entering and exiting from the well-circumscribed mass. Plexiform neurofibromas are large lesions affecting large segments of a nerve, resulting in multinodular tangles (Figure 13-4C) or a thick convoluted mass, like a bag of worms. The microscopic appearances of the three forms of neurofibroma differ to varying degrees. Basically, neurofibromas consist of widely spaced, spindle (Schwann) cells and fibroblasts with variable amounts of collagenous fibers and myxoid matrix (Figure 13-4D). The spindle cells are intimately associated with coarse, collagen bundles like "shredded carrots." In diffuse and localized cutaneous neurofibromas, tumor cells infiltrate around normal structures, such as skin adnexa and blood vessels, and may extend into adipose tissue. The stroma may contain mast cells and lymphocytes. Early lesions of plexiform neurofibroma show expanded endoneurium with myxoid material, and at later stages, tumor cells spill out of the nerve into the soft tissue, which resembles areas of diffuse neurofibroma. Residual nerve fibers are commonly found in plexiform neurofibroma. Neurofibromas may show significantly increased cellularity (cellular neurofibroma) or nuclear atypia. Focal or diffuse nuclear atypia is not only associated with malignancy. Immunohistochemically, neurofibromas exhibit a mixed population of cells that are reactive for S100 protein, EMA/human erythrocyte glucose transporter 1 (Glut1), and CD34, indicating a heterogeneous composition of the constituents.[35] Neurofilament-positive axons are frequently present in neurofibromas, particularly plexiform neurofibromas.

Malignant Change in Neurofibroma

MPNSTs can arise in NF-1-associated neurofibroma, typically a deep-seated plexiform neurofibroma with an incidence of 5%.[36] Neurofibroma with atypical features is reserved for tumors that exhibit any combination of atypical features (cellularity, atypia, or mitotic activity) that fall

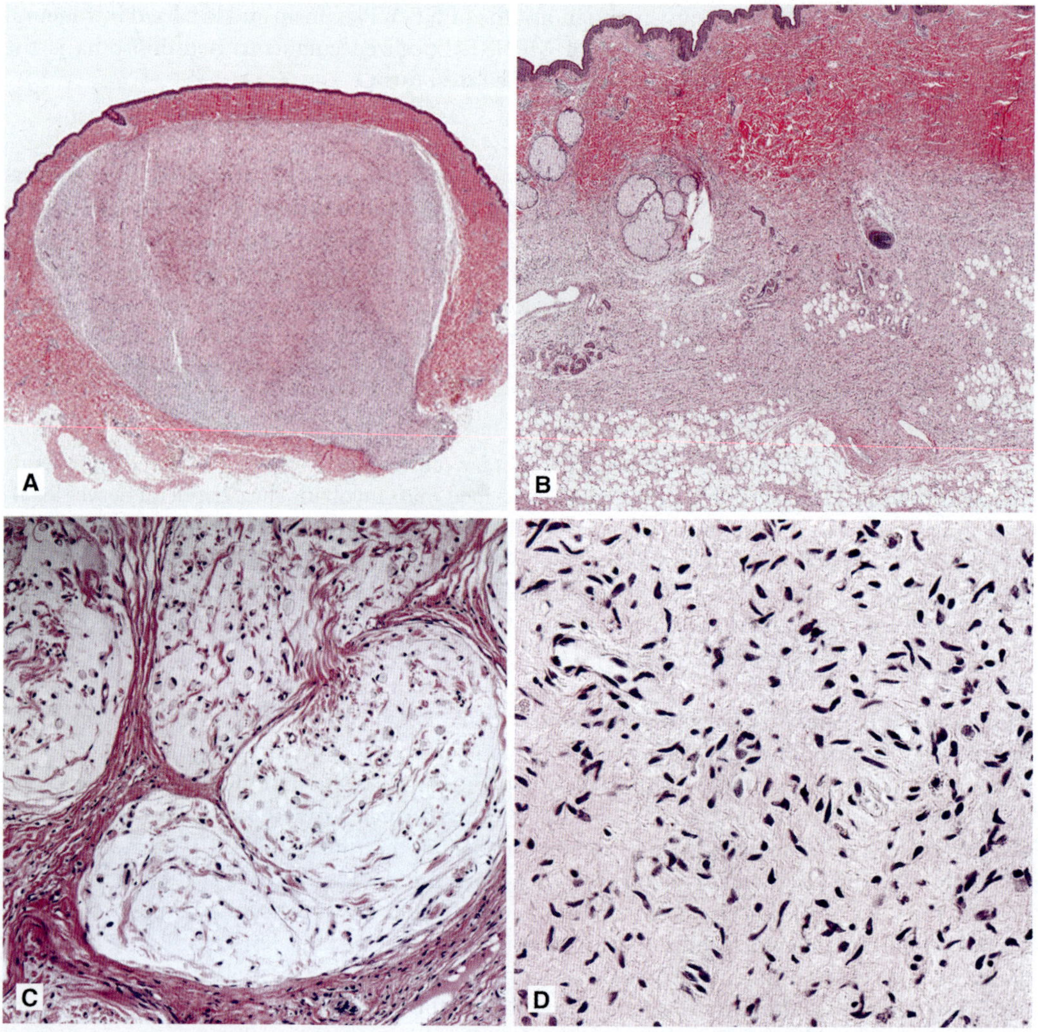

FIGURE 13-4: Neurofibroma. Low-power view of localized cutaneous neurofibroma (**A**), diffuse cutaneous neurofibroma (**B**), and plexiform neurofibroma (**C**). Note widely spaced, small, and curved cells in collagenous stroma (**D**).

short of the minimum criteria for a diagnosis of low-grade MPNST.[37] Low-grade MPNST arising in neurofibroma is diagnosed when there is generalized nuclear atypia (at least three times the size of neurofibroma nuclei), hyperchromasia, and definite cellular crowding.[38] In differential diagnosis with a low-grade MPNST, immunohistochemistry to detect loss of tumor suppressor gene proteins may be helpful. p16 is expressed in neurofibromas, while it is lost in MPNSTs.[39] p53 is significantly overexpressed in over half of MPNSTs and cellular neurofibromas, but not in neurofibromas.[40] The reactivity to Ki-67 is much higher in MPNSTs (mean 38.0%) than in atypical and cellular neurofibromas (mean 2.5%).[41]

PERINEURIOMA

Perineurioma is an uncommon peripheral nerve sheath tumor composed exclusively of neoplastic perineurial cells. Perineuriomas have been classified into intra- and extraneural forms according to tumor location. Extraneural tumors occur in soft tissue and skin, and are more common than are intraneural ones. Intraneural perineuriomas correspond histologically to WHO grade 1.

Soft tissue perineuriomas range from benign (WHO grade I) to variably malignant, corresponding to WHO grades II to III.[2]

Genetics

Cytogenetic studies have shown abnormalities of the chromosome 22, mainly monosomy or deletion of the 22q11-q13.1 bands,[42] and deletions and point mutations of the *NF2* gene on 22q12.[43] A loss of chromosome 13,[44] and rearrangements and/or deletions of 10q24 have also been identified.[45]

Intraneural Perineurioma

Intraneural perineurioma has been described as localized hypertrophic neuropathy, hypertrophic mononeuropathy, localized hypertrophic neurofibroma, intraneural neurofibroma, and hypertrophic interstitial neuritis.[46] Emory et al.[42] in 1995 confirmed its neoplastic nature by demonstrating cytogenetic abnormalities on chromosome 22 and coined the term "intraneural perineurioma." Tumors typically occur in adolescents or young adults (median, 20 years) as a slow-growing, painless mononeuropathy with motor and/or sensory deficits.[46] The male-to-female ratio was 0.8. This tumor mainly affects peripheral nerves and, rarely, cranial nerves.[47] The tumor appears as a fusiform, segmental enlargement of affected nerves. Histologically, it is characterized by an "onion bulb"–like arrangement of perineurial cells around axons and their Schwann sheaths. Immunohistochemically, tumor cells show positive membranous staining with EMA and negative staining for S100 protein. Claudin-1 and Glut1 are not specific, but useful, especially in difficult cases.[48] Neurofilament-positive residual axons can be seen in the concentric whorls. Ultrastructurally, pseudo-onion bulbs consist of concentric layers of perineurial cells.

Soft Tissue Perineurioma

This tumor is common in middle-aged men and women, and presents as a subcutaneous, painless mass in the extremities, limb girdle, and trunk. Deep soft tissues and visceral locations have been also described.[49] Tumors rarely recur, but do not metastasize. Grossly, most tumors are well circumscribed, and the cut surface is firm and rubbery, and yellow to white tan (Figure 13-5A). Central necrosis or infarction may be seen. Histologically, tumors show a morphologic spectrum, ranging from hypercellular lesions with collagenous stroma to hypocellular tumors with myxoid stroma. Tumor cells are spindled with wavy, tapering nuclei and thin elongated, and bipolar cytoplasmic processes. They are arranged predominantly in a storiform, and focally in a whorled or fascicular pattern (Figure 13-5B). Degenerative nuclear atypia can be found. Tumors exhibit a membranous staining with EMA (Figure 13-5C). Other positive markers include claudin-1 (~30%), CD34 (65%), smooth muscle actin (20%), and at least focal staining of S100 protein (5%). Ultrastructurally, tumor cells have long tapering nuclei and extremely thin, bipolar cytoplasmic processes with prominent pinocytotic vesicles, discontinuous external lamina, and occasional tight junctions in a collagen-rich matrix (Figure 13-5D). Soft tissue perineuriomas frequently have a storiform pattern, with high cellularity, similar to a dermatofibrosarcoma protuberance, but immunostaining for EMA can separate the two entities. Other differential diagnoses include low-grade fibromyxoid sarcoma (LGFMS) and low-grade myxofibrosarcoma. EMA can be positive in up to 30% of LGFMS.[49] But alternating fibrous and myxoid areas and the curvilinear small vessels of LGFMS are not seen in perineuriomas. The typical vascular pattern of elongated, thin curvilinear vessels, and pseudolipoblasts of myxofibrosarcoma are absent in perineuriomas.

HYBRID PERIPHERAL NERVE SHEATH TUMORS

Peripheral nerve sheath tumors may show characteristic histology of perineuriomas and schwannomas or neurofibromas within a single lesion.[50,51] Hybrid tumors are generally biphasic with abrupt transitions between the components. Hybrid schwannomas and perineuriomas are the

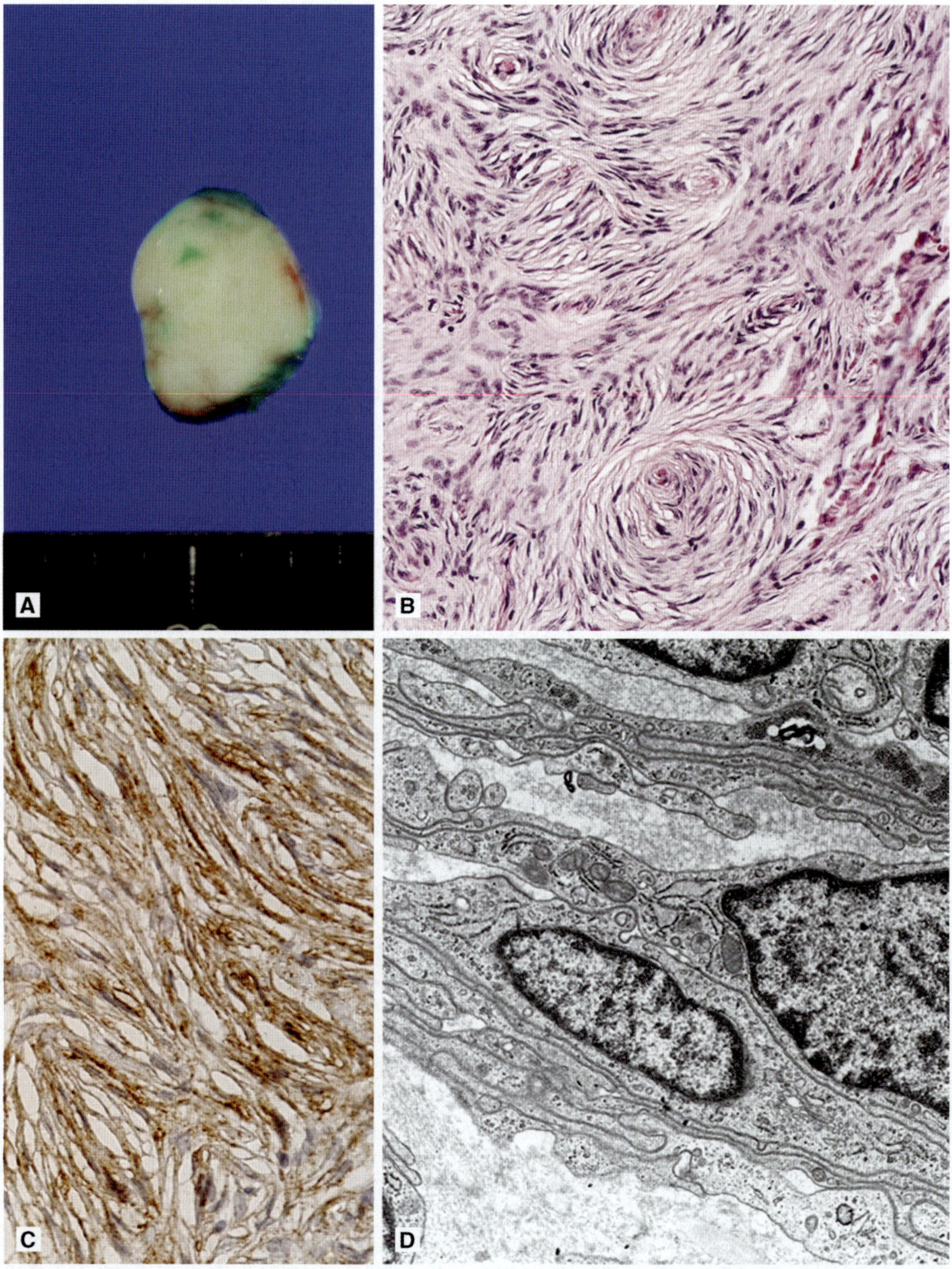

FIGURE 13-5: Soft tissue perineurioma. Note a well-circumscribed, whitish mass (**A**), a whorled or storiform arrangement of spindle cells (**B**), and membranous immunoreactivity for epithelial membrane antigen (**C**). Ultrastructure showing thin, bipolar cell processes with pinocytotic vesicles, discontinuous external lamina, and intercellular junctions in a collagen-rich matrix (**D**).

most common, and usually arise in the dermis and subcutis.[51] This tumor has no association with NF and seems to recur rarely. Grossly, the tumors are well circumscribed but not encapsulated. Histologically, hybrid schwannomas/perineuriomas shows storiform, lamellar, or whorled growth in a collagenous stroma, typical of perineurioma, but predominantly schwannian cytology.[50]

Immunohistochemically, tumors contain biphasic S100- and EMA- or CD34-positive cells. Most cases express GFAP, claudin-1, and Glut1.

NERVE SHEATH MYXOMA

Nerve sheath myxoma is a superficial, highly myxoid, multinodular, or multilobulated mass with a fibrous border. Clinicopathologic and immunohistochemical studies suggested that this tumor is of true nerve sheath origin, which has been confirmed by a molecular genetic study.[52,53] Tumors occurs at any age (range 8 to 72, mean 36 years) and in males and females equally. The extremities are the most common sites, particularly in the fingers and knee. Spinal and intracranial locations have been rarely reported.[54,55] The local recurrence rate is relatively high when managed by simple local excision. Microscopically, tumors are typically myxoid, multinodular with a peripheral fibrous border (Figure 13-6A). Tumor cells consist of spindled, stellate-shaped, ring-shaped, and epithelioid Schwann cells (Figure 13-6B). Tumor cells express S100 protein, GFAP, CD57, and neuron-specific enolase (NSE). EMA-positive perineurial cells and CD34-positive fibroblasts are observed rarely at the periphery of tumors.

GRANULAR CELL TUMOR

Granular cell tumor (GCT) is a benign tumor, characterized by large granular cells with abundant intracytoplasmic lysosomes. They occur in both benign and malignant forms, although the latter are very rare.[1] Currently, GCTs are considered to be of nerve sheath origin.[2] GCTs occur in adults, predominantly females, and present with small, painless nodules in the dermis or subcutis. This tumor occurs mostly with a single lesion but at multiple locations (15% to 20%).[37] GCTs are also encountered in the peripheral nervous system, including a digital nerve.[56] Intracranial GCTs are usually found in the posterior hypophysis, and rarely in cranial nerves,[57] or cerebral hemispheres.[58] GCTs at the region of the infundibulum are a well-recognized entity,[59] but cerebral

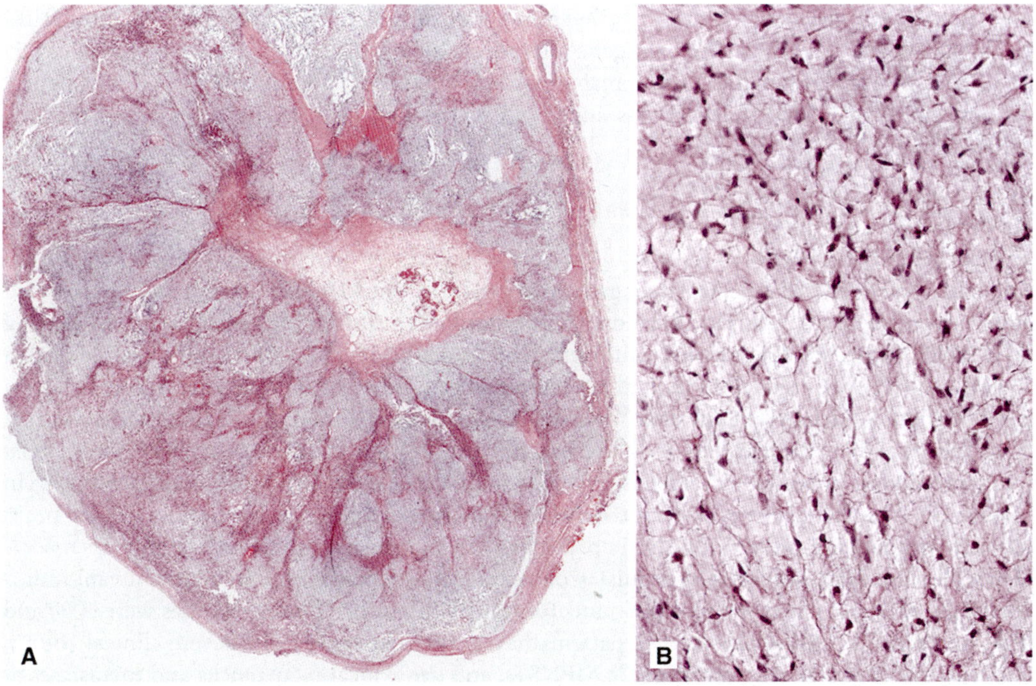

FIGURE 13-6: Spinal nerve sheath myxoma. Note a myxoid, multilobulated mass with a fibrous border (**A**), and spindled or stellate-shaped tumor cells in myxoid matrix (**B**).

GCTs exhibit histologic features, suggesting an astrocytic origin.[58,60] They usually show foci of transition from high-grade astrocytomas, GFAP expression, and glial filaments in tumor cells by electron microscopy. Local surgical excision is curative in noncerebral tumors. Grossly, this tumor is poorly circumscribed, and the cut surface is gray-white to yellow and firm. Histologically, tumors consist of round or elongated cells with dark small to large vesicular nuclei and abundant granular cytoplasm. The cytoplasmic granules are periodic acid–Schiff-positive and diastase-resistant lysosomes. Tumor cells express S100 protein, NSE, laminin, myelin proteins (P0 and P2), CD68, and inhibin-α. Ultrastructurally, tumor cells contain a large number of secondary lysosomes. The Ki-67-labeling index is less than 1%, and p53 is not expressed.[61] Malignant GCTs are mostly similar to their benign counterparts except for their larger size,[37] a high rate of metastasis (50%), and short survival. The diagnosis of malignant GCT should be restricted to neoplasms that are histologically similar to benign ones but that have three or more of the following histologic features: necrosis, spindling, vesicular nucleoli, mitotic activity (>2/10 HPF), high nucleocytoplasmic ratio, and pleomorphism.[61]

MALIGNANT PERIPHERAL NERVE SHEATH TUMORS

MPNSTs are defined by the WHO as malignant tumors, arising from the peripheral nerves or soft tissue neoplasms with differentiation into components of the nerve sheath, such as Schwann cells, fibroblasts, and perineurial cells.[2] MPNSTs can be graded as II, III, or IV according to WHO classification. MPNST is derived from Schwann cells or pluripotent cells of the neural crest.[50] More than half of MPNSTs occur in association with NF-1.[62] Malignant transformation from schwannomas is extremely rare, but it is relatively common in intracranial or cranial nerve MPNSTs.[63] Approximately 10% of tumors may occur in sites of previous radiation exposure, and develop after a latent period.[64]

Genetics

Cytogenetic studies have shown that MPNSTs have remarkably complex karyotypes with a wide spectrum of chromosomal alterations, including translocations, duplications, and numerical gains and losses.[65] The most frequent gene alterations include loss of *NF1* on 17q11 and of *p53* on 17q13. The molecular basis for transformation of neurofibroma to MPNST is still poorly understood. *CDKN2A/B* deletion was suggested as the first step in the progression towards MPNST.[66]

Malignant Peripheral Nerve Sheath Tumors, Conventional Type

Clinical Findings

An incidence of MPNST is 0.0001% in general population, but 4.6% among patients with NF-1.[36] NF-1 patients with internal plexiform neurofibromas have a 20-fold increased risk of developing an MPNST versus NF-1 individuals without such tumors.[67] MPNSTs affect adults mainly, with a roughly equal gender distribution, and a wide age range. However, intracranial MPNSTs have a much higher incidence (80%) in men.[68,69] When associated with NF-1, MPNSTs tend to present at a younger age (28 to 36 years) than do the sporadic cases (40 to 44 years).[62] MPNSTs occur most frequently in the proximal extremities, followed by the trunk and head and neck. Most arise in major nerve trunks, such as the sciatic nerve. MPNSTs occur rarely in the cranial nerves, brain parenchyma, and the dura.[68,70] MPNSTs present with a painful or rapidly enlarging mass associated with neurologic deficits. The mainstay of treatment is radical resection with adjuvant radiotherapy. A recent study revealed that 5- and 10-year disease-specific survival rates were 60% and 45%, respectively.[71] MPNSTs in NF-1 patients have larger masses, a more severe clinical course, and a shorter survival than do sporadic MPNSTs, and show local recurrences and metastases at a significantly earlier stage. Poor prognosis of cranial MPNSTs is attributed to the inaccessibility and subtotal resections, and metastasis to the spinal cord is most frequent.[72]

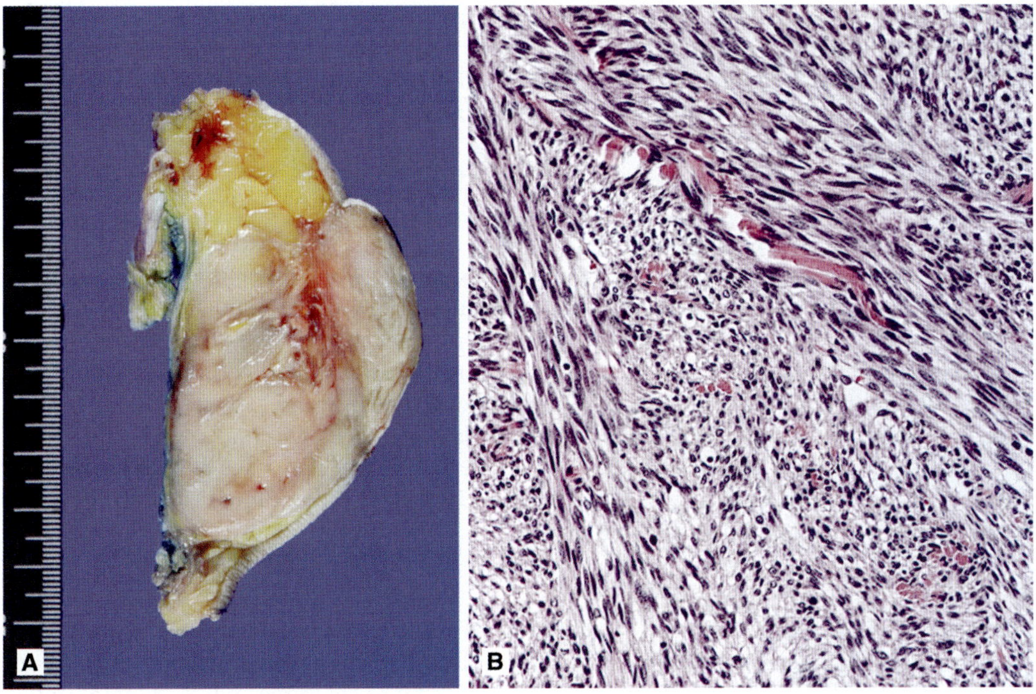

FIGURE 13-7: Malignant peripheral nerve sheath tumor. Note a lobulated, gray-tan, fleshy mass with foci of hemorrhage and necrosis (**A**). Note densely cellular fascicles of spindle cells with hyperchromatic, wavy, and buckled nuclei (**B**).

Pathologic Findings

Grossly, MPNSTs resemble neurofibromas, ranging from well-circumscribed, fusiform, or globular enlargement of a nerve to a lesion unassociated with a nerve and showing more infiltrative soft tissue extension. The cut surface is white tan, fleshy, and firm, with areas of hemorrhage and necrosis (Figure 13-7A). Microscopically, MPNSTs shows a marble appearance with densely cellular fascicles alternating with less cellular myxoid areas. Dense cellular fascicles resemble the herringbone pattern of fibrosarcoma (Figure 13-7B). Tumor cells are spindle to fusiform with elongated wavy and buckled nuclei and indistinct eosinophilic cytoplasm. A nodular or whorled pattern and nuclear palisading may also be found. Perineural and intraneural spread of tumor cells are common. Heterologous elements may be present in 10% to 15% of MPNST, and include mature bone, cartilage islands, skeletal muscle fibers, mucin-secreting glands, and squamous elements. Tumors focally express S100 protein (50% to 90%), and the S100 positivity depends on the degree of schwannian differentiation.[73] Recently, Sox-10 (SRY-related HMG box 10) is identified as a more specific marker for MPNST than is S100 protein.[74] p53, CD57 (Leu-7), collagen type IV, laminin, CD34, cytokeratin, and GFAP are expressed variably.[75]

Differential Diagnosis

Because MPNST shows morphologic heterogeneity and a lack of specific immunohistochemical or molecular markers, histologic diagnosis is challenging. Diagnosis of MPNST requires a clinical history of NF-1 with or without preexisting plexiform neurofibroma, and the exclusion of histologic mimickers by immunohistochemistry with or without a molecular genetic analysis. Synovial sarcoma, especially the monophasic variant, and MPNST have morphologic, immunophenotypical, and clinical similarities. Synovial sarcoma shows a more uniform fascicular pattern with focal expression of cytokeratin or EMA, but both antigens are generally negative in MPNSTs. Transducin-like enhancer protein (TLE1) expression is typically diffuse and strong in synovial sarcomas, but may also be present in a somewhat weaker, more variable pattern in some

MPNSTs.[76] SOX10 is a specific (93%) but not very sensitive (67%) marker to make a diagnosis of MPNST over synovial sarcoma.[74] The histology of fibrosarcoma may be nearly identical to that of MPNST, but S100 protein and Leu-7 are negative in fibrosarcoma. Low-grade MPNST should be differentiated from atypical or cellular neurofibromas, and cellular schwannoma (discussed in malignant change in neurofibroma).

MPNST with Rhabdomyoblastic Differentiation (Malignant Triton Tumor)

MPNSTs may show divergent differentiation: focal epithelial or mesenchymal differentiation. Epithelial elements are histologically benign, whereas mesenchymal differentiation is malignant (rhabdomyosarcoma, osteosarcoma, or chondrosarcoma). The most common heterologous component is a rhabdomyosarcoma.[77] MPNST with rhabdomyoblastic differentiation is also known as a "malignant triton tumor" (MTT), and approximately 60% of MTTs occur in patients with NF-1. The tumor develops most commonly in the fourth decade and can affect any soft tissue sites. Rare examples of intracranial MTTs have been documented.[78] This tumor has a worse prognosis than does the classical MPNST. The histologic hallmark is the presence of rhabdomyoblasts scattered throughout the ordinary MPNST (Figure 13-8). They are readily detected by immunoreactivity for desmin, MyoD1, and myogenin.

MPNST with Glandular Differentiation

Almost all of these tumors occur in patients with NF-1. Tumors usually involve major nerves, including the spinal nerve. This tumor has characteristically heterologous elements, such as cartilage, bone, and glands. The glands are lined with cuboidal or columnar cells, and often contain goblet cells or neuroendocrine cells. The glands may appear to be malignant. Benign schwannoma with glandular elements can be distinguished by a strong, diffuse S100 protein immunoreactivity, in contrast to focal positive or negative staining in MPNSTs.

Epithelioid MPNST

Epithelioid MPNST is composed predominantly or exclusively of epithelioid Schwann cells. Tumors occur mostly from 20 to 50 years of age, with a slight male predominance. This tumor appears either as a superficial cutaneous mass or as a deep soft tissue mass in the extremities.[79] Most of the tumors affect major nerves. This tumor is less often associated with NF-1.[80] The superficial tumors are smaller, easier to excise, and associated with a better prognosis. Histologically, tumors show a striking multinodular growth pattern with intervening fibrous septation.[81] Tumors consist of round, eosinophilic, or amphophilic epithelioid cells with vesicular nuclei and a prominent nucleolus, resembling malignant melanoma (Figure 13-9A). Spindle cells typical of MPNST often coexist. Tumors show a diffuse, strong positivity for S100 protein, and often cytokeratin, EMA, or collagen type IV expression. About half of the tumors show loss of nuclear staining for SMARCB1/INI-1[82] (Figure 13-9B).

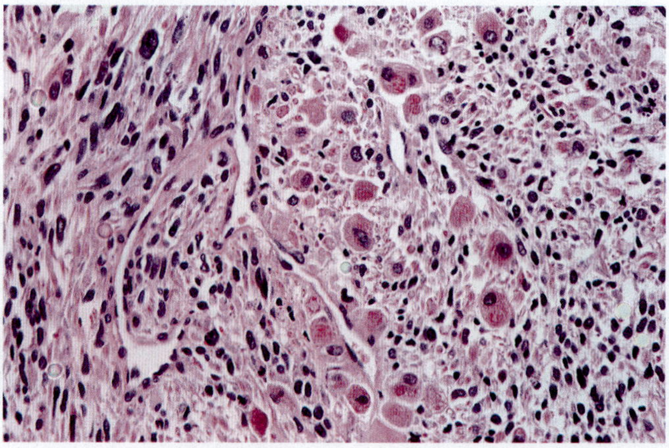

FIGURE 13-8: Malignant peripheral nerve sheath tumor with rhabdomyoblastic differentiation. Note round rhabdomyoblasts with abundant eosinophilic cytoplasm.

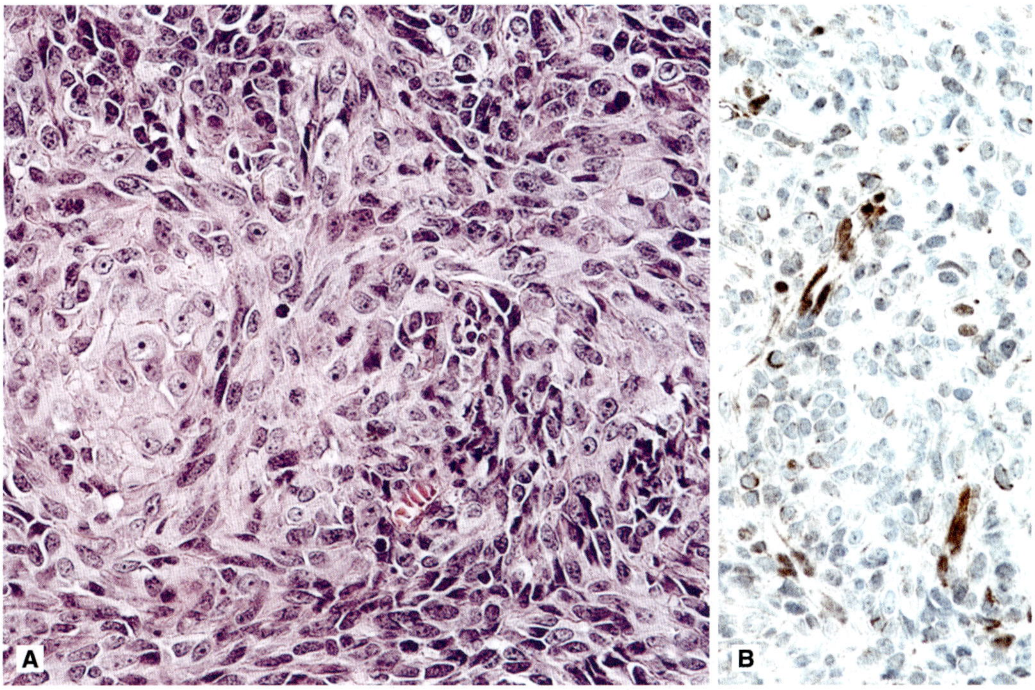

FIGURE 13-9: Epithelioid malignant peripheral nerve sheath tumor. Note a nodular growth of epithelioid cells with prominent nuclei (**A**), and loss of INI-1 (**B**), in contrast to a nuclear staining in normal endothelial cells.

References

1. Perry A, Brat DJ. *Practical Surgical Neuropathology a Diagnostic Approach*. Philadelphia, PA: Churchill Livingstone/Elsevier; 2010.
2. Louis DN; International Agency for Research on Cancer. *WHO Classification of Tumours of the Central Nervous System*. Lyon, France: International Agency for Research on Cancer; 2007.
3. Suh YL, Koo H, Kim TS, et al. Tumors of the central nervous system in Korea: a multicenter study of 3221 cases. *J Neurooncol* 2002;56:251–259.
4. Chandler CL, Ramsden RT. Acoustic schwannoma. *Br J Hosp Med* 1993;49:335–343.
5. McCormick PC, Bello JA, Post KD. Trigeminal schwannoma. Surgical series of 14 cases with review of the literature. *J Neurosurg* 1988;69:850–860.
6. Kim NR, Suh YL, Shin HJ. Thoracic pediatric intramedullary schwannoma: report of a case. *Pediatr Neurosurg* 2009;45:396–401.
7. Ramos AA, Vega MA, Valencia HS, et al. Intraparenchymal schwannoma involving the brainstem in a young woman. *Pediatr Neurol* 2013;48:472–474.
8. Jacoby LB, MacCollin M, Barone R, et al. Frequency and distribution of NF2 mutations in schwannomas. *Genes Chromosomes Cancer* 1996;17:45–55.
9. Louis DN, Ramesh V, Gusella JF. Neuropathology and molecular genetics of neurofibromatosis 2 and related tumors. *Brain Pathol* 1995;5:163–172.
10. Stemmer-Rachamimov AO, Xu L, Gonzalez-Agosti C, et al. Universal absence of merlin, but not other ERM family members, in schwannomas. *Am J Pathol* 1997;151:1649–1654.
11. Smith MJ, Wallace AJ, Bowers NL, et al. Frequency of SMARCB1 mutations in familial and sporadic schwannomatosis. *Neurogenetics* 2012;13:141–145.
12. Piotrowski A, Xie J, Liu YF, et al. Germline loss-of-function mutations in LZTR1 predispose to an inherited disorder of multiple schwannomas. *Nat Genet* 2014;46:182–187.
13. Huang HY, Park N, Erlandson RA, et al. Immunohistochemical and ultrastructural comparative study of external lamina structure in 31 cases of cellular, classical, and melanotic schwannomas. *Appl Immunohistochem Mol Morphol* 2004;12:50–58.

14. Dickersin GR. *Diagnostic Electron Microscopy a Text/Atlas*. New York, NY: Springer; 2005.
15. Casadei GP, Scheithauer BW, Hirose T, et al. Cellular schwannoma. A clinicopathologic, DNA flow cytometric, and proliferation marker study of 70 patients. *Cancer* 1995;75:1109–1119.
16. White W, Shiu MH, Rosenblum MK, et al. Cellular schwannoma. A clinicopathologic study of 57 patients and 58 tumors. *Cancer* 1990;66:1266–1275.
17. Rongioletti F, Drago F, Rebora A. Multiple cutaneous plexiform schwannomas with tumors of the central nervous system. *Arch Dermatol* 1989;125:431–432.
18. Berg JC, Scheithauer BW, Spinner RJ, et al. Plexiform schwannoma: a clinicopathologic overview with emphasis on the head and neck region. *Hum Pathol* 2008;39:633–640.
19. Agaram NP, Prakash S, Antonescu CR. Deep-seated plexiform schwannoma: a pathologic study of 16 cases and comparative analysis with the superficial variety. *Am J Surg Pathol* 2005;29:1042–1048.
20. Ioannou M, Papanastassiou I, Iakowidou I, et al. Plexiform schwannoma of the posterior tibial nerve: a case report. *Cases J* 2009;2:8392.
21. Reith JD, Goldblum JR. Multiple cutaneous plexiform schwannomas. Report of a case and review of the literature with particular reference to the association with types 1 and 2 neurofibromatosis and schwannomatosis. *Arch Pathol Lab Med* 1996;120:399–401.
22. Tassano E, Sementa AR, Tavella E, et al. Trisomy 17 in congenital plexiform (multinodular) cellular schwannoma. *Cancer Genet Cytogenet* 2010;203:313–315.
23. Woodruff JM, Scheithauer BW, Kurtkaya-Yapicier O, et al. Congenital and childhood plexiform (multinodular) cellular schwannoma: a troublesome mimic of malignant peripheral nerve sheath tumor. *Am J Surg Pathol* 2003;27:1321–1329.
24. Zhang HY, Yang GH, Chen HJ, et al. Clinicopathological, immunohistochemical, and ultrastructural study of 13 cases of melanotic schwannoma. *Chin Med J (Engl)* 2005;118:1451–1461.
25. Torres-Mora J, Dry S, Li X, et al. Malignant melanotic schwannian tumor: a clinicopathologic, immunohistochemical, and gene expression profiling study of 40 cases, with a proposal for the reclassification of "melanotic schwannoma." *Am J Surg Pathol* 2014;38:94–105.
26. Gonzalvo A, Fowler A, Cook RJ, et al. Schwannomatosis, sporadic schwannomatosis, and familial schwannomatosis: a surgical series with long-term follow-up. Clinical article. *J Neurosurg* 2011;114:756–762.
27. Merker VL, Esparza S, Smith MJ, et al. Clinical features of schwannomatosis: a retrospective analysis of 87 patients. *Oncologist* 2012;17:1317–1322.
28. Baser ME, Friedman JM, Evans DG. Increasing the specificity of diagnostic criteria for schwannomatosis. *Neurology* 2006;66:730–732.
29. Woodruff JM. Pathology of tumors of the peripheral nerve sheath in type 1 neurofibromatosis. *Am J Med Genet* 1999;89:23–30.
30. Skuse GR, Kosciolek BA, Rowley PT. The neurofibroma in von Recklinghausen neurofibromatosis has a unicellular origin. *Am J Hum Genet* 1991;49:600–607.
31. Perry A, Roth KA, Banerjee R, et al. NF1 deletions in S-100 protein-positive and negative cells of sporadic and neurofibromatosis 1 (NF1)-associated plexiform neurofibromas and malignant peripheral nerve sheath tumors. *Am J Pathol* 2001;159:57–61.
32. Serra E, Puig S, Otero D, et al. Confirmation of a double-hit model for the NF1 gene in benign neurofibromas. *Am J Hum Genet* 1997;61:512–519.
33. Storlazzi CT, Von Steyern FV, Domanski HA, et al. Biallelic somatic inactivation of the NF1 gene through chromosomal translocations in a sporadic neurofibroma. *Int J Cancer* 2005;117:1055–1057.
34. Koga T, Iwasaki H, Ishiguro M, et al. Losses in chromosomes 17, 19, and 22q in neurofibromatosis type 1 and sporadic neurofibromas: a comparative genomic hybridization analysis. *Cancer Genet Cytogenet* 2002;136:113–120.
35. Hirose T, Tani T, Shimada T, et al. Immunohistochemical demonstration of EMA/Glut1-positive perineurial cells and CD34-positive fibroblastic cells in peripheral nerve sheath tumors. *Mod Pathol* 2003;16: 293–298.
36. Ducatman BS, Scheithauer BW, Piepgras DG, et al. Malignant peripheral nerve sheath tumors. A clinicopathologic study of 120 cases. *Cancer* 1986;57:2006–2021.
37. Weiss SW, Goldblum JR, Enzinger FM. *Enzinger and Weiss's Soft Tissue Tumors*. St. Louis, MO: Mosby; 2014.
38. Burger PC, Scheithauer BW; American Registry of Pathology Armed Forces Institute of Pathology. *Tumors of the Central Nervous System*. Washington, DC: American Registry of Pathology in Collaboration with the Armed Forces Institute of Pathology; 2007.
39. Nielsen GP, Stemmer-Rachamimov AO, Ino Y, et al. Malignant transformation of neurofibromas in neurofibromatosis 1 is associated with CDKN2A/p16 inactivation. *Am J Pathol* 1999;155:1879–1884.

40. Halling KC, Scheithauer BW, Halling AC, et al. p53 expression in neurofibroma and malignant peripheral nerve sheath tumor. An immunohistochemical study of sporadic and NF1-associated tumors. *Am J Clin Pathol* 1996;106:282–288.
41. Lin BT, Weiss LM, Medeiros LJ. Neurofibroma and cellular neurofibroma with atypia: a report of 14 tumors. *Am J Surg Pathol* 1997;21:1443–1449.
42. Emory TS, Scheithauer BW, Hirose T, et al. Intraneural perineurioma. A clonal neoplasm associated with abnormalities of chromosome 22. *Am J Clin Pathol* 1995;103:696–704.
43. Lasota J, Fetsch JF, Wozniak A, et al. The neurofibromatosis type 2 gene is mutated in perineurial cell tumors: a molecular genetic study of eight cases. *Am J Pathol* 2001;158:1223–1229.
44. Mott RT, Goodman BK, Burchette JL, et al. Loss of chromosome 13 in a case of soft tissue perineurioma. *Clin Neuropathol* 2005;24:69–76.
45. Brock JE, Perez-Atayde AR, Kozakewich HP, et al. Cytogenetic aberrations in perineurioma: variation with subtype. *Am J Surg Pathol* 2005;29:1164–1169.
46. Boyanton BL Jr, Jones JK, Shenaq SM, et al. Intraneural perineurioma: a systematic review with illustrative cases. *Arch Pathol Lab Med* 2007;131:1382–1392.
47. Christoforidis M, Buhl R, Paulus W, et al. Intraneural perineurioma of the VIIIth cranial nerve: case report. *Neurosurgery* 2007;61:E652; discussion E652.
48. Macarenco RS, Ellinger F, Oliveira AM. Perineurioma: a distinctive and underrecognized peripheral nerve sheath neoplasm. *Arch Pathol Lab Med* 2007;131:625–636.
49. Hornick JL, Fletcher CD. Soft tissue perineurioma: clinicopathologic analysis of 81 cases including those with atypical histologic features. *Am J Surg Pathol* 2005;29:845–858.
50. Rodriguez FJ, Folpe AL, Giannini C, et al. Pathology of peripheral nerve sheath tumors: diagnostic overview and update on selected diagnostic problems. *Acta Neuropathol* 2012;123:295–319.
51. Hornick JL, Bundock EA, Fletcher CD. Hybrid schwannoma/perineurioma: clinicopathologic analysis of 42 distinctive benign nerve sheath tumors. *Am J Surg Pathol* 2009;33:1554–1561.
52. Fetsch JF, Laskin WB, Miettinen M. Nerve sheath myxoma: a clinicopathologic and immunohistochemical analysis of 57 morphologically distinctive, S-100 protein- and GFAP-positive, myxoid peripheral nerve sheath tumors with a predilection for the extremities and a high local recurrence rate. *Am J Surg Pathol* 2005;29:1615–1624.
53. Sheth S, Li X, Binder S, et al. Differential gene expression profiles of neurothekeomas and nerve sheath myxomas by microarray analysis. *Mod Pathol* 2011;24:343–354.
54. Paulus W, Warmuth-Metz M, Sorensen N. Intracranial neurothekeoma (nerve-sheath myxoma). Case report. *J Neurosurg* 1993;79:280–282.
55. Lee D, Suh YL, Han J, et al. Spinal nerve sheath myxoma (neurothekeoma). *Pathol Int* 2006;56:144–149.
56. Ha SY, Suh YL, Sung CO. Granular cell tumour arising in a digital nerve. *J Hand Surg Eur Vol* 2011;36:249–250.
57. Chimelli L, Symon L, Scaravilli F. Granular cell tumor of the fifth cranial nerve: further evidence for Schwann cell origin. *J Neuropathol Exp Neurol* 1984;43:634–642.
58. Lee D, Suh YL, Nam do H. Cerebral granular cell tumor. *Neuropathology* 2008;28:417–421.
59. Geddes JF, Thom M, Robinson SF, et al. Granular cell change in astrocytic tumors. *Am J Surg Pathol* 1996;20:55–63.
60. Dickson DW, Suzuki KI, Kanner R, et al. Cerebral granular cell tumor: immunohistochemical and electron microscopic study. *J Neuropathol Exp Neurol* 1986;45:304–314.
61. Fanburg-Smith JC, Meis-Kindblom JM, Fante R, et al. Malignant granular cell tumor of soft tissue: diagnostic criteria and clinicopathologic correlation. *Am J Surg Pathol* 1998;22:779–794.
62. Hagel C, Zils U, Peiper M, et al. Histopathology and clinical outcome of NF1-associated vs. sporadic malignant peripheral nerve sheath tumors. *J Neurooncol* 2007;82:187–192.
63. Endo M, Yamamoto H, Harimaya K, et al. Conventional spindle cell-type malignant peripheral nerve sheath tumor arising in a sporadic schwannoma. *Hum Pathol* 2013;44:2845–2848.
64. Foley KM, Woodruff JM, Ellis FT, et al. Radiation-induced malignant and atypical peripheral nerve sheath tumors. *Ann Neurol* 1980;7:311–318.
65. Thway K, Fisher C. Malignant peripheral nerve sheath tumor: pathology and genetics. *Ann Diagn Pathol* 2014;18:109–116.
66. Beert E, Brems H, Daniels B, et al. Atypical neurofibromas in neurofibromatosis type 1 are premalignant tumors. *Genes Chromosomes Cancer* 2011;50:1021–1032.
67. Tucker T, Wolkenstein P, Revuz J, et al. Association between benign and malignant peripheral nerve sheath tumors in NF1. *Neurology* 2005;65:205–211.

68. Scheithauer BW, Erdogan S, Rodriguez FJ, et al. Malignant peripheral nerve sheath tumors of cranial nerves and intracranial contents: a clinicopathologic study of 17 cases. *Am J Surg Pathol* 2009;33:325–338.
69. Ziadi A, Saliba I. Malignant peripheral nerve sheath tumor of intracranial nerve: a case series review. *Auris Nasus Larynx* 2010;37:539–545.
70. Albayrak BS, Gorgulu A, Kose T. A case of intra-dural malignant peripheral nerve sheath tumor in thoracic spine associated with neurofibromatosis type 1. *J Neurooncol* 2006;78:187–190.
71. Stucky CC, Johnson KN, Gray RJ, et al. Malignant peripheral nerve sheath tumors (MPNST): the Mayo Clinic experience. *Ann Surg Oncol* 2012;19:878–885.
72. Schmidt RF, Yick F, Boghani Z, et al. Malignant peripheral nerve sheath tumors of the trigeminal nerve: a systematic review of 36 cases. *Neurosurg Focus* 2013;34:E5.
73. Zhou H, Coffin CM, Perkins SL, et al. Malignant peripheral nerve sheath tumor: a comparison of grade, immunophenotype, and cell cycle/growth activation marker expression in sporadic and neurofibromatosis 1-related lesions. *Am J Surg Pathol* 2003;27:1337–1345.
74. Kang Y, Pekmezci M, Folpe AL, et al. Diagnostic utility of SOX10 to distinguish malignant peripheral nerve sheath tumor from synovial sarcoma, including intraneural synovial sarcoma. *Mod Pathol* 2014;27:55–61.
75. Gray MH, Rosenberg AE, Dickersin GR, et al. Glial fibrillary acidic protein and keratin expression by benign and malignant nerve sheath tumors. *Hum Pathol* 1989;20:1089–1096.
76. Valente AL, Tull J, Zhang S. Specificity of TLE1 expression in unclassified high-grade sarcomas for the diagnosis of synovial sarcoma. *Appl Immunohistochem Mol Morphol* 2013;21:408–413.
77. Stasik CJ, Tawfik O. Malignant peripheral nerve sheath tumor with rhabdomyosarcomatous differentiation (malignant triton tumor). *Arch Pathol Lab Med* 2006;130:1878–1881.
78. Han DH, Kim DG, Chi JG, et al. Malignant triton tumor of the acoustic nerve. Case report. *J Neurosurg* 1992;76:874–877.
79. Lodding P, Kindblom LG, Angervall L. Epithelioid malignant schwannoma. A study of 14 cases. *Virchows Arch A Pathol Anat Histopathol* 1986;409:433–451.
80. Laskin WB, Weiss SW, Bratthauer GL. Epithelioid variant of malignant peripheral nerve sheath tumor (malignant epithelioid schwannoma). *Am J Surg Pathol* 1991;15:1136–1145.
81. McMenamin ME, Fletcher CD. Expanding the spectrum of malignant change in schwannomas: epithelioid malignant change, epithelioid malignant peripheral nerve sheath tumor, and epithelioid angiosarcoma: a study of 17 cases. *Am J Surg Pathol* 2001;25:13–25.
82. Hornick JL, Dal Cin P, Fletcher CD. Loss of INI1 expression is characteristic of both conventional and proximal-type epithelioid sarcoma. *Am J Surg Pathol* 2009;33:542–550.

Hematolymphoid and Histiocytic Tumors

14

Xinmin Zhang
Jian Yi Li

PRIMARY CENTRAL NERVOUS SYSTEM LYMPHOMA

Definition

Primary central nervous system lymphoma (PCNSL) is a malignant lymphoma involving the parenchyma of brain or spinal cord in the absence of lymphoma outside the central nervous system (CNS) at initial diagnosis.

Historical Background

PCNSL was first reported as "perithelial sarcoma" by Bailey in 1929. At least 12 synonyms including "adventitial sarcoma" and "reticulum cell sarcoma" have been used in the preimmunohistochemistry era.[1] The mystery was resolved during the modern classification of lymphomas. The PCNSL has been designated as a distinct entity.

Clinical Features

PCNSL is a rare tumor of the CNS, constituting 0.8% to 6.6% of all primary CNS tumors.[1] Most of the PCNSLs (95%) are diffuse large B-cell lymphomas (DLBCL).[1] The remaining are low-grade B-cell lymphoma, Burkitt lymphoma, and peripheral T-cell lymphoma (PTCL). An Epstein-Barr virus (EBV)-related genome can be detected in virtually all PCNSLs in patients with acquired immunodeficiency syndrome (AIDS). However, PCNSL is generally not associated with EBV in immunocompetent patients. So far there are no clear risk factors for PCNSL in immunocompetent patients. PCNSLs in immunocompetent patients affect predominantly adults, with a median age in the sixth decade and a slight male preponderance while the median age of AIDS patients with PCNSL is 35 years.

Neuroimaging Findings

PCNSL in immunocompetent patients typically presents as a solitary homogeneously enhancing parenchymal mass and less frequently as multifocal solid enhancing lesions (Figure 14-1A, B, and F). PCNSL in immunodeficient patients often presents as multifocal lesions, which commonly show irregular ring enhancement (Figure 14-1E). Peritumoral edema is less prominent than that in malignant gliomas or metastases. Most lesions are located in central hemispheric or periventricular white matter. The most common location is frontal lobe, followed by basal ganglia, cerebellum, brainstem, and spinal cord. Diffusion-weighted imaging (DWI) measures the diffusion of water molecules in the tissue. Since the water diffusion is restricted in PCNSL due to hypercellularity, the lesions appear hyperintense on DWI and hypointense on apparent diffusion coefficient (ADC) maps (Figure 14-1C and D).

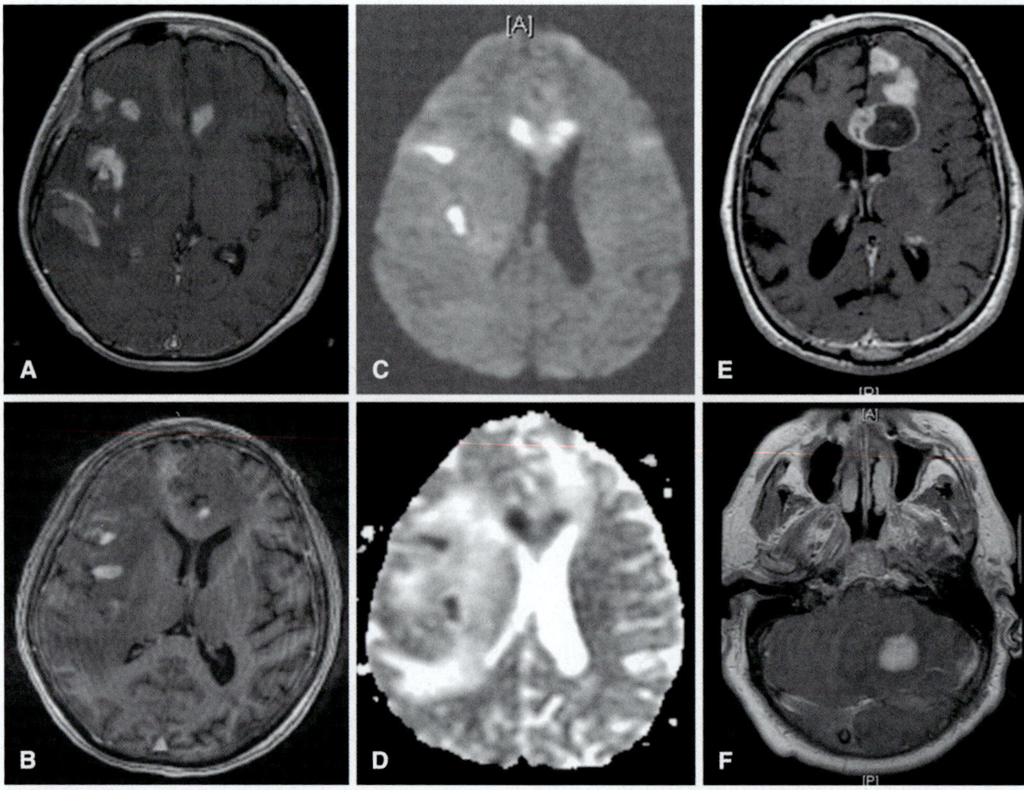

FIGURE 14-1: Characteristic findings of PCNSL on MRI. Axial, T1 postcontrast, multiple solid contrast-enhanced lesions in immunocompetent patients with PCNSL (**A**). Axial, T1 postcontrast, after 4 days of treatment with steroid, sizes of multiple contrast-enhanced lesions are decreased (**A** and **B** from the same patient) (**B**). Axial, diffusion-weighted imaging (DWI) reveals restricted diffusion within the tumor with high signal intensity on DWI (**C**) and corresponding low signal intensity on the ADC map (**D**). Axial, T1 postcontrast, two solid contrast-enhanced lesions and one ring enhanced lesion in AIDS PCNSL (**E**). Axial, T1 postcontrast, a solid contrast-enhanced cerebellar lesion in the patient with primary CNS T-cell lymphoma (**F**).

Pathologic Features

Intraoperative Consultation

Stereotactic brain biopsy is the most reliable method for the diagnosis of PCNSL. During the intraoperative consultation, both smears (squash preparations) and touch imprints can be prepared: First, use one slide to touch all the pieces of tissue from brain biopsy to make one touch imprint; and second, cut tiny teeny tissue from each end of the cores and use them to prepare multiple smears. H&E staining of these cytologic preparations reveals numerous relatively monotonous, discohesive large cells with scant cytoplasm and prominent nucleoli in a background of prominent lymphoglandular bodies (Figure 14-2A). Mitoses are easily seen. Nuclear crush artifact can be seen on squash preparations. Occasionally, tingible body macrophages also can be seen (Figure 14-2A). Touch preparation is very useful in differentiating lymphoma from high-grade glioma because high-grade glioma is less discohesive and as a result, the touch imprint usually is much less cellular. It is unnecessary to perform frozen section, if a diagnosis of lymphoma can be made based on cytologic evaluation. On frozen section, PCNSL exhibits intense perivascular clustering of large atypical lymphoid cells with prominent nucleoli that infiltrate into the surrounding brain parenchyma (Figure 14-2B). Unlike high-grade gliomas, PCNSL lacks microvascular proliferation or pseudopalisading necrosis.

Histology on Permanent Section

PCNSL is characterized by perivascular and angiocentric lymphoid infiltrate composed of a monotonous population of large lymphocytes with prominent nucleoli, which is accompanied

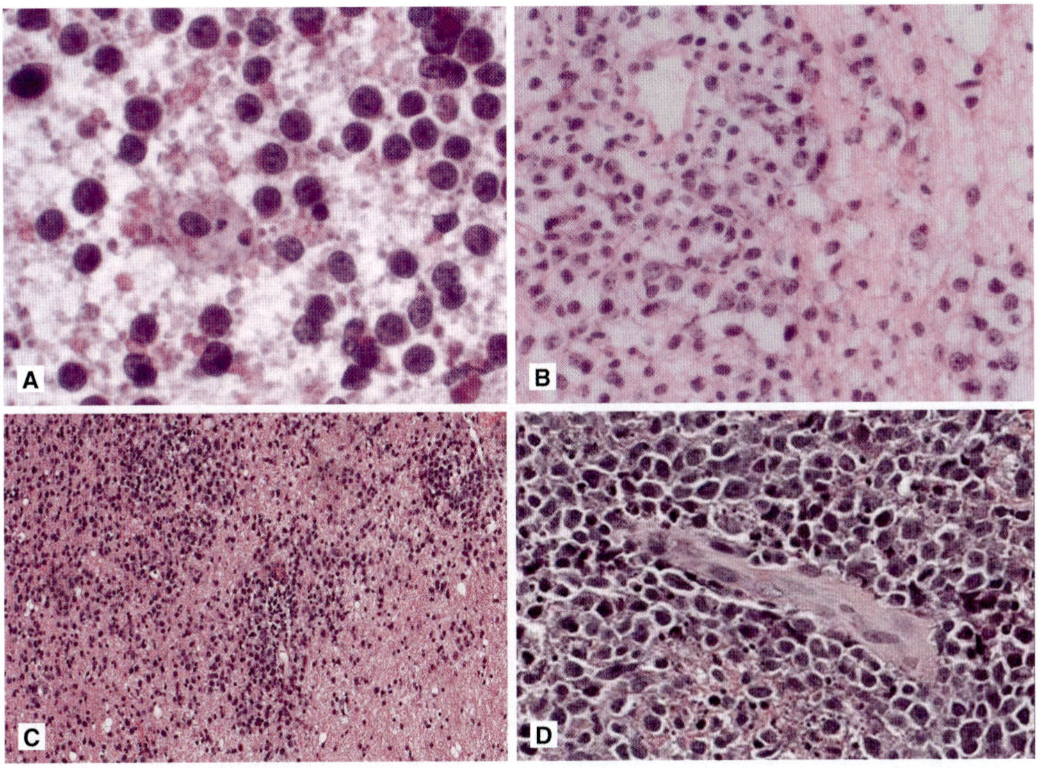

FIGURE 14-2: Primary CNS diffuse large B-cell lymphoma (DLBCL). Smear during intraoperative consultation shows numerous relatively monotonous large, discohesive cells with scant cytoplasm and prominent nucleoli, prominent lymphoglandular bodies in the background, and a tingible body macrophage (*center*) (**A**). Frozen section shows obvious perivascular clustering of large atypical lymphoma cells with prominent nucleoli and infiltration into the adjacent brain parenchyma (**B**). At low power, DLBCL exhibits an angiocentric growth pattern and diffuse infiltration of brain parenchyma (**C**). At high power, DLBCL has an angiocentric growth pattern (**D**).

by extensive infiltration in brain parenchyma (Figure 14-2C and D). Reticulin stain highlights concentric deposition of reticulin around the involved vessels, which are infiltrated and dissected by lymphoma cells imparting an "onion bulb" appearance.

DLBCL is the most common type of PCNSL. DCBCLs are positive for B-cell markers (CD20, CD79a, PAX-5), but negative for T-cell markers (CD3, CD2, CD4, CD8), although rare CD5-positive cases have been reported. Leukocyte common antigen (CD45) is not reliable for the diagnosis of CNS DLBCLs because it can be negative or only focally positive. An algorithm based on a panel of immunohistochemical markers (CD10, BCL-6, and MUM-1) has been developed to subclassify DLBCLs into two major subtypes: activated B cell like (ABC) (positive for MUM-1 and negative for CD10) (Figure 14-3A) and germinal center B cell like (GCB) (either positive for CD10 or positive for BCL-6 while negative for MUM-1) (Figure 14-3B and C).[2–5] Two studies have shown that in the CNS, GCB DLBCLs might have a better prognosis than do ABC DLBCLs.[6,7] However, several other studies did not reveal significant difference in overall survival between these two groups.[8–11] Anaplastic variant of DLBCL is extremely rare characterized by large to very large round, oval, or polygonal cells with bizarre pleomorphic nuclei, extensive necrosis, and many mitotic figures, mimicking undifferentiated carcinoma or melanoma (Figure 14-3D). *In situ* hybridization for Epstein-Barr virus–encoded small RNAs (EBERs) is positive in primary CNS DLBCLs in patients with AIDS.

PTCL, not otherwise specified (NOS), can present as PCNSL. Lymphoma cells are intermediate and/or large in size, admixed with reactive small T and B lymphocytes and histiocytes. They can express some or all pan T-cell markers such as CD2, CD3, CD5, and CD7 with or without

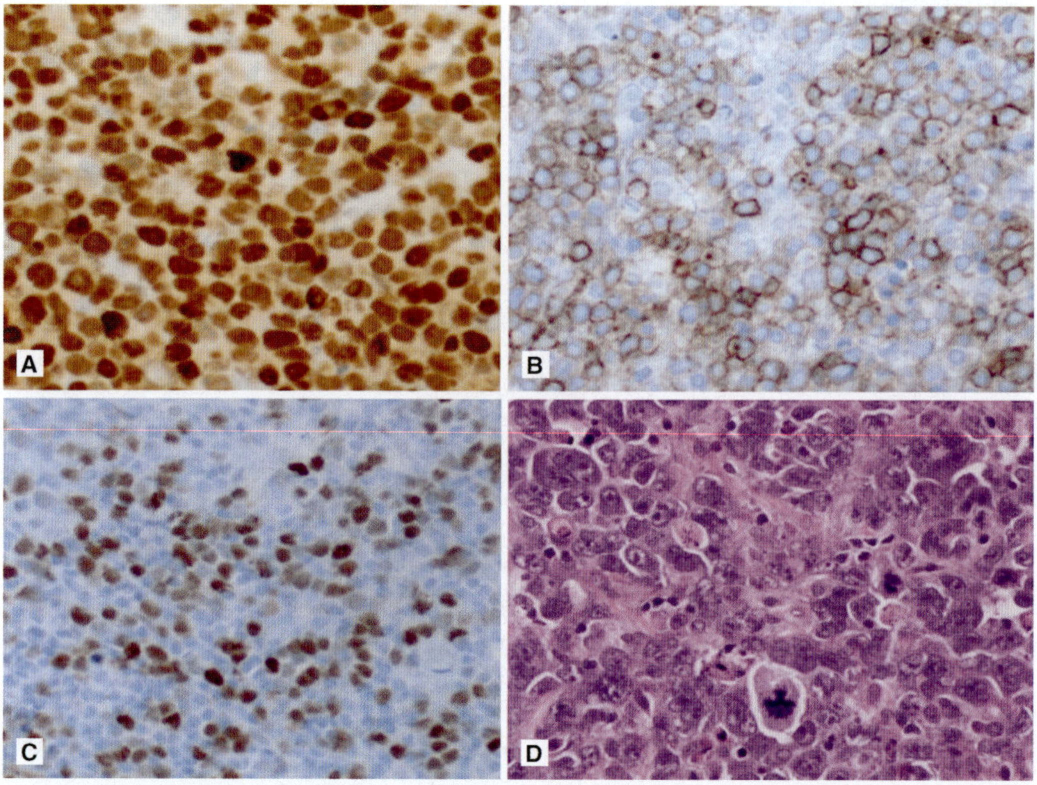

FIGURE 14-3: Primary CNS diffuse large B-cell lymphoma (DLBCL). Activated B-cell like subtype. Lymphoma cell nuclei are positive for MUM-1 (lymphoma cells are negative for CD10, data not shown) (**A**). Germinal central B-cell like subtype. Lymphoma cells are positive for CD10 with membranous staining pattern (lymphoma cells are negative for MUM-1, data not shown) (**B**). Lymphoma cell nuclei are positive for BCL-6 (**C**). Primary CNS DLBCL, anaplastic variant, with undifferentiated polymorphic tumor cells, multinucleated giant cells, and conspicuous mitotic activity (**D**).

CD4 or CD8 positivity (Figure 14-4A and B). The Ki-67 labeling index is markedly elevated in these lymphoma cells (Figure 14-4C). For difficult cases, PCR for T-cell receptor gene arrangement should be performed to confirm the diagnosis of PTCL, NOS.

Anaplastic large cell lymphoma (ALCL) rarely occurs in the CNS. Cytologic evaluation of the smear reveals many large pleomorphic cells with abundant cytoplasm, horseshoe- or wreath-shaped nuclei, and prominent nucleoli. Eosinophils can be seen in the background. Histologically, ALCL is characterized by scattered large pleomorphic cells admixed with histiocytes, small lymphocytes, and eosinophils (Figure 14-4D). The large atypical cells are strongly positive for CD30 (Figure 14-4E) with or without ALK-1 expression. The tumor cells exhibit high proliferation index.

Lastly, other types of lymphomas, such as Hodgkin lymphoma, Burkitt lymphoma, and low-grade B-cell lymphoma rarely present as PCNSL.

The Effect of Corticosteroids on the Diagnosis of PCNSL

If the stereotactic biopsy is applied, it must be done before the glucocorticoid therapy. The administration of steroid has a direct antitumor effect on lymphoma, resulting in apoptosis and lysis of tumor cells, and can cause dramatic reduction in MRI abnormalities (Figure 14-1A and B). In some cases, the malignant B cells may vanish, which makes the diagnosis of lymphoma on brain biopsy impossible. In other cases, only scattered residual malignant B cells are present in the biopsy. In order to make a diagnosis of B-cell lymphoma, it is necessary to demonstrate that the large atypical cells are positive for CD20, while the Ki-67 labeling index is extremely high in these large atypical cells (often >50%) (Figure 14-5). However, CD20 expression alone without the high proliferation index is not enough to make a definitive diagnosis of B-cell lymphoma.

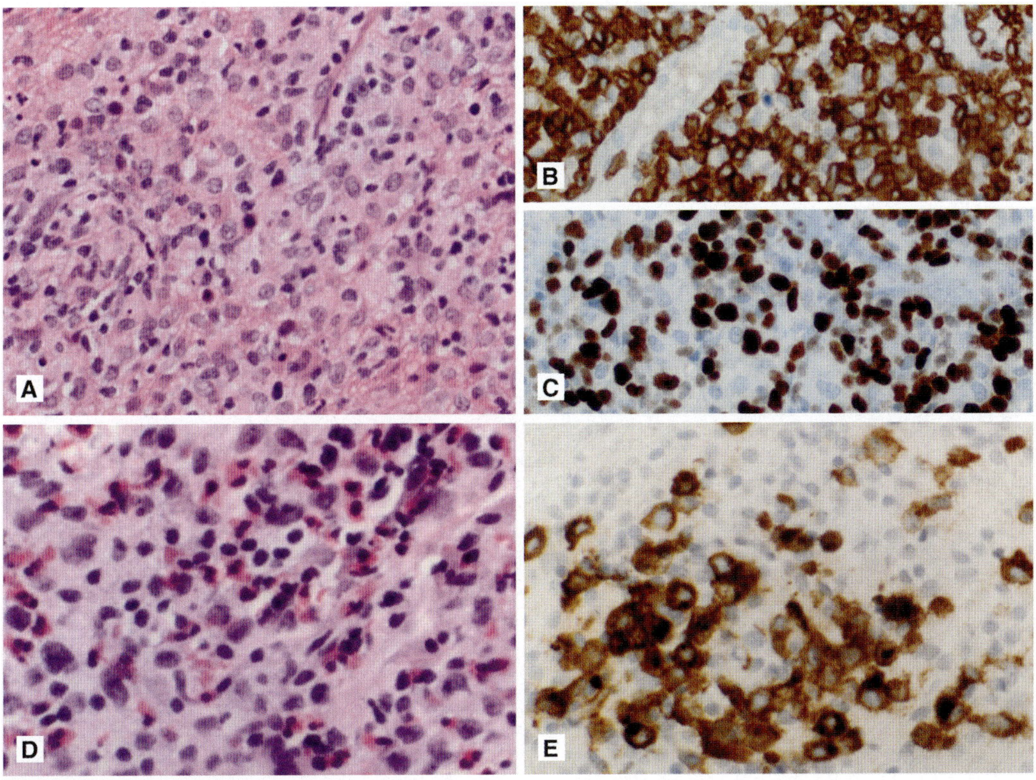

FIGURE 14-4: Primary CNS T-cell lymphoma. Primary CNS T-cell lymphoma in cerebellum (**A–C**). Brain tissue infiltrated with numerous large atypical lymphoma cells admixed with reactive small lymphocytes and histiocytes (**A**). Large atypical lymphoma cells are strongly and diffusely positive for CD3 in membranous staining pattern (**B**). The Ki-67 labeling index is markedly elevated (>80%) in large atypical lymphoma cells (**C**). ALCL in brain. H&E-stained slide demonstrates scattered large pleomorphic cells admixed with some histiocytes, small lymphocytes, and eosinophils (**D**). Large atypical cells are positive for CD30 (**E**).

The expression of MUM-1, BCL-6, or CD10 in the large atypical cells is very helpful for the diagnosis of B-cell lymphoma in this setting although a very small subset of CNS lymphomas can be CD20+, MUM-1(−), BCL-6(−), and CD10(−).

Treatment

Systemic administration of high-dose methotrexate can achieve therapeutic levels in brain parenchyma and is the single most effective chemotherapeutic agent for PCNSL. Although the combination of chemotherapy and radiation therapy has more than doubled the survival time in PCNSL patients, over 50% of the patients who survive more than 18 months on chemoradiation therapy will develop dementia. Radiation therapy is probably the best second-line treatment option for PCNSL.

Prognosis

Methotrexate-based chemotherapy as the sole treatment for immunocompetent patients can result in a median survival time of 21 to 48 months. Patients with AIDS have a 4-month median survival duration with radiation therapy alone and 10 to 18-month median survival with the combination of chemotherapy and whole-brain radiotherapy.

Prognostic and Diagnostic Biomarkers

It has been initially shown that GCB type of CNS DLBCL might have a better prognosis than does ABC type of DLBCL.[7] However, several recent studies did not reveal any significant difference in overall survival between these two groups.[12] BCL-6 as a prognostic marker for PCNSL is still controversial. Two studies have shown that overexpression of BCL-6 was associated with improved

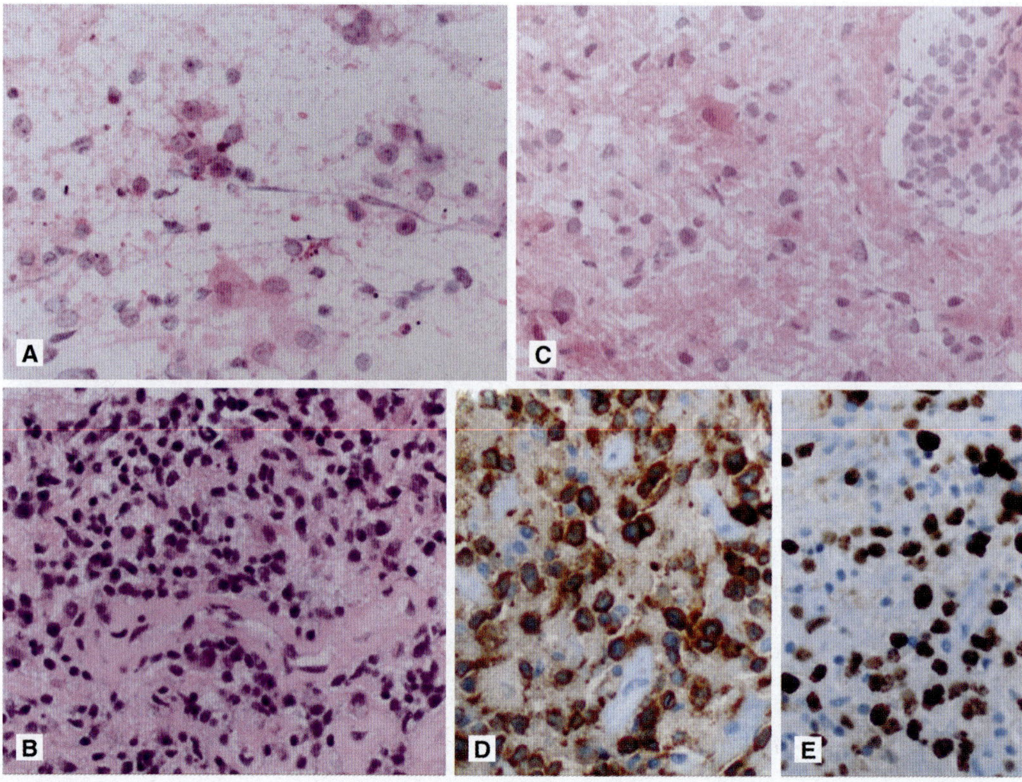

FIGURE 14-5: Steroid-treated PCNSL. Intraoperative consultation smear demonstrates rare large atypical cells with prominent nuclei as well as scattered reactive astrocytes, small lymphocytes, and histiocytes (**A**). Frozen section shows rare perivascular lymphocytic cuffing and rare large atypical cells in the brain parenchyma while there are numerous reactive astrocytes, histiocytes, and small lymphocytes (**B**). Permanent section shows lymphohistiocytic infiltrate in the brain parenchyma (**C**). Scattered larger atypical cells are positive for CD20 (**D**) and Ki-67 (**E**).

survival in PCNSL.[13,14] In contrast, three other studies demonstrated that BCL-6 expression by tumor cells was an independent predictor of poorer overall survival.[10,15,16] Other studies did not reveal any difference in survival between the two groups.[12] BCL-2 was found to be expressed by tumor cells in 49% to 80.9% of primary CNS DLBCL patients.[12,17] So far there was no statistically survival difference between BCL-2 positive and negative DLBCLs.[12]

Recently, efforts have been made to identify potential biomarkers in the serum and CSF in PCNSL patients. One study has shown that the serum levels of YKL-40 and MMP-9 were correlated with CNS lymphoma disease status, radiographic appearance, and length of survival. They concluded that the serum YKL-40 and MMP-9 levels were good indicators for the tumor burden.[18] Other studies have shown that the levels of CXCL13, IL-10, miR-21, miR-19, and miR-92a were significantly increased in CSF samples from PCNSL patients compared with controls with inflammatory CNS disease or other neurologic disorders.[19–21] Besides brain biopsy, these biomarkers may become alternative tools for the diagnosis of PCNSLs in the near future.

LYMPHOMAS INVOLVING THE CNS AND OTHER MULTIPLE ORGANS

Lymphomatoid Granulomatosis

Lymphomatoid granulomatosis (LYG) is a very rare type of B-cell lymphoproliferative disorder that is EBV driven. It almost always involves the lungs presenting with multiple bilateral pulmonary nodules and commonly affects the skin and CNS at multiple foci. The liver and kidney also can

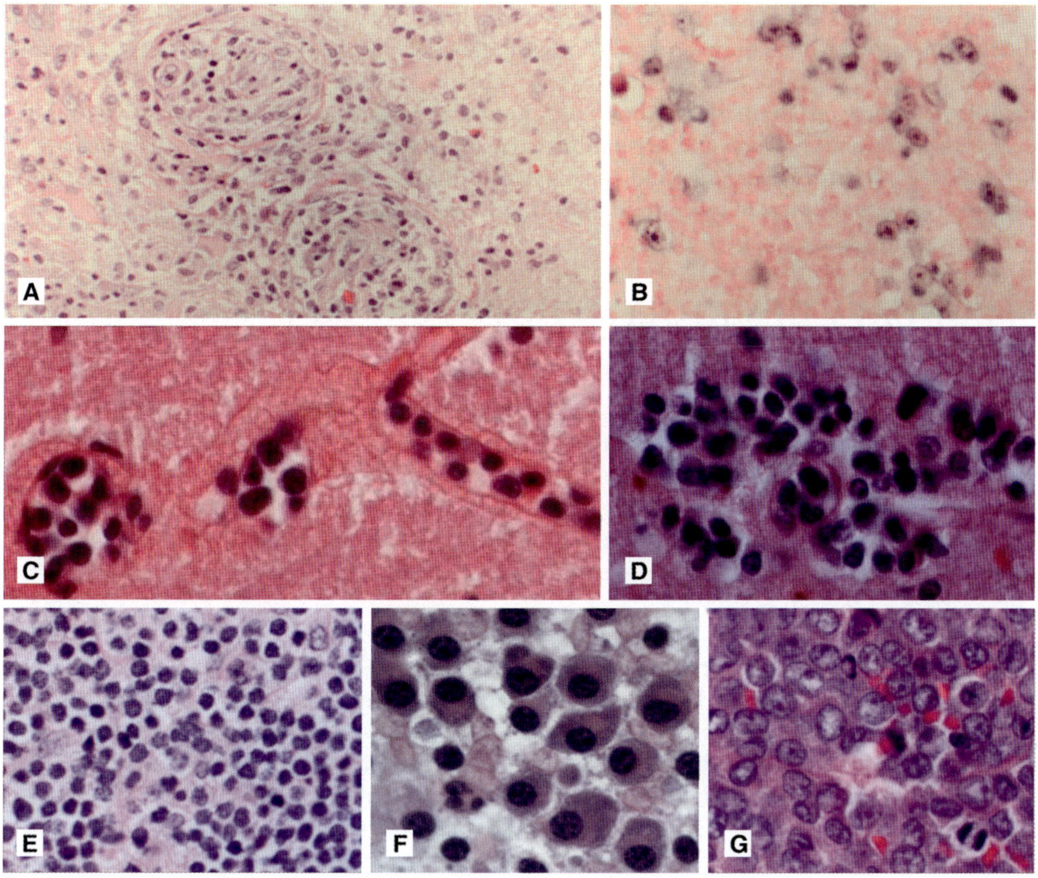

FIGURE 14-6: Lymphomatoid granulomatosis. H&E-stained slide reveals an angiocentric and angiodestructive accumulation of small lymphocytes, histiocytes, plasma cells, and large atypical lymphocytes with prominent nucleoli (**A**). EBER *in situ* hybridization demonstrates the nuclei of large atypical lymphocytes are positive (**B**). IVL in brain. H&E-stained slide shows large atypical lymphoma cells in the cerebral capillaries without intraparenchymal involvement (**C**). CNS involvement by acute monocytic leukemia. H&E-stained slide demonstrates that leukemia cells migrate through and damage intraparenchymal blood vessels (**D**). Primary dural MZL (mucosa-associated lymphoid tissue lymphoma). H&E-stained slide shows sheets of small-sized monotonous lymphocytes (**E**). Plasmacytoma. Intraoperative consultation smear demonstrates tumor cells with abundant cytoplasm and eccentric nuclei with heterochromatin in a characteristic clock-face arrangement (**F**). MS (myelomonocytic type). H&E-stained slide, at high power, demonstrates sheets of large atypical tumor cells with open chromatin, prominent nucleoli, and certain amount of basophilic cytoplasm (**G**).

be involved. Brain tissue sections show an angiocentric and angiodestructive accumulation of a variable number of clonal EBV-positive B cells admixed with small lymphocytes, histiocytes, and plasma cells (Figure 14-6A). Perivascular geographic necrosis and hemorrhage are very common in LYG. In order to make a diagnosis of LYG, *in situ* hybridization for EBV should be positive in these large atypical B cells (Figure 14-6B). LYG can progress to EBV-positive DLBCL; so it is considered as a malignant B-cell lymphoma by the majority of pathologists.[22] LYG can be graded into three groups based on the proportion of EBV-positive B cells relative to the reactive lymphocyte background: grade I, EBV-positive cells are infrequently identified; grade II, EBV-positive cells readily detected and usually number 5 to 20/high-power field by *in situ* hybridization; and grade III, numerous atypical B cells and EBV-positive cells.[22] The treatment for high-grade LG is similar to that for DLBCL.

Intravascular Lymphomatosis

Intravascular lymphomatosis (IVL) is a rare lymphoproliferative disorder characterized by the neoplastic lymphoid cells being mainly lodged in the lumens of small or intermediate vessels with no or minimal intraparenchymal involvement. Although IVL can rarely present as pure CNS disease, it usually involves brain and many other organs such as the skin, kidney, heart, lung, and adrenal gland. The clinical presentation can be variable ranging from rash to focal or diffuse neurologic symptoms. Brain biopsy shows intravascular proliferation of larger atypical lymphoid cells with prominent nucleoli and brisk mitoses (Figure 14-6C). The vast majority of IVL are of B-cell lineage. It is very aggressive and usually fatal without treatment. IVL temporally responds to steroid and can be treated by combination chemotherapy (i.e., rituximab, cyclophosphamide, Adriamycin, Oncovin, and prednisone).[23]

SECONDARY HEMATOLYMPHOID TUMORS

Secondary Lymphoma

Secondary involvement of the CNS by systemic lymphoma now becomes less common due to the successful systemic chemotherapy and targeted therapy. By far, B-cell lymphomas, especially high-grade ones such as DLBCL and Burkitt lymphoma, more commonly metastasize to CNS compared to Hodgkin lymphoma or PTCLs. Typically, secondary lymphomas first involve leptomeninges, cranial and spinal nerve root, and Virchow-Robin spaces (VRS), and then invade into brain parenchyma. At the late stage, by histology alone, PCNSL and secondary lymphoma are indistinguishable.

Secondary Leukemia

Due to aggressive treatment for acute leukemia, including CNS prophylaxis, the incidence of the secondary involvement of CNS by acute leukemia appears to have decreased. Acute lymphoblastic leukemia (ALL) has the highest incidence to develop secondary CNS involvement. Histologically, ALL exhibits similar features to high-grade B-cell lymphoma. Acute myeloid leukemia, acute myelomonocytic leukemia, or acute monocytic leukemia also can develop secondary CNS involvement; leukemia cells migrate through and damage intraparenchymal small blood vessels (Figure 14-6D), which cause microhemorrhage around these blood vessels. In the late phase, the patient develops intraparenchymal hematoma.

OTHER HEMATOLYMPHOID AND HISTIOCYTIC TUMORS

Primary Dural Lymphoma

Definition

Primary dural lymphoma (PDL) is a rare type of lymphoma that arises from the dura mater. PDL usually is a low-grade marginal zone lymphoma (MZL).

Clinical Features

PDL is a rare type of lymphoma and the incidence is unknown. PDL occurs in middle-age patients with a female predilection (the female/male ratio is 3 to 4:1).[24,25] The most common clinical presentations for intracranial PDL are headaches, seizures, focal sensory or motor deficits, visual disturbances, nausea, vomiting, and ataxia. Spinal cord PDL commonly causes radicular pain and paraparesis.[26]

Neuroimaging Findings

On MRI, PDL usually exhibits homogeneous solid contrast enhancing single or multiple extra-axial masses, which mimics meningioma. Dural tail sign, brain vasogenic edema, calvarial hyperostosis, and bone erosion can be seen. Cerebral convexities are the most common location followed by falx, tentorium, sellar/parasellar region, intraventricular, or spinal cord.

Pathologic Features

Intraoperative consultation cytologic preparations from PDL (MZL) show hypercellular smear with small- to medium-sized monomorphic lymphocytes. On frozen section and permanent sections, the lymphoma consists of mostly small- to medium-sized lymphocytes with monocytoid morphology, plasma cells, and occasional large transformed cells (Figure 14-6E). The lymphoma cells express B-cell markers (CD20 and CD79a), but are negative for CD10, CD5, and CD23. CD43 is positive in a subset of cases. In difficult cases, PCR for immunoglobulin gene arrangement should be performed for the confirmation of the diagnosis of MZL lymphoma. Very rarely, high-grade non-Hodgkin lymphoma, follicular lymphoma, Hodgkin lymphoma, or ALCL can present as PDL.[26–32]

Treatment and Prognosis

The treatment for PDL is surgical resection with or without radiation therapy. If gross total resection is achieved, no additional treatment is needed. For most cases in which tumors are subtotally resected, the patients should be treated with local radiation therapy or systemic chemotherapy. PDL (MZL) responds well to therapies, is more indolent, and has a better prognosis than parenchymal PCNSL. However, systemic relapses/recurrences can occur several years after the initial diagnosis of PDL.[33] Long-term clinical follow-up is recommended for all patients.

Plasmacytoma

It is well known that multiple myeloma occasionally involves skull, intracranial soft tissue, or brain parenchyma. Solitary extraosseous intracranial plasmacytoma is a very rare entity, which commonly presents as a nodular or a plaque-like dural mass and mimics meningioma (Figure 14-7A). A few cases of intrasellar plasmacytoma and rare cases of pure intraparenchymal plasmacytoma have been reported.

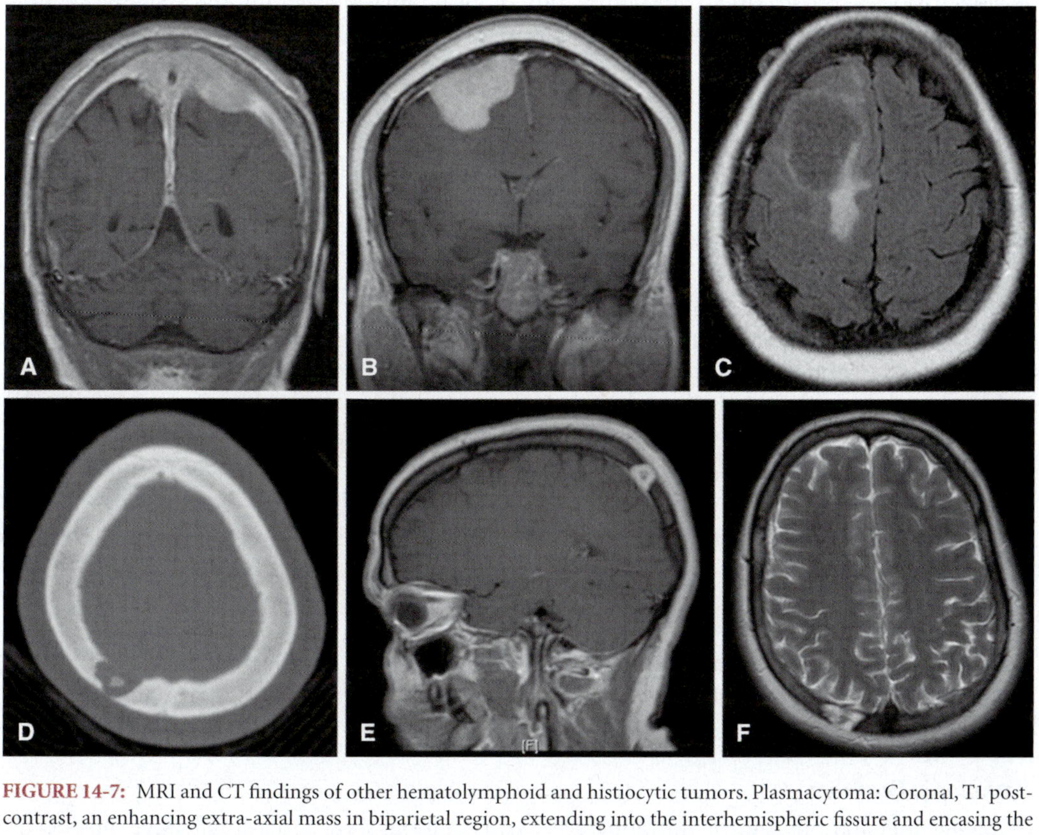

FIGURE 14-7: MRI and CT findings of other hematolymphoid and histiocytic tumors. Plasmacytoma: Coronal, T1 postcontrast, an enhancing extra-axial mass in biparietal region, extending into the interhemispheric fissure and encasing the superior sagittal sinus (**A**). Rosai-Dorfman disease: Coronal, T1 postcontrast, an enhancing extra-axial dura-based mass in right frontoparietal region (**B**). Axial, fluid attenuated inversion recovery, peritumoral brain edema (**C**). LCH: CT, Axial, a lytic lesion in the high right parietal calvarium (**D**). Sagittal, T1 postcontrast, an enhancing lesion at right parietal involving calvarium and dura (**E**). Axial, T2, hyperintense signal on T2 (**F**).

Cytologic preparations during intraoperative consultation demonstrate a cellular smear containing tumor cells with abundant cytoplasm and eccentric nuclei. The nuclear chromatin shows the characteristic clock-face arrangement (Figure 14-6F). There are occasional binucleated and multinucleated cells. The cytologic preparation is much superior to the frozen section. H&E-stained slides show sheets of tumor cells with abundant basophilic cytoplasm and eccentric nuclei with heterochromatin in a clock-face arrangement. Plasmacytoma cells are positive for CD138, CD38, EMA, and MUM-1 but negative for CD45. Both immunohistochemistry and *in situ* hybridization for kappa and lambda light chains can be used to evaluate the clonality. *In situ* hybridization shows low background staining and is much more reliable compared to immunohistochemistry. The main differential diagnosis is plasma cell granuloma, which has intermixed reactive lymphocytes, histiocytes, other inflammatory cells, vascular hyperplasia, and fibrosis. In addition, plasma cell granuloma lacks the restricted expression of light chains.

Surgical resection is the choice of treatment. Local radiation therapy can be used for residual or recurrent disease. Solitary intracranial plasmacytoma is indolent and has a good prognosis if it is not associated with multiple myeloma.

Myeloid Sarcoma

Myeloid sarcoma (MS) is an extramedullary manifestation of acute myeloid leukemia and is also called as granulocytic sarcoma or chloroma. Rarely, MS can occur in brain, spinal cord, or leptomeninges/dura. Histologically, there are sheets of large atypical cells with pleomorphic nuclei and abundant cytoplasm (Figure 14-6G). High-grade lymphoma is the main differential diagnosis. MS is positive for some of the myeloid or monocytic markers such as CD117, CD33, CD15, CD68, myeloperoxidase, or lysozyme. The combination of local radiation therapy and systemic chemotherapy is used to treat MS. However, the prognosis is grave with 6-month median survival.

Rosai-Dorfman Disease

Definition

Rosai-Dorfman disease (Aka: sinus histiocytosis with massive lymphadenopathy) is a benign histiocytic proliferative disorder that often involves lymph nodes and presents as massive lymphadenopathy with sinus histiocytosis.

Historical Background and Clinical Features

Rosai-Dorfman disease was first reported in 1969 in a young black male with sinus histiocytosis and massive lymphadenopathy.[34] Rosai-Dorfman disease predominantly occurs in children and young adults with a mean age of 20.6 years and a slight male predilection.[35,36] Extranodal involvement is reported in 43% of the cases and the most common extranodal sites are skin, nasal cavity, paranasal sinus, eyelid, orbit, bone, salivary gland, and CNS.[35–38] The CNS involvement (predominantly affecting dura/leptomeninges) is only seen in less than 5% of cases.[39–41] CNS Rosai-Dorfman disease usually affects middle-aged patients with a mean age of 39.4-year old and has a male predilection.[42]

Neuroimaging Findings

Rosai-Dorfman disease typically exhibits a homogeneous solid contrast-enhancing extra-axial mass on MRI that mimics meningioma (Figure 14-7B and C). Dural tail sign or brain vasogenic edema can be seen.[43,44]

Pathologic Features

Cytologic preparations during intraoperative consultation show occasional large histiocytes engulfing small lymphocytes or plasma cells (emperipolesis) (Figure 14-8A). Scattered small lymphocytes and other inflammatory cells are seen in the background. At low power, the frozen section and permanent section reveal scattered pale nodules or islands in a fibrotic background

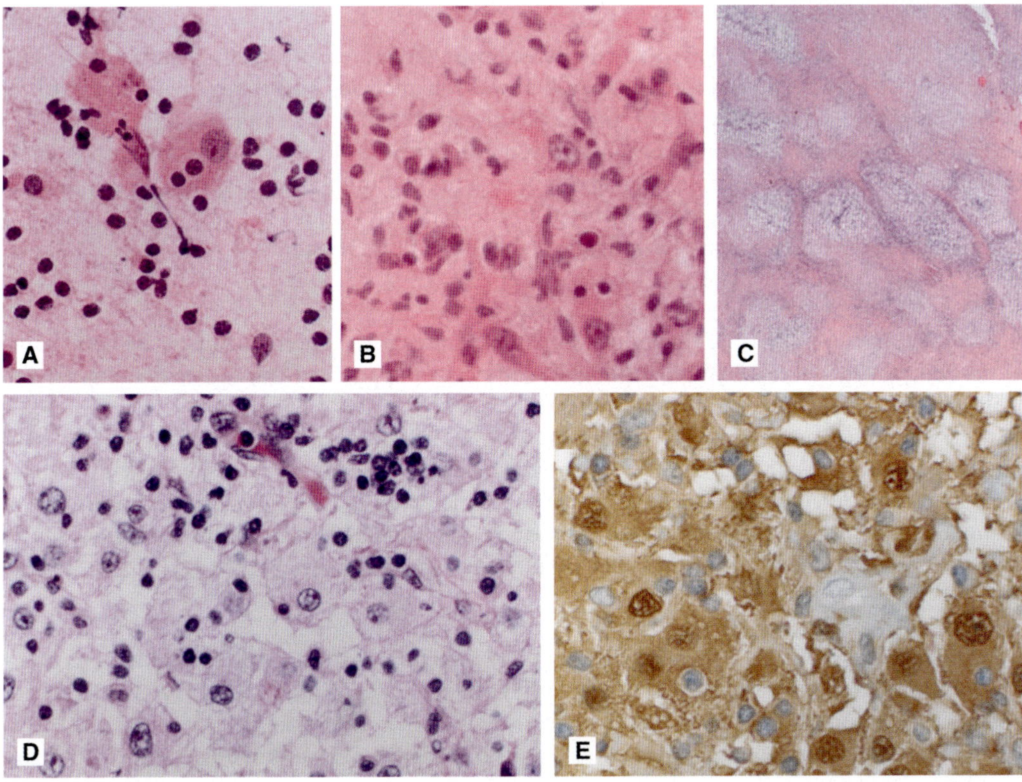

FIGURE 14-8: Rosai-Dorfman disease. Intraoperative consultation smear demonstrates occasional histiocytes with small lymphocytes in their cytoplasm (emperipolesis). Scattered small lymphocytes are in the background (**A**). Frozen section shows epithelioid histiocytes with small lymphocytes in their cytoplasm while chronic inflammatory cells are in the background (**B**). H&E-stained slide shows pale nodules or islands in the fibrotic background at low power (**C**). H&E-stained slide, at high power, demonstrates sheets of epithelioid histiocytes with pale to eosinophilic cytoplasm admixed with lymphocytes and other inflammatory cells (**D**). Lymphocytes and other inflammatory cells present within the cytoplasm of these histiocytes (emperipolesis). These histiocytes are positive for S100 protein while lymphocytes within these histiocytes are negative for S100 protein (**E**).

(Figure 14-8C). At high power, there are sheets of epithelioid histiocytes with pale to eosinophilic cytoplasm intermixed with lymphocytes and other inflammatory cells (Figure 14-8B and D). Within the cytoplasm of these epithelioid histiocytes are lymphocytes, plasma cells, and red blood cells (emperipolesis). The nuclei of these histiocytes are round or oval, with vesicular chromatin and single small nucleolus. Rare histiocytes are multinucleated. The histiocytes express S100 protein, CD68, and HAM 56, but are negative for CD1a. Emperipolesis is much better appreciated on S100 protein stain since lymphocytes within these S100 protein–positive histiocytes are negative for S100 protein (Figure 14-8E).

Treatment and Prognosis

Rosai-Dorfman disease can be treated by gross total or subtotal resection. Residual or recurrent lesions can be successfully treated with local radiation therapy or systemic corticosteroid. However, data on the long-term outcomes of patients with CNS Rosai-Dorfman disease are still very limited.

Langerhans Cell Histiocytosis

Definition

Langerhans cell histiocytosis (LCH) is a group of neoplastic diseases characterized by the clonal proliferation of bone marrow–derived dendritic Langerhans cells.

Historical Background

Hand-Schüller-Christian disease, Abt-Letterer-Siwe disease, eosinophilic granuloma, and histiocytosis X have been used for this disease. It was renamed as Langerhans cell histiocytosis in 1985 by the Histiocyte Society. According to the disease extent, LCH can be subclassified as follows: (i) single-system LCH, single organ involvement, can be unifocal or multifocal and (ii) multisystem LCH, involving multiple organs, can be in a limited number of organs or disseminated. CNS involvement in LCH has been reported in the very early published cases of the disease.[45] Recently, more CNS lesions have been diagnosed by MRI in LCH patients.[46,47]

Clinical Features

The annual incidence for LCH ranges from 0.5 to 5.4 cases per million persons. LCH commonly affects children aged 0 to 15 years, although it can occur in patients from the neonatal period to adulthood. Male and female are equally affected.

The most common clinical presentations in CNS LCH are diabetes insipidus and anterior pituitary hormone deficiency due to the involvement of the hypothalamic/pituitary region. Neurodegenerative changes due to diffuse intraparenchymal LCH lesions are the second most frequent clinical presentation. The manifestation related to LCH lesions in the extra-axial spaces (i.e., the meninges, pineal gland, and choroid plexus) is less frequent.[45,47]

Neuroimaging Findings

Computed tomographic (CT) scan can reveal these lytic lesions in calvarium (Figure 14-7D).

According to the Histiocyte Society (http://dx.doi.org/10.1594/ecr2014/C-1293), the radiologic manifestations of LCH in the CNS can be classified into two groups: (1) intracranial extra-axial lesions: (a) hypothalamic–pituitary axis and (b) other locations (meninges, choroid plexus, pineal gland); and (2) intracranial intra-axial lesions: (a) intraparenchymal lesions, (b) neurodegenerative disease, and (c) other findings: dilated VRS.

MRI findings of patients with diabetes insipidus include thickening and enhancement of the pituitary stalk, accompanied by lack of the normal T1WI shortening in the posterior pituitary, and the atrophy of the stalk in the late phase of LCH. Meningeal lesions show iso- or hyperintense on T1 and hyperintense on T2WI with moderate or marked, homogeneous contrast enhancement (Figure 14-7E and F). Choroid plexus or pineal gland lesions demonstrate homogeneous contrast enhancement and a marked signal intensity loss on T2WI, suggesting calcification.

Intraparenchymal lesions or tumor-like lesions exhibit rounded masses with iso- or hypointense on T1 and hyperintense on T2WI, intense contrast enhancement and have well-demarcated edges with surrounding brain edema and mass effect.

For neurodegenerative disease, dentate nuclei appears as moderate T2 hypointense and T1 hyperintense signal while the white matter of the cerebellum appears as symmetrical hyperintense on T2 and fluid attenuated inversion recovery without contrast enhancement. In severe cases, the abnormal signal can spread to the cerebellar peduncles and pons. Basal ganglia (especially globus pallidus) show bilateral, symmetrical hyperintense on T1WI, variable signal intensities on T2WI, and no contrast enhancement. Leukoencephalopathy-like pattern (poorly defined hyperintense areas on T2WI in the cerebral periventricular white matter, pons and cerebellar white matter, without mass effect or enhancement) has been described.

Cerebellar and supratentorial atrophy and dilated VRS can be seen in CNS LCH.

Pathologic Features

Smears during intraoperative consultation demonstrate scattered histiocytes with coffee bean-shaped nuclei (Figure 14-9A). Frozen section shows sheets of histiocytes with coffee bean-shaped nuclei. Occasional eosinophils can be seen on smears and frozen sections, which might lack granular cytoplasm (Figure 14-9B). However, bi-lobar nuclei are a key feature to recognize eosinophils on smears and frozen sections. At low power, permanent sections show small granulomatous nodules in the fibrotic tissue (Figure 14-9C). At high power, there are sheets of Langerhans cells with distinct

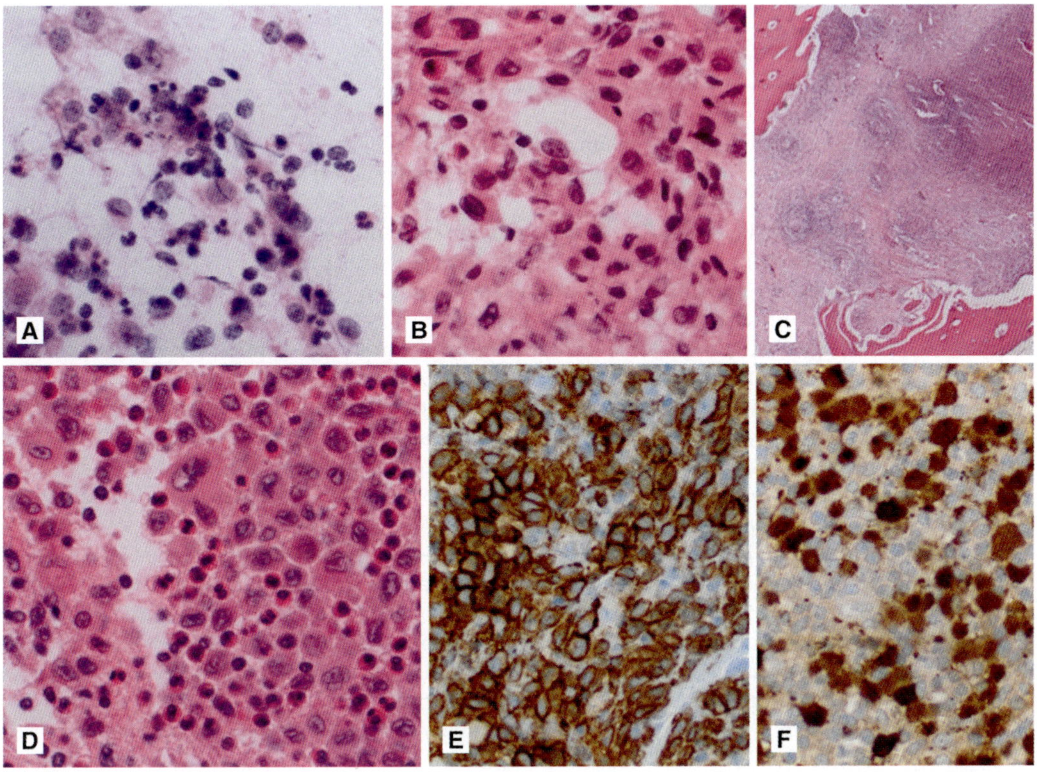

FIGURE 14-9: Langerhans cell histiocytosis. Intraoperative consultation smear demonstrates scattered histiocytes with coffee bean–shaped nuclei. Scattered eosinophils are in the background (**A**). Frozen section shows sheets of histiocytes with coffee bean–shaped nuclei while rare eosinophils are in the background (**B**). H&E-stained slide shows small nodules in the fibrotic tissue within the calvarium at low power, which mimic granulomas (**C**). H&E-stained slide, at high power, demonstrates sheets of Langerhans cells with distinct cell margin and pink granular cytoplasm are admixed with numerous eosinophils (**D**). Langerhans cells are positive for CD1a (**E**). Langerhans cells are positive for S100 protein (**F**).

cell border, pink granular cytoplasm, and coffee bean-shaped nuclei with longitudinal grooves, which are intermixed with numerous eosinophils (Figure 14-9D). Immunohistochemically, Langerhans cells are positive for CD68, S100 protein, CD1a, and CD207 (langerin) (Figure 14-9E and F). CD207 (langerin), a C-type lectin, is selectively expressed by Langerhans cells. CD207 (langerin) immunostain for the diagnosis of LCH is superior to CD1a and S100 protein. Electron microscopy demonstrates Birbeck granules in the cytoplasm of these Langerhans cells.

Recently, the recurrent oncogenic *BRAF V600E* mutation are identified in more than 50% of LCH,[48–51] which indicates that LCH is a neoplastic process and may respond to BRAF pathway inhibitors.

Treatment and Prognosis

The treatment for single skull lesion is curettage only, curettage plus injection of methylprednisolone, or radiation therapy.

For LCH patients with mass lesions in the hypothalamic–pituitary region, choroid plexus, gray matter, or white matter, chemotherapy such as vinblastine with or without corticosteroids, cladribine (2-CdA), or cytarabine, can be effective.[52–54]

The patients with neurodegenerative disease have been treated with dexamethasone, 2-CdA, retinoic acid, intravenous immunoglobulin, infliximab, or cytarabine with or without vincristine.[55–59]

The prognosis depends on the extent of organ involvement. The patients with a single-focus disease have an excellent prognosis. More than half of patients with multifocal disease have a chronic course. The patients with disseminated disease have the worst prognosis.

References

1. Deckert M, Paulus W. Malignant lymphomas. In: Louis DN, Ohgaki H, Wiestler OD, et al., eds. *WHO Classification of Tumour of the Central Nervous System*. Lyon, France: International Agency for Research on Cancer; 2007.
2. Berglund M, Thunberg U, Amini RM, et al. Evaluation of immunophenotype in diffuse large B-cell lymphoma and its impact on prognosis. *Mod Pathol* 2005;18:1113–1120.
3. Alizadeh AA, Eisen MB, Davis RE, et al. Distinct types of diffuse large B-cell lymphoma identified by gene expression profiling. *Nature* 2000;403:503–511.
4. Rosenwald A, Wright G, Chan WC, et al. The use of molecular profiling to predict survival after chemotherapy for diffuse large-B-cell lymphoma. *N Engl J Med* 2002;346:1937–1947.
5. Hans CP, Weisenburger DD, Greiner TC, et al. Confirmation of the molecular classification of diffuse large B-cell lymphoma by immunohistochemistry using a tissue microarray. *Blood* 2004;103:275–282.
6. Lin CH, Kuo KT, Chuang SS, et al. Comparison of the expression and prognostic significance of differentiation markers between diffuse large B-cell lymphoma of central nervous system origin and peripheral nodal origin. *Clin Cancer Res* 2006;12:1152–1156.
7. Bhagavathi S, Sharathkumar A, Hunter S, et al. Activated B-cell immunophenotype might be associated with poor prognosis of primary central nervous system lymphomas. *Clin Neuropathol* 2008;27:13–20.
8. Imai H, Shimada K, Shimada S, et al. Comparative clinicopathological study of primary CNS diffuse large B-cell lymphoma and intravascular large B-cell lymphoma. *Pathol Int* 2009;59:431–437.
9. Raoux D, Duband S, Forest F, et al. Primary central nervous system lymphoma: immunohistochemical profile and prognostic significance. *Neuropathology* 2010;30:232–240.
10. Hattab EM, Martin SE, Al Khatib SM, et al. Most primary central nervous system diffuse large B-cell lymphomas occurring in immunocompetent individuals belong to the nongerminal center subtype: a retrospective analysis of 31 cases. *Mod Pathol* 2010;23:235–243.
11. Camilleri-Broet S, Criniere E, Broet P, et al. A uniform activated B-cell-like immunophenotype might explain the poor prognosis of primary central nervous system lymphomas: analysis of 83 cases. *Blood* 2006;107:190–196.
12. Zhang X, Chen QH, Farmer P, et al. Central nervous system lymphoma in immunocompetent patients: the North Shore-Long Island Jewish Health System experience. *J Clin Neurosci* 2013;20:75–79.
13. Braaten KM, Betensky RA, de Leval L, et al. BCL-6 expression predicts improved survival in patients with primary central nervous system lymphoma. *Clin Cancer Res* 2003;9:1063–1069.
14. Song MK, Chung JS, Joo YD, et al. Clinical importance of Bcl-6-positive non-deep-site involvement in non-HIV-related primary central nervous system diffuse large B-cell lymphoma. *J Neurooncol* 2011;104: 825–831.
15. Chang CC, Kampalath B, Schultz C, et al. Expression of p53, c-Myc, or Bcl-6 suggests a poor prognosis in primary central nervous system diffuse large B-cell lymphoma among immunocompetent individuals. *Arch Pathol Lab Med* 2003;127:208–212.
16. Rubenstein JL, Hsi ED, Johnson JL, et al. Intensive chemotherapy and immunotherapy in patients with newly diagnosed primary CNS lymphoma: CALGB 50202 (Alliance 50202). *J Clin Oncol* 2013;31: 3061–3068.
17. Deckert-Schluter M, Rang A, Wiestler OD. Apoptosis and apoptosis-related gene products in primary non-Hodgkin's lymphoma of the central nervous system. *Acta Neuropathol* 1998;96:157–162.
18. Hottinger AF, Iwamoto FM, Karimi S, et al. YKL-40 and MMP-9 as serum markers for patients with primary central nervous system lymphoma. *Ann Neurol* 2011;70:163–169.
19. Rubenstein JL, Wong VS, Kadoch C, et al. CXCL13 plus interleukin 10 is highly specific for the diagnosis of CNS lymphoma. *Blood* 2013;121:4740–4748.
20. Baraniskin A, Kuhnhenn J, Schlegel U, et al. MicroRNAs in cerebrospinal fluid as biomarker for disease course monitoring in primary central nervous system lymphoma. *J Neurooncol* 2012;109:239–244.
21. Baraniskin A, Kuhnhenn J, Schlegel U, et al. Identification of microRNAs in the cerebrospinal fluid as marker for primary diffuse large B-cell lymphoma of the central nervous system. *Blood* 2011;117: 3140–3146.
22. Dunleavy K, Roschewski M, Wilson WH. Lymphomatoid granulomatosis and other Epstein-Barr virus associated lymphoproliferative processes. *Curr Hematol Malig Rep* 2012;7:208–215.

23. Orwat DE, Batalis NI. Intravascular large B-cell lymphoma. *Arch Pathol Lab Med* 2012;136:333–338.
24. Iwamoto FM, Abrey LE. Primary dural lymphomas: a review. *Neurosurg Focus* 2006;21:E5.
25. Tu PH, Giannini C, Judkins AR, et al. Clinicopathologic and genetic profile of intracranial marginal zone lymphoma: a primary low-grade CNS lymphoma that mimics meningioma. *J Clin Oncol* 2005;23: 5718–5727.
26. Miranda RN, Glantz LK, Myint MA, et al. Stage IE non-Hodgkin's lymphoma involving the dura: a clinicopathologic study of five cases. *Arch Pathol Lab Med* 1996;120:254–260.
27. Abdullah S, Morgensztern D, Rosado MF, et al. Primary lymphoblastic B-cell lymphoma of the cranial dura mater: a case report and review of the literature. *Leuk Lymphoma* 2005;46:1651–1657.
28. Johnson MD, Kinney MC, Scheithauer BW, et al. Primary intracerebral Hodgkin's disease mimicking meningioma: case report. *Neurosurgery* 2000;47:454–456.
29. Beriwal S, Hou JS, Miyamoto C, et al. Primary dural low grade BCL-2 negative follicular lymphoma: a case report. *J Neurooncol* 2003;61:23–25.
30. Tandon R, Mukherjee U, Abrari A, et al. Primary dural follicular lymphoma masquerading as meningioma: a case report. *Br J Neurosurg* 2012;26:905–906.
31. Brito AB, Reis F, de Souza CA, et al. Intracranial primary dural diffuse large B-cell lymphoma successfully treated with chemotherapy. *Int J Clin Exp Med* 2014;7:456–460.
32. Kim MK, Cho CH, Sung WJ, et al. Primary anaplastic large cell lymphoma in the dura of the brain: case report and prediction of a favorable prognosis. *Int J Clin Exp Pathol* 2013;6:1643–1651.
33. Assaf C, Coupland SE, Hummel M, et al. Relapse of primary extranodal marginal-zone B-cell lymphoma of the dura mater. *Lancet Oncol* 2005;6:187–189.
34. Rosai J, Dorfman RF. Sinus histiocytosis with massive lymphadenopathy. A newly recognized benign clinicopathological entity. *Arch Pathol* 1969;87:63–70.
35. Fukushima T, Yachi K, Ogino A, et al. Isolated intracranial Rosai-Dorfman disease without dural attachment—case report. *Neurol Med Chir (Tokyo)* 2011;51:136–140.
36. Walid MS, Grigorian AA. Ethmo-spheno-intracranial Rosai-Dorfman disease. *Indian J Cancer* 2010;47: 80–81.
37. Foucar E, Rosai J, Dorfman R. Sinus histiocytosis with massive lymphadenopathy (Rosai-Dorfman disease): review of the entity. *Semin Diagn Pathol* 1990;7:19–73.
38. Vemuganti GK, Naik MN, Honavar SG. Rosai Dorfman disease of the orbit. *J Hematol Oncol* 2008;1:7.
39. Andriko JA, Morrison A, Colegial CH, et al. Rosai-Dorfman disease isolated to the central nervous system: a report of 11 cases. *Mod Pathol* 2001;14:172–178.
40. Wu M, Anderson AE, Kahn LB. A report of intracranial Rosai-Dorfman disease with literature review. *Ann Diagn Pathol* 2001;5:96–102.
41. Kattner KA, Stroink AR, Roth TC, et al. Rosai-Dorfman disease mimicking parasagittal meningioma: case presentation and review of literature. *Surg Neurol* 2000;53:452–457.
42. Mahzoni P, Zavareh MH, Bagheri M, et al. Intracranial Rosai-Dorfman disease. *J Res Med Sci* 2012;17: 304–307.
43. Forest F, N'guyen AT, Fesselet J, et al. Meningeal Rosai-Dorfman disease mimicking meningioma. *Ann Hematol* 2013;93:937–940.
44. Hingwala D, Neelima R, Kesavadas C, et al. Advanced MRI in Rosai-Dorfman disease: correlation with histopathology. *J Neuroradiol* 2010;38:113–117.
45. Grois N, Prayer D, Prosch H, et al. Neuropathology of CNS disease in Langerhans cell histiocytosis. *Brain* 2005;128:829–838.
46. Barthez MA, Araujo E, Donadieu J. Langerhans cell histiocytosis and the central nervous system in childhood: evolution and prognostic factors. Results of a collaborative study. *J Child Neurol* 2000;15:150–156.
47. Prayer D, Grois N, Prosch H, et al. MR imaging presentation of intracranial disease associated with Langerhans cell histiocytosis. *AJNR Am J Neuroradiol* 2004;25:880–891.
48. Badalian-Very G, Vergilio JA, Degar BA, et al. Recurrent BRAF mutations in Langerhans cell histiocytosis. *Blood* 2010;116:1919–1923.
49. Bates SV, Lakshmanan A, Green AL, et al. BRAF V600E-positive multisite Langerhans cell histiocytosis in a preterm neonate. *AJP Rep* 2013;3:63–66.
50. Roden AC, Hu X, Kip S, et al. BRAF V600E expression in Langerhans cell histiocytosis: clinical and immunohistochemical study on 25 pulmonary and 54 extrapulmonary cases. *Am J Surg Pathol* 2014;38:548–551.
51. Satoh T, Smith A, Sarde A, et al. B-RAF mutant alleles associated with Langerhans cell histiocytosis, a granulomatous pediatric disease. *PLoS One* 2012;7:e33891.

52. Buchler T, Cervinek L, Belohlavek O, et al. Langerhans cell histiocytosis with central nervous system involvement: follow-up by FDG-PET during treatment with cladribine. *Pediatr Blood Cancer* 2005;44: 286–288.
53. Grois N, Fahrner B, Arceci RJ, et al. Central nervous system disease in Langerhans cell histiocytosis. *J Pediatr* 2010;156:873–881.
54. Ng Wing TS, Martin-Duverneuil N, Idbaih A, et al. Efficacy of vinblastine in central nervous system Langerhans cell histiocytosis: a nationwide retrospective study. *Orphanet J Rare Dis* 2011;6:83.
55. Imashuku S, Okazaki N, Nakayama M, et al. Treatment of neurodegenerative CNS disease in Langerhans cell histiocytosis with a combination of intravenous immunoglobulin and chemotherapy. *Pediatr Blood Cancer* 2008;50:308–311.
56. Imashuku S, Ishida S, Koike K, et al. Cerebellar ataxia in pediatric patients with Langerhans cell histiocytosis. *J Pediatr Hematol Oncol* 2004;26:735–739.
57. Idbaih A, Donadieu J, Barthez MA, et al. Retinoic acid therapy in "degenerative-like" neuro-Langerhans cell histiocytosis: a prospective pilot study. *Pediatr Blood Cancer* 2004;43:55–58.
58. Allen CE, Flores R, Rauch R, et al. Neurodegenerative central nervous system Langerhans cell histiocytosis and coincident hydrocephalus treated with vincristine/cytosine arabinoside. *Pediatr Blood Cancer* 2010;54:416–423.
59. Chohan G, Barnett Y, Gibson J, et al. Langerhans cell histiocytosis with refractory central nervous system involvement responsive to infliximab. *J Neurol Neurosurg Psychiatry* 2012;83:573–575.

15 Central Nervous System Metastasis

Fumi Kawakami
Hidehiro Takei

INTRODUCTION

Metastases are the most common tumors of the central nervous system (CNS) and are associated with major morbidity and mortality in patients with malignant tumor of various locations. About 25% of patients who succumbed to cancer were reported to have CNS metastases detected at autopsy.[1] Although both single and multiple metastases are common, it is reported that 70% of patients have three or fewer metastases in a large series,[2] and those lesions may be treated by local excision and radiosurgery. Of malignancies causing CNS metastasis, carcinomas are most common. Brain is considered to be a protected organ from metastases given the presence of blood–brain barrier (BBB). However, once metastasis is established *via* hematogenous spread, CNS becomes a "sanctuary" or "safe haven" for the primary malignancy since BBB shelters metastatic foci from chemotherapeutic agents. Brain metastasis has been thought to be associated with an extremely poor prognosis. However, recent outstanding progress in systemic therapy and technologic advances in radiation therapy have contributed to improve the quality of life and survival for patients with CNS metastasis.[3]

CLINICAL FEATURES

CNS metastases can cause a wide variety of symptoms, which are usually related to the location of the tumor. The common symptoms include new-onset headaches; cognitive, personality, and behavioral changes; seizures; ataxia; nausea and vomiting; and motor dysfunction. CNS metastases may appear as the initial presentation leading to detection of the primary malignancy.

Brain metastases arise most commonly from primary lung carcinoma, breast cancer, melanoma, and renal cell carcinoma (RCC).[4] Although nearly every single malignancy has the potential for intracranial involvement, brain metastases from ovary, prostate, and thyroid are less common, and their incidence has been reported to be less than 1%.[5–7] Brain metastases in sarcomas are rather rare with the reported incidence of 1% to 8%.[8] Although the available literature is limited mainly to small case series, undifferentiated pleomorphic sarcoma, uterine leiomyosarcoma, and alveolar soft part sarcoma are common histologies of sarcoma with brain metastasis.[9]

Brain metastases can arise at any age of patients, but are much more commonly seen in aged individuals. On the other hand, osteosarcoma and Ewing sarcoma are the major primary solid tumors among pediatric CNS metastases.[10]

RADIOLOGIC FEATURES

Computed tomography (CT) of brain metastasis demonstrates solitary or multiple, hyper- to hypodense mass lesions compared to the background brain with variable surrounding edema.[11] Magnetic resonance imaging (MRI) is a sensitive screening test for brain metastasis. In general, metastases are usually iso- or hypointense on T1-weighted image (WI), hyperintense on T2 WI, and

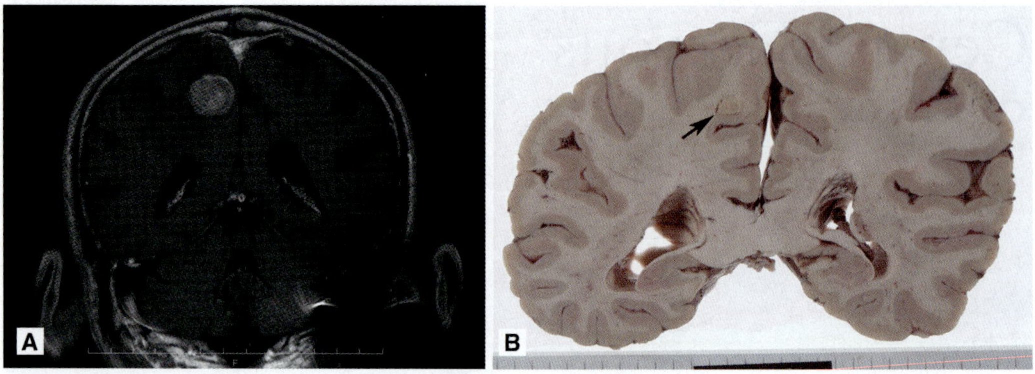

FIGURE 15-1: Metastatic pulmonary carcinoma. Coronal T1-weighted MRI with contrast enhancement showing an enhancing metastatic lesion at gray–white junction with peritumoral edema in the frontoparietal area (**A**). Gross feature of the corresponding metastatic focus (*arrow*) treated with gamma knife surgery 8 months prior to the autopsy (**B**).

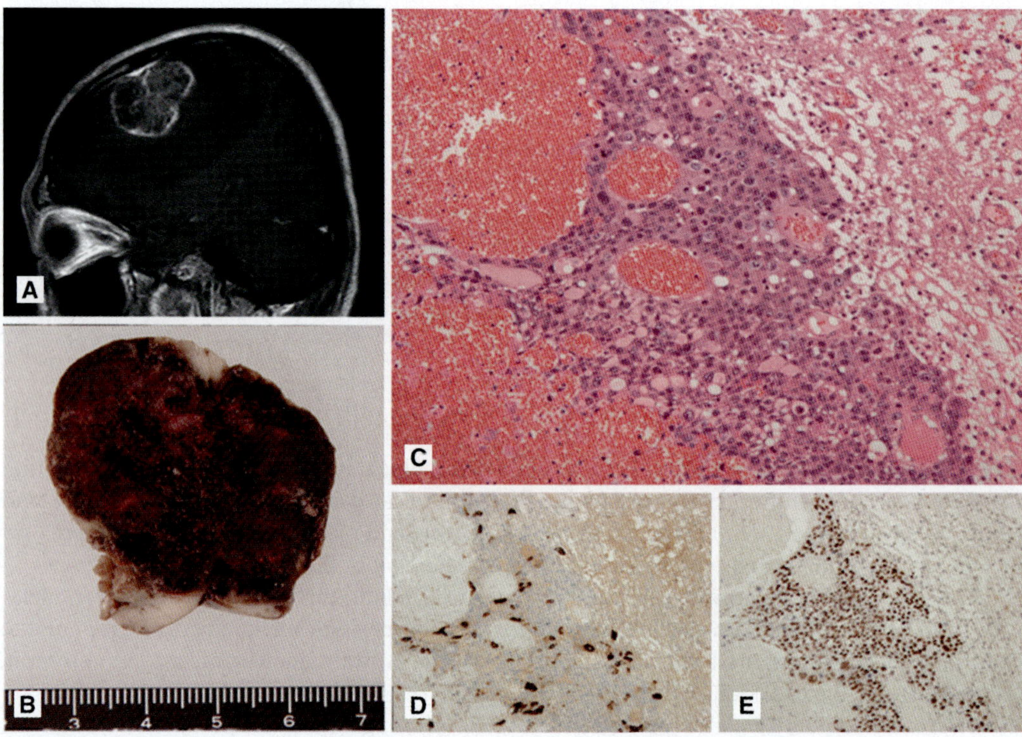

FIGURE 15-2: Metastatic choriocarcinoma. Sagittal T1-weighted MRI with contrast enhancement showing a homogenously enhancing mass lesion with prominent peritumoral edema (**A**). Gross feature of resected mass lesion showing predominantly massive hemorrhage (**B**). Microscopic feature showing epithelioid malignant tumor with prominent recent hemorrhage (**C**). hCG IHC showing focal positivity (**D**). SALL-4 IHC showing diffuse positivity (**E**).

exhibit remarkable enhancement with substantial peritumoral edema on MRI (Figures 15-1A and 15-2A). Melanin within the tumor and intratumoral hemorrhage affects their intensity.[12]

The vast majority of brain metastases occur in the cerebral hemispheres, followed by the cerebellum (15%) and basal nuclei (3%).[11,13] Interestingly, a certain cancer may preferentially metastasize to a certain location of CNS (i.e., site specificity), and the number of metastatic foci in CNS may also be characteristic of a primary site. For example, non–small cell lung cancer and breast cancer tend to show multiple brain metastases. Occipital lobe and cerebellum are predominantly involved by non–small cell lung cancers, while cerebellum and brainstem are the common metastatic sites for breast cancers.[14,15] About a half of the cases of brain metastases from gastrointestinal carcinomas are isolated lesions, and those lesions are observed most often in the cerebellum.[16]

PATHOLOGIC FEATURES

Gross Findings

Within the brain, metastatic foci are most commonly found in the cerebral gray–white junction, especially in the territory of middle cerebral artery (MCA), due to luminal narrowing and acute angle branching of vessels at this point (Figure 15-1B). Brain metastases also commonly involve the terminal "watershed" areas of arterial circulations, especially in the territory between MCA and posterior cerebral artery.[17] The gross appearance is largely nonspecific with the exception of its tendency to have sharp borders in contrast to primary brain tumors. Metastatic melanoma can display black discoloration due to melanin pigments. Metastatic mucin-producing adenocarcinoma may show a shiny mucoid appearance. Hemorrhagic intracranial metastasis is not uncommon, and the following primary tumors are known for hemorrhagic presentation: melanoma, RCC, choriocarcinoma (Figure 15-2B), thyroid carcinoma (papillary carcinoma), breast carcinoma, and bronchogenic carcinoma (mnemonic MR CT BB). The differential diagnosis includes primary hemorrhagic brain tumors (most commonly, glioblastoma).

Microscopic and Immunohistochemical Findings

Not only grossly but also microscopically, metastatic tumors are characteristically sharply demarcated from the surrounding brain. In most cases, its metastatic nature is histologically and cytologically evident and primary glial neoplasms can be easily excluded. Sometimes, hemorrhagic metastasis (e.g., melanoma and choriocarcinoma) causes massive bleeding that is severe enough to obscure the tumor cells (Figure 15-2C). Metastatic cancer tends to retain their inherent morphology of its origin. However, it is sometimes difficult to identify the site of origin of the metastasis based only on the histology, although clinical and radiologic information is crucial for this purpose. In order to identify as well as to confirm the site of origin, immunohistochemistry (IHC) is of great help (Figure 15-2D and E). Given that no IHC antibodies with absolute sensitivity and specificity exist, using a panel of antibodies is necessary. To identify the nature of tumor cells, *pancytokeratin (panCK)* for carcinoma, *melanoma cocktail* for malignant melanoma, *glial fibrillary acidic protein (GFAP)* for primary glial tumor, and *leukocyte common antigen* for malignant lymphoma should be used as the first-line panel. In cases of metastatic carcinoma, combined use of *CK7* and *CK20* is informative to narrow down its origin. Commonly used organ-"specific" markers that are of help in identification and confirmation of the site of origin are illustrated in Table 15-1. Sometimes, differential diagnosis between high-grade gliomas and metastasis is difficult (especially, epithelioid glioblastoma vs. amelanotic melanoma vs. undifferentiated carcinoma; gliosarcoma vs. sarcoma). Interestingly, a significant proportion of metastatic melanomas in the brain are amelanotic/pauci-melanotic, mimicking epithelioid malignancies. *GFAP* usually labels epithelioid glioblastoma and glioma component of gliosarcoma and is useful for the differential diagnosis. Of note is that glioblastomas frequently show obvious immunoreactivity for *panCK cocktails (AE1/AE3)* probably due to cross-reactivity in intermediate filaments (i.e., cytokeratin and GFAP). In this setting, low molecular weight cytokeratin cocktails (e.g., *CK CAM 5.2*) can be used to confirm the epithelial nature of metastasis. In cases suggestive of metastatic melanoma, specific melanocytic markers (e.g., *HMB45*, *Melan A*, *microphthalmia-associated transcription factor*) are needed for the diagnosis and differentiation from high-grade glioma. *SOX10* is relatively newly introduced pan-schwannian and melanocytic marker. It is positive in both metastatic melanoma and primary CNS glial tumors.[18] Another challenging and important differential diagnosis that is occasionally encountered in a practice is metastatic RCC versus hemangioblastoma (this issue is discussed in Chapter 12). IHC is also of help in identification of cancer cells in a background of massive hemorrhage (i.e., hemorrhagic metastasis).

Table 15-1 Immunohistochemical Profile of Metastatic CNS Tumors

Primary Tumor	Positive	Negative
Lung adenocarcinoma	CK7, TTF-1, napsin A	CK20
Lung small cell carcinoma	TTF-1, synaptophysin, chromogranin A, CD56	
Breast carcinoma	CK7, GCDFP-15, mammaglobin, ER, PgR, GATA3	CK20
Renal cell carcinoma	CD10, vimentin, PAX-2, PAX-8	
Colonic adenocarcinoma	CK20, CDX-2	CK7
Ovarian cancer	CK7, PAX8	
Prostatic cancer	PSA	CK7, CK20
Thyroidal cancer	TTF-1, thyroglobulin	
Choriocarcinoma	hCG, SALL4	
Squamous cell carcinoma	CK 5/6, p63, p40	
Leiomyosarcoma	α-SMA, desmin, caldesmon, HHF35	
Alveolar soft part sarcoma	TFE-3	
Ewing sarcoma	CD99, FLI-1, NKX2.2	
Neuroblastoma	Neurofilament protein, chromogranin A, synaptophysin	
Malignant melanoma	S100 protein, HMB-45, melan A, SOX-10	

CK, cytokeratin; TTF-1, thyroid transcription factor-1; GCDFP-15, gross cystic disease fluid protein-15; ER, estrogen receptor; PgR, progesterone receptor; hCG, human chorionic gonadotropin; TFE-3, transcription factor E3.

DISTINCT PATHOLOGIC FORMS OF CNS METASTASIS

Tumor-to-Tumor Metastasis

Tumor-to-tumor metastasis in CNS most commonly occurs from an aggressive systemic malignancy such as melanoma, lung cancer, or breast cancer to a slow-growing primary CNS tumor such as pituitary adenoma or meningioma (Figure 15-3).[19,20] The most common donor is breast cancer, and the most common recipient is meningioma in tumor-to-CNS tumor metastasis. As with other rare situations, hemangioblastoma harboring metastatic RCC in the setting of von Hippel-Lindau (VHL) disease, astrocytoma and ependymoma with metastatic lung cancer (adenocarcinoma and small cell carcinoma), and oligodendroglioma and acoustic neuroma with metastatic breast cancer have been reported.[21–24] Given the rapid progression with short survival of high-grade gliomas, cases of glioblastoma harboring metastatic carcinoma have not been reported to date.

Leptomeningeal Carcinomatosis

Although most cases with CNS metastasis involve the brain parenchyma, metastatic disease can occur in any CNS compartments, including the skull bone, meninges, epidural space, and spine. Leptomeningeal dissemination and subarachnoid space involvement of cancer cells is referred to as leptomeningeal carcinomatosis (LC). Its incidence is around 1% to 5% of patients with solid tumors.[25,26] Breast cancer (triple-negative biologic subtype and lobular histologic type), lung cancer (adenocarcinoma and small cell carcinoma), and melanoma are the representative primary malignancies causing LC.[25,27–30] LC is a rare complication of gastric cancer but it can be seen especially in south-eastern Asia.[31] Although the prognosis is considered to be dismal, with

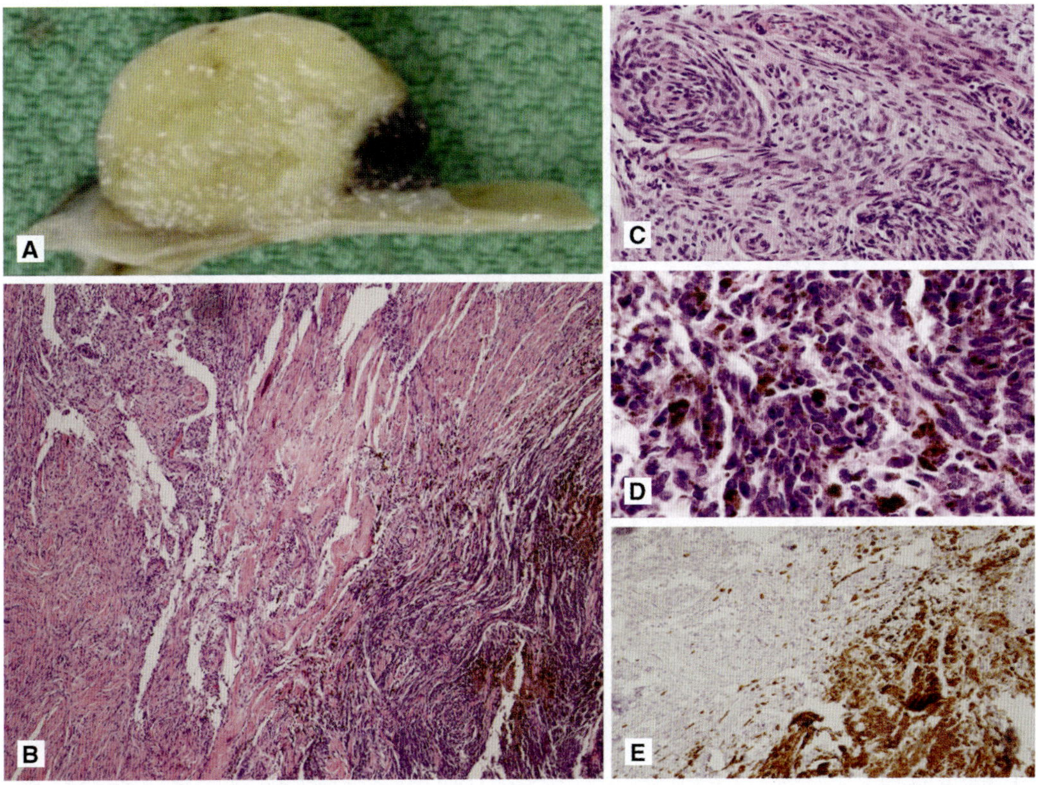

FIGURE 15-3: Tumor-to-tumor (melanoma-to-meningioma) metastasis. Gross feature of cross section of the tumor. A dura-based tumor contains an area of black discoloration (**A**). Low-power microscopic view at an interface between melanoma (***right***) and meningioma (***left***) (**B**). Intermediate-power microscopic view of meningioma. Syncytial spindled tumor cell proliferation with focal whorl formation (***left upper***) is seen (**C**). Intermediate-power microscopic view of melanoma. Cellular proliferation of atypical hyperchromatic tumor cells is noted. Scattered melanin-containing tumor cells are identified (**D**). Melan A immunohistochemistry (**E**) on **B**. Metastatic melanoma (***right***) is highlighted, while meningioma (***left***) is not immunoreactive.

a reported median survival of 4 to 6 weeks in untreated cases, recent advances in diagnostic technology for earlier detection and in therapy have contributed to longer survival for some of the patients with LC.[25–27,32] Postmortem brains with LC often show subtle gross findings (e.g., congestion, mildly thickening, and/or slightly increased opacification of the leptomeninges) (Figure 15-4A). The standard and most specific diagnostic test for LC is cerebrospinal fluid (CSF) cytology to identify malignant cells (Figure 15-4B).[33] Cytologically, presence of any large cells in CSF should be considered to be metastatic carcinoma, regardless of degree of cytologic atypia, until proven otherwise. Repeated examination of CSF is strongly recommended because of its low sensitivity.[34] Radiologically, focal or diffuse contrast enhancement on meninges, ependyma, tentorium, basal cistern, and sulci in the brain and spinal cord is considered to be positive for a diagnosis of LC in gadolinium-enhanced MRI.[34] Although enhanced MRI has approximately 30% false-negative results,[35,36] MRI plays an important role to diagnose LC even in CSF cytology-negative cases.[35,37] Postmortem histologic examination reveals cancer cells diffusely infiltrating into the leptomeninges (usually with involvement of Virchow-Robin spaces) (Figure 15-4C and D).

Prognosis and Treatment

Malignant tumor with CNS metastasis is not curable, and in general, the outcome is fairly poor. Death usually occurs within 2 years.[38,39] The prognosis of those patients may depend on the primary site of the tumor, histologic type of neoplasm, and extent of the disease.

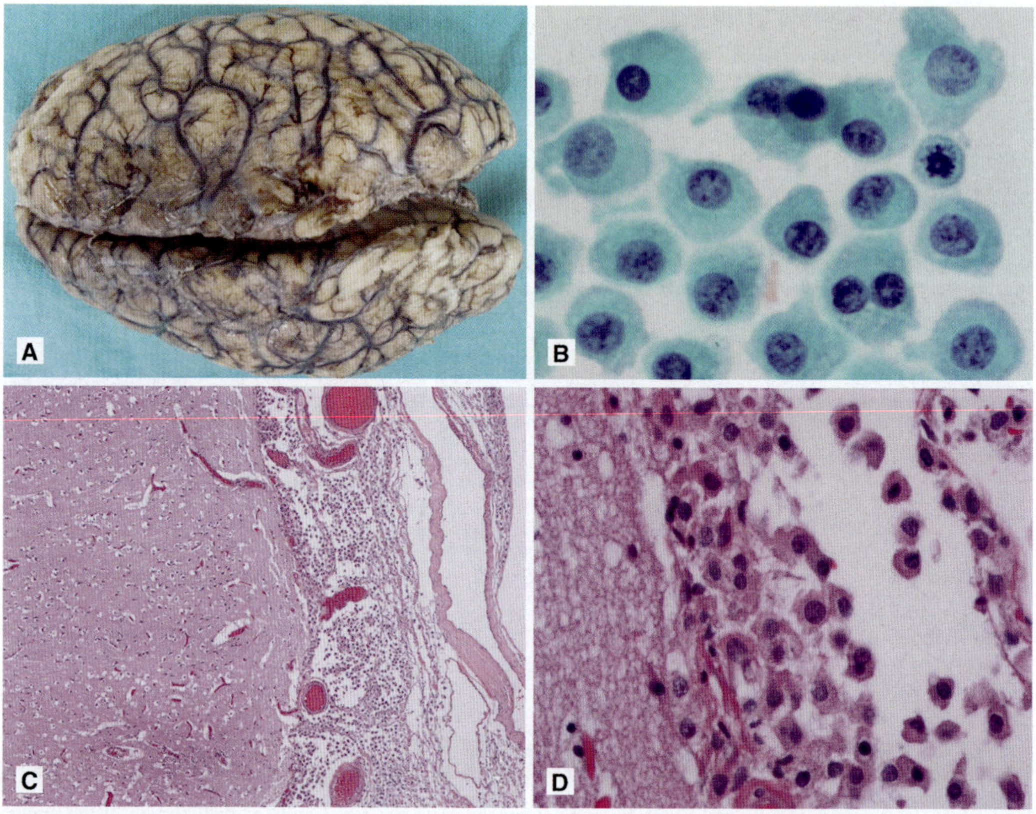

FIGURE 15-4: Leptomeningeal carcinomatosis (metastatic breast ductal carcinoma). Gross feature of autopsy brain. Slightly thickened, congested leptomeninges over the convexities. Of note, gross alteration is very subtle (**A**). CSF cytology (premortem examination): Monomorphic large plasmacytoid tumor cells are noted (Papanicolaou stain) (**B**). Low-power microscopic view of cerebral cortex (*left*) and overlying congested leptomeninges, which are thickened and hypercellular (**C**). High-power microscopic view showing cancer cells diffusely infiltrating in the leptomeninges with no obvious involvement of the underlying cortex (*left*) (**D**).

The mainstays of therapy at the time of the initial diagnosis of brain metastases include surgery, whole-brain radiation therapy (WBRT), and stereotactic radiosurgery (Figure 15-1B), alone or in combination.[40] Some reports showed efficacy of salvage radiosurgery after prior WBRT for recurrent CNS metastases.[3,41,42]

References

1. Gavrilovic IT, Posner JB. Brain metastases: epidemiology and pathophysiology. *J Neurooncol* 2005; 75:5–14.
2. Delattre J-Y, Krol G, Thaler HT, et al. Distribution of brain metastases. *Arch Neurol* 1988;45:741–744.
3. Kurtz G, Zadeh G, Gingras-Hill G, et al. Salvage radiosurgery for brain metastases: prognostic factors to consider in patient selection. *Int J Radiat Oncol Biol Phys* 2014;88:137–142.
4. Schouten LJ, Rutten J, Huveneers HAM, et al. Incidence of brain metastases in a cohort of patients with carcinoma of the breast, colon, kidney, and lung and melanoma. *Cancer* 2002;94:2698–2705.
5. Kolomainen DF, Larkin JM, Badran M, et al. Epithelial ovarian cancer metastasizing to the brain: a late manifestation of the disease with an increasing incidence. *J Clin Oncol* 2002;20:982–986.
6. Tremont-Lukats IW, Bobustuc G, Lagos GK, et al. Brain metastasis from prostate carcinoma: The M. D. Anderson Cancer Center experience. *Cancer* 2003;98:363–368.

7. Hjiyiannakis P, Jefferies S, Harmer CL. Brain metastases in patients with differentiated thyroid carcinoma. *Clin Oncol (R Coll Radiol)* 1996;8:327–330.
8. Fox BD, Patel A, Suki D, et al. Surgical management of metastatic sarcoma to the brain. *J Neurosurg* 2009;110:181–186.
9. Chua C, Raaj J, Pan S, et al. Brain metastasis in sarcoma: does metastasectomy or aggressive multi-disciplinary treatment improve survival outcomes. *Asia Pac J Clin Oncol* 2013;13. [Epub ahead of print].
10. Kebudi R, Ayan I, Görgün O, et al. Brain metastasis in pediatric extracranial solid tumors: survey and literature review. *J Neurooncol* 2005;71:43–48.
11. Potts DG, Abbott GF, von Sneidern JV. National Cancer Institute study evaluation of computed tomography in the diagnosis of intracranial neoplasms. III. Metastatic tumors. *Radiology* 1980;136:657–664.
12. Fink KR, Fink JR. Imaging of brain metastases. *Surg Neurol Int* 2013;4(suppl 4):S209–S219.
13. Osborn AG. Section 6 neoplasms, metastatic tumors and remote effects of cancer, parenchymal metastases. In: Osborn AG, Salzman KL, Barkovich AJ, eds. *Diagnostic Imaging, Brain.* 2nd ed. Salt Lake City, UT: Amirsys; 2009:I-6-174–I-6-177.
14. Graf AH, Buchberger W, Langmayr H, et al. Site preference of metastatic tumors of the brain. *Virchows Arch A Pathol Anat Histopathol* 1988;412:493–498.
15. Tsukada Y, Fouad A, Pickren JW, et al. Central nervous system metastasis from breast carcinoma. Autopsy study. *Cancer* 1983;52:2349–2354.
16. Bartelt S, Momm F, Weissenberger C, et al. Patients with brain metastases from gastrointestinal tract cancer treated with whole brain radiation therapy: prognostic factors and survival. *World J Gastroenterol* 2004;10:3345–3348.
17. Hwang TL, Close TP, Grego JM, et al. Predilection of brain metastasis in gray and white matter junction and vascular border zones. *Cancer* 1996;77:1551–1555.
18. Nonaka D, Chiriboga L, Rubin BP. Sox10: a pan-schwannian and melanocytic marker. *Am J Surg Pathol* 2008;32:1291–1298.
19. Takei H, Powell SZ. Tumor-to-tumor metastasis to the central nervous system. *Neuropathology* 2009; 29:303–308.
20. Caroli E, Salvati M, Giangaspero F, et al. Intrameningioma metastasis as first clinical manifestation of occult primary breast carcinoma. *Neurosurg Rev* 2006;29:49–54.
21. Mottolese C, Stan H, Giordano F, et al. Metastasis of clear-cell renal carcinoma to cerebellar hemangioblastoma in von Hippel Lindau disease: rare or not investigated. *Acta Neurochir (Wien)* 2001;143:1059–1063.
22. Mork SJ, Rubinstein LJ. Metastatic carcinoma to glioma: a report of three cases with a critical review of the literature. *J Neurol Neurosurg Psychiatry* 1988;51:256–259.
23. Strang RR. Metastasis of breast carcinoma to an intracerebral oligodendroglioma. *Zentralbl Neurochir* 1965;25:206–209.
24. Wong TW, Bennington JL. Metastasis of a mammary carcinoma to an acoustic neuroma. Report of a case. *J Neurosurg* 1962;19:1088–1093.
25. Jaeckle KA. Neoplastic meningitis from systemic malignancies: diagnosis, prognosis and treatment. *Semin Oncol* 2006;33:312–323.
26. Blaney SM, Poplack DG. Neoplastic meningitis: diagnosis and treatment considerations. *Med Oncol* 2000;17:151–162.
27. Wasserstrom WR, Glass JP, Posner JB. Diagnosis and treatment of leptomeningeal metastases from solid tumors: experience with 90 patients. *Cancer* 1982;49:759–772.
28. Kaplan JG, DeSouza TG, Farkash A, et al. Leptomeningeal metastases: comparison of clinical features and laboratory data of solid tumors, lymphomas and leukemias. *J Neurooncol* 1990;9:225–229.
29. Amer MH, Al-Sarraf M, Baker LH, et al. Malignant melanoma and central nervous system metastases: incidence, diagnosis, treatment and survival. *Cancer* 1978;42:660–668.
30. Niwi ska A, Rudnicka H, Murawska M. Breast cancer leptomeningeal metastasis: propensity of breast cancer subtypes for leptomeninges and the analysis of factors influencing survival. *Med Oncol* 2013; 30:408.
31. Tomita H, Yasui H, Boku N, et al. Leptomeningeal carcinomatosis associated with gastric cancer. *Int J Clin Oncol* 2012;17:361–366.
32. Shapiro WR, Johanson CE, Boogerd W. Treatment modalities for leptomeningeal metastases. *Semin Oncol* 2009;36:S46–S54.
33. Kolmel HW. Cytology of neoplastic meningosis. *J Neurooncol* 1998;38:121–125.
34. Jung TY, Chung WK, Oh IJ. The prognostic significance of surgically treated hydrocephalus in leptomeningeal metastases. *Clin Neurol Neurosurg* 2014;119:80–83.

35. Freilich RJ, Krol G, DeAngelis LM. Neuroimaging and cerebrospinal fluid cytology in the diagnosis of leptomeningeal metastasis. *Ann Neurol* 1995;38:51–57.
36. Chamberlain MC. Comparative spine imaging in leptomeningeal metastases. *J Neurooncol* 1995;23: 233–238.
37. Rodesch G, Van Bogaert P, Mavroudakis N, et al. Neuroradiologic findings in leptomeningeal carcinomatosis: the value interest of gadolinium-enhanced MRI. *Neuroradiology* 1990;32:26–32.
38. Gaspar L, Scott C, Rotman M, et al. Recursive partitioning analysis (RPA) of prognostic factors in three radiation therapy oncology group (RTOG) brain metastases trials. *Int J Radiat Oncol Biol Phys* 1997;37:745–751.
39. Lutterbach J, Bartelt S, Ostertag C. Long-term survival in patients with brain metastases. *J Cancer Res Clin Oncol* 2002;128:417–425.
40. Tsao MN, Wades D, Wirth A, et al. Radiotherapeutic and surgical management for newly diagnosed brain metastasis(es): an American Society for Radiation Oncology evidence-based guideline. *Pract Radiat Oncol* 2002;2:210–225.
41. Caballero JA, Sneed PK, Lamborn KR, et al. Prognostic factors for survival in patients treated with stereotactic radiosurgery for recurrent brain metastases after prior whole brain radiotherapy. *Int J Radiat Oncol Biol Phys* 2012;83:303–309.
42. Chao ST, Barnett GH, Vogelbaum MA, et al. Salvage stereotactic radiosurgery effectively treats recurrences from whole-brain radiation therapy. 2008;113:2198–2204.

SECTION

III

Imaging

▸ CHAPTER 16: Correlation of Imaging with Pathology

Correlation of Imaging with Pathology

16

▶ Steve Huntz Fung
▶ Sanjay K. Singh

Medical imaging relies on the use of energy that is capable of penetrating tissues to obtain information deep within the human body. Visible light, while useful for direct visual observation as in light microscopy, does not penetrate deeply within tissues because of rapid scatter and absorption by biologic molecules within the body. Medical imaging uses instead parts of the electromagnetic spectrum outside of visible light such as x-rays in computed tomography (CT), radiofrequency (RF) energy in magnetic resonance imaging (MRI), and gamma rays in nuclear medicine to probe local properties of tissue. Except for nuclear medicine, all medical imaging modalities require energy that penetrates the body to also interact with tissue to obtain useful information about the tissue environment and surrounding anatomy. For example, x-rays are attenuated by scatter and absorption in tissue that is dependent on local volumetric mass density and atomic number of constituent elements. With MRI, RF energy is absorbed and reemitted after a delay by protons (hydrogen nuclei in water and organic molecules) with signal dependent on local biochemical, microstructural, and physiologic properties. In nuclear medicine imaging, gamma rays are emitted by radioactive tracers that accumulate in parts of the body dependent on local physiology. All medical imaging modalities provide spatial information about anatomy with displayed regional image intensity (brightness) generally dependent on local tissue properties that the imaging modality is sensitive for.

The objectives of medical imaging in the evaluation of patients with known or suspected brain tumors are to localize and characterize the pathologic lesion, to provide a reasonable differential diagnosis; to guide further diagnostic, imaging, and treatment planning; to determine adequacy of surgical resection; and to monitor therapeutic response and complications. Providing a reasonable differential diagnosis requires a systematic approach that includes knowledge of the patient's age, location of the lesion, single or multiple lesions, and imaging characteristics. The first goal in localization is determining if the lesion is intra-axial (within brain parenchyma) or extra-axial (outside brain parenchyma), which is of utmost importance because it absolutely determines the correct differential diagnosis, treatment planning, and prognosis. Differential diagnosis also depends on specific anatomical areas involved, for example, supratentorial or infratentorial, cortical or deep parenchymal, intraventricular, skull base, sellar–suprasellar, cerebellopontine angle, or pineal location. Multiple lesions usually indicate metastatic disease, although primary brain tumors such as lymphoma, multicentric glioblastoma, and gliomatosis cerebri as well as tumors associated with phakomatoses and oncogene/tumor suppressor gene mutations can present with multifocal lesions. Many benign tumor-like lesions such as microvascular disease, vasculitis, demyelinating disease (e.g., multiple sclerosis), and infection (e.g., cerebral abscesses) can also be multifocal. Various tumors and tumor-like lesions tend to have certain imaging characteristics such as presence or absence of contrast enhancement, calcification, hemorrhage, fat, cyst, and necrosis. Information from diffusion-weighted imaging (DWI), perfusion imaging, magnetic resonance spectroscopy (MRS), and metabolism imaging such as from ^{18}F-fluorodeoxyglucose (FDG) positron emission tomography can further help narrow the differential diagnosis.

The purpose of this chapter is to review some basic imaging modalities commonly used to image patients with known or suspected brain tumor, to introduce imaging terms often associated with each modality, and to provide limited examples of imaging characteristics of lesions that can be correlated with findings on pathology.

IMAGING MODALITIES

Computed Tomography

CT scanning uses an array of detectors and an x-ray beam to form a reconstructed picture of the body. CT allows rapid assessment of patients because it is readily available and has few contradictions. It is still the primary method for detection of calcification[1] and acute hemorrhage. Brain tumors can present acutely due to a number of causes including hemorrhage and hydrocephalus. Hydrocephalus can be caused by a focal mass in the ventricular system (Figure 16-1). Fatty tumors can easily be detected by CT scanning (Figure 16-2).

Magnetic Resonance Imaging

MRI relies on the interaction of biologic tissue with RF waves and magnetic fields. The various MRI sequences (experiments) allow different qualities of tissues to be visualized. One sequence ("T1-weighted" or T1W) shows normal fat tissue as high signal (bright), but water (e.g., cerebrospinal fluid) as low signal (dark). Another sequence ("T2-weighted" or T2W) shows CSF as brighter than fat. This range of tissue qualities on MRI is much wider than the differences revealed by CT scanning (relying on density differences in tissue). Unfortunately, the typical MRI scan (with many sequences) takes much longer to perform than does a CT scan. An MRI of the brain can require 30 to 40 minutes compared to 1 to 3 minutes for a CT scan of the brain.

Intravascular contrast in MRI studies generally has relied on the T1 shortening effect of paramagnetic compounds containing gadolinium. This leads to higher signal on T1-weighted MR images where gadolinium compounds concentrate (areas of blood–brain barrier breakdown). This high signal of an area of brain compared to the appearance before gadolinium contrast injection (on T1W images) is "enhancement."

The traditional role of imaging has been to define the anatomic location of an abnormality. Are masses within the brain (intra-axial) or outside the brain parenchyma (extra-axial)? In the white matter or in the gray matter or both? Extra-axial masses have a more limited set of possible histologic diagnoses with meningiomas and dural metastases heading the list (in adults).

FIGURE 16-1: CT image shows subependymal nodule with calcification (*arrow*) in a tuberous sclerosis patient with a giant cell astrocytoma (*arrowhead*) causing hydrocephalus.

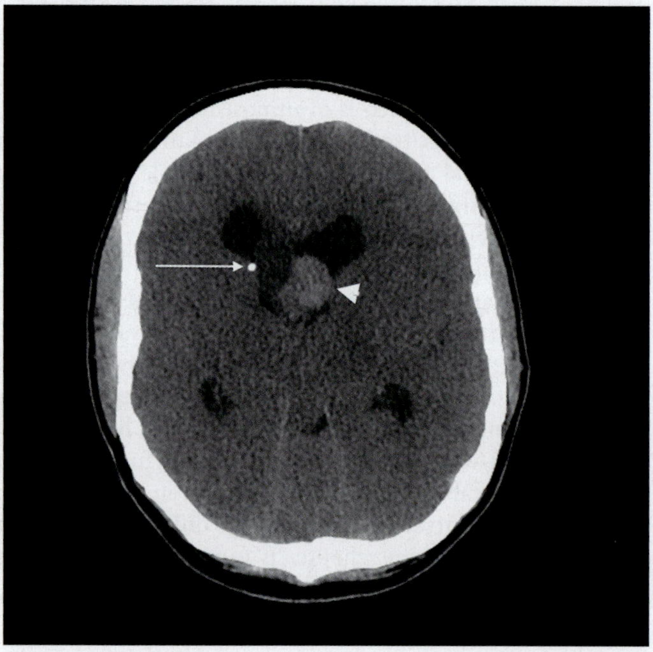

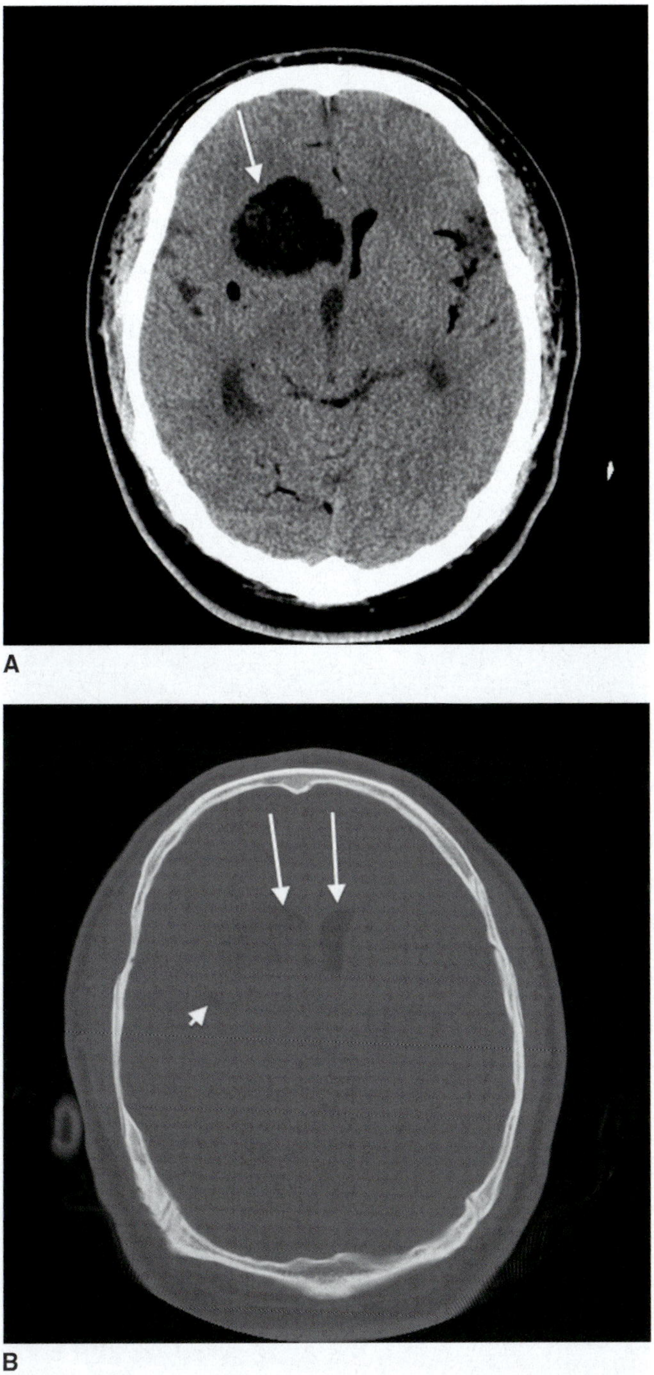

FIGURE 16-2: CT images in soft tissue (**A**) and bone (**B**) windows show a large right-sided dermoid (*arrow* in **A**) with subarachnoid (*short arrow* in **B**) and intraventricular rupture (*long arrow* in **B**).

The secondary goal of imaging has been to use the intrinsic MRI features of brain tumors to diagnose the neoplasm before surgery. These features include how well defined a mass appears, whether a part of the mass enhances, etc. Different MRI sequences help in this process.

Most brain neoplasms are easier to identify on T2W images. Both the neoplasm and especially any surrounding edema are typically higher in signal than the normal brain tissue (Figure 16-3A). However, if the mass is near the bright CSF, the suppression of fluid signal can make the tumor easier to identify. Fluid attenuated inversion recovery (FLAIR) sequences help in this regard (Figure 16-3B). The diseases involving the fluid of the subarachnoid space such as infectious meningitis and leptomeningeal metastasis are also easier to identify using FLAIR images.[2]

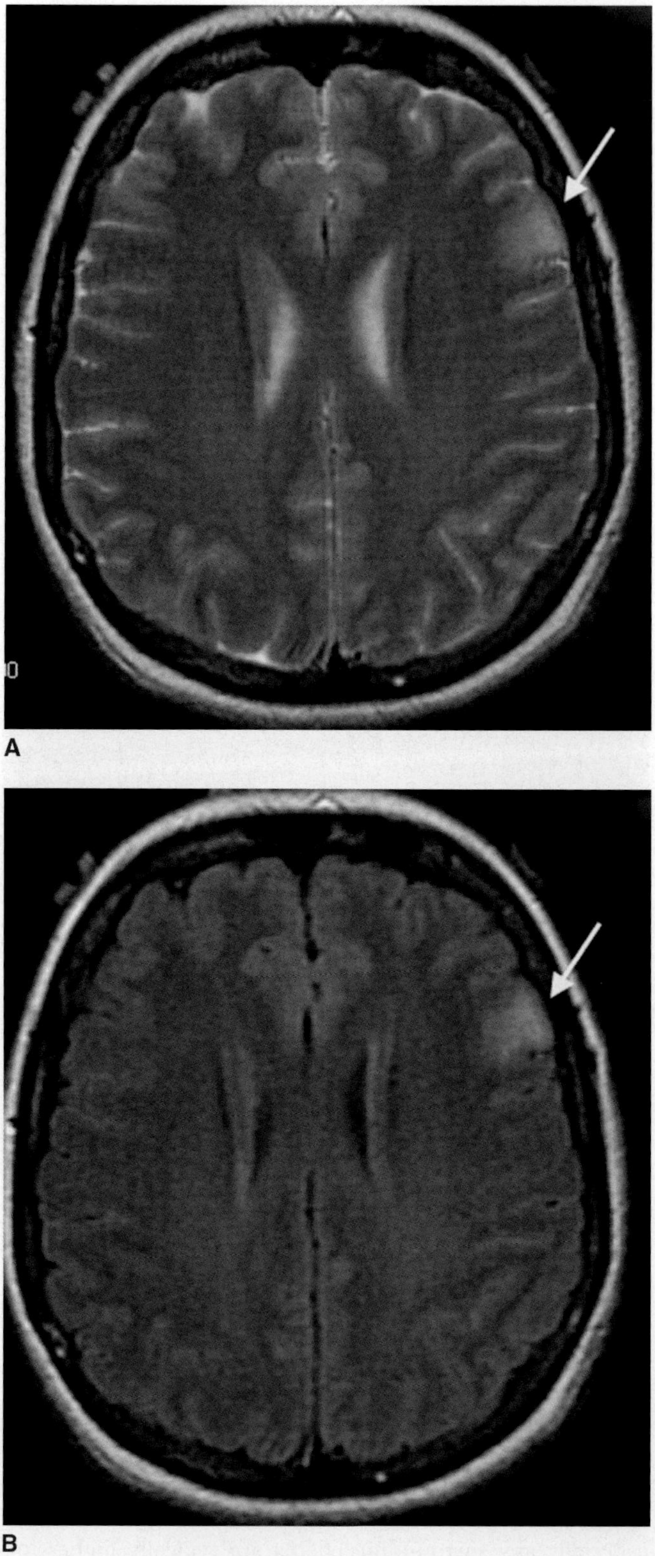

FIGURE 16-3: Axial T2W image shows a hyperintense lesion (*arrow*) at the left frontal lobe that is near the hyperintense fluid of the subarachnoid space (**A**). Axial FLAIR image suppresses the fluid and makes this low-grade fibrillary astrocytoma (*arrow*) easier to identify (**B**).

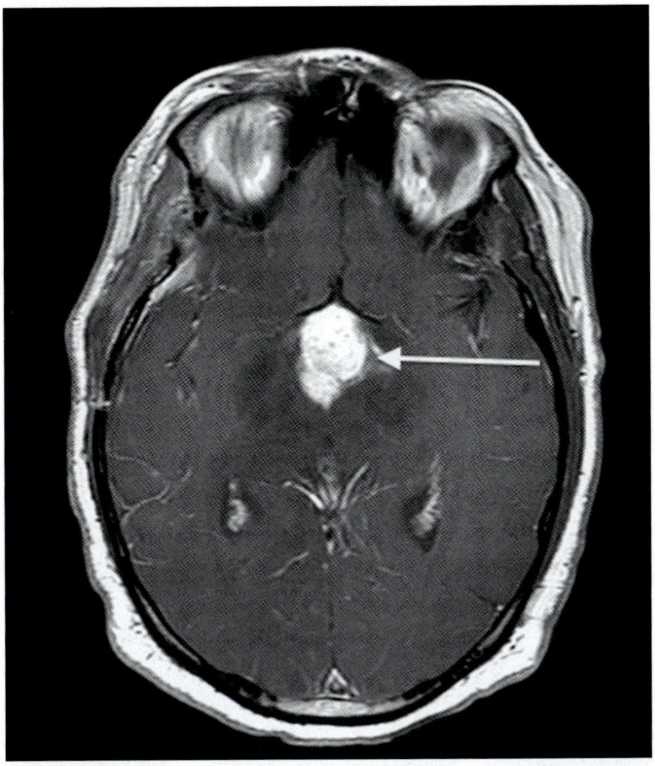

FIGURE 16-4: Axial T1W image after intravenous contrast injection shows enhancement (*arrow*) in a chordoid glioma.

Contrast enhancement on MRI studies of brain neoplasms has been correlated with tumor neovascularity.[3] Higher-grade fibrillary astrocytomas tend to have more enhancement than do low-grade ones (Figure 16-4). A glioblastoma invariably has enhancement, as well as irregular margins. Unfortunately, the correlation between enhancement and the grade of gliomas has limits: In one study, 40% of nonenhancing gliomas were anaplastic rather than low grade.[4]

MRI techniques measure the motion of molecules in biologic tissue. This dispersion of water molecules is diffusion and is dependent upon the state of the brain tissue in question. There is less ability for diffusion where water molecules are confined within a cell membrane as opposed to the extracellular fluid. If the proportion of intracellular volume to extracellular volume increases (as in a highly cellular neoplasm), there is overall less diffusion of water molecules. The DWI and apparent diffusion coefficient (ADC) images reflect these diffusion changes in abnormal tissue. ADC values allow differentiation of pilocytic astrocytomas from medulloblastomas due to the higher cellularity (lower ADC) in the latter relative to the former.[5]

MRI can also assess the amount of certain chemical compounds within a particular volume of tissue. This proton spectroscopy (MRS) in brain tissue allows evaluation of choline (Cho), creatine, and *N*-acetylaspartate (NAA) levels. Cho is felt to reflect membrane turnover and is often elevated in aggressive neoplasms with respect to NAA, which is seen in normal neurons.[6]

Imaging Approach in Specific Cases

An example of the imaging approach to analyzing intracranial masses is the case of a 55-year-old female with an extra-axial mass. This mass lies between the frontal lobes and shows uniform enhancement (Figure 16-5). The most likely diagnosis is a meningioma. However, the location also contains the pericallosal arteries. In addition, careful examination of the MRI images reveals the presence of pulsation artifact (arrowheads). A digital subtraction angiogram shows a dissecting (pseudo) aneurysm (Figure 16-6). This was treated with endovascular obliteration.

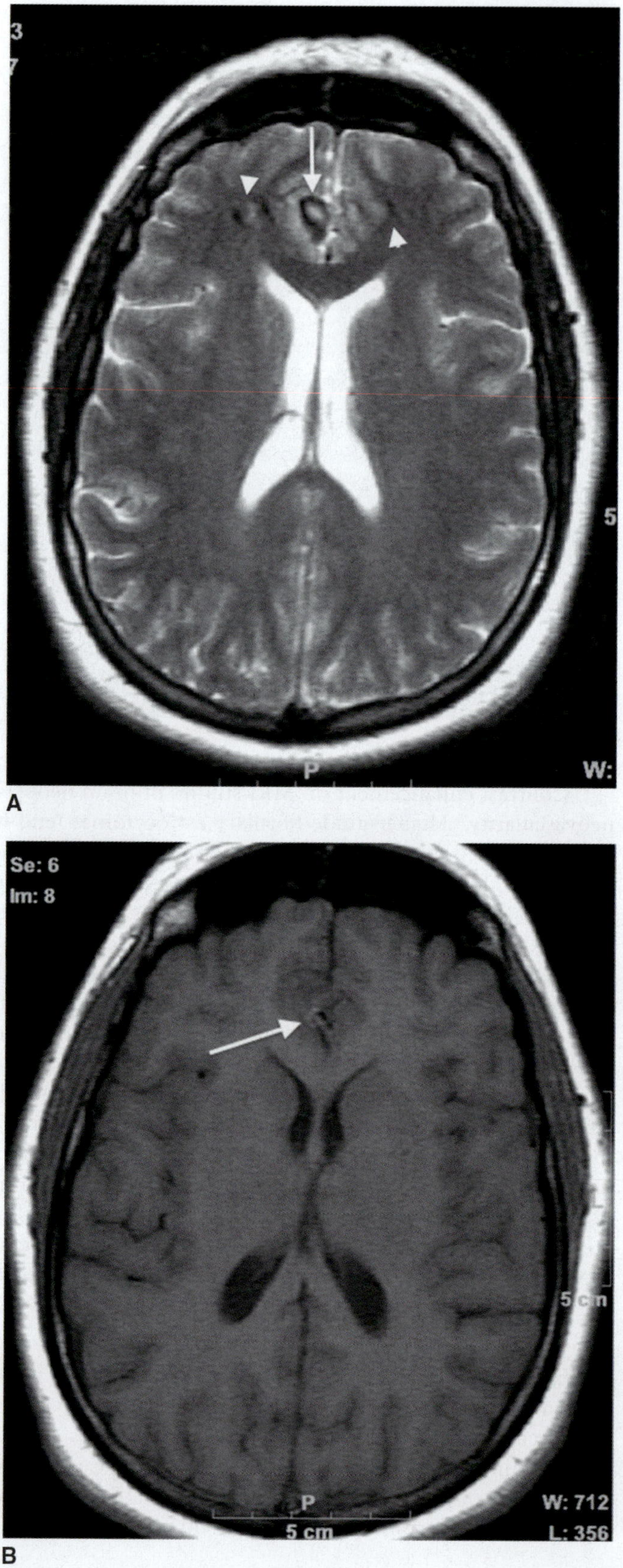

FIGURE 16-5: Axial T2W image shows dark-rimmed (*arrow*) mass between the frontal lobes. Pulsation artifact is present (*arrowheads*) (**A**). Axial T1W image without intravenous contrast shows minimal bright signal (*arrow*) in the mass (**B**).

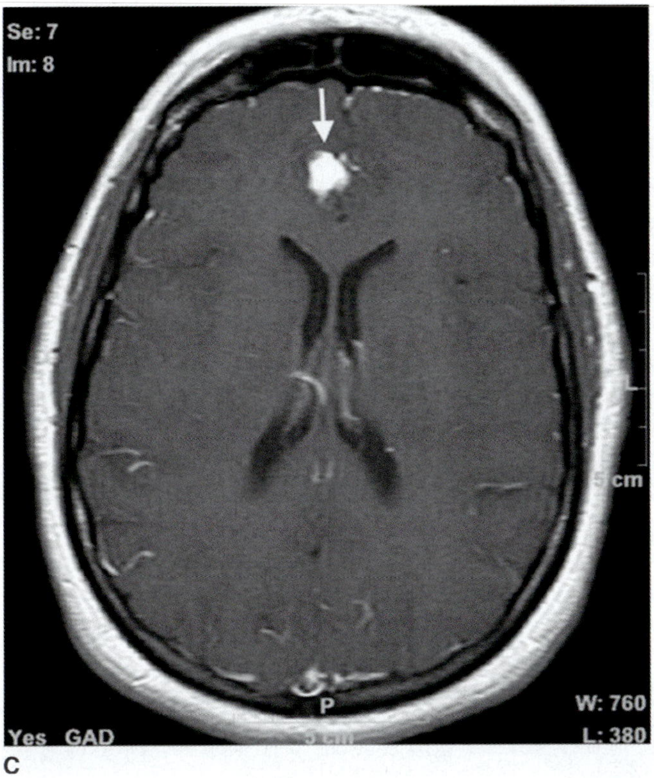

FIGURE 16-5: *(Continued)* Axial T1W image after intravenous contrast injection shows definite enhancement (*arrow*) in the mass (**C**).

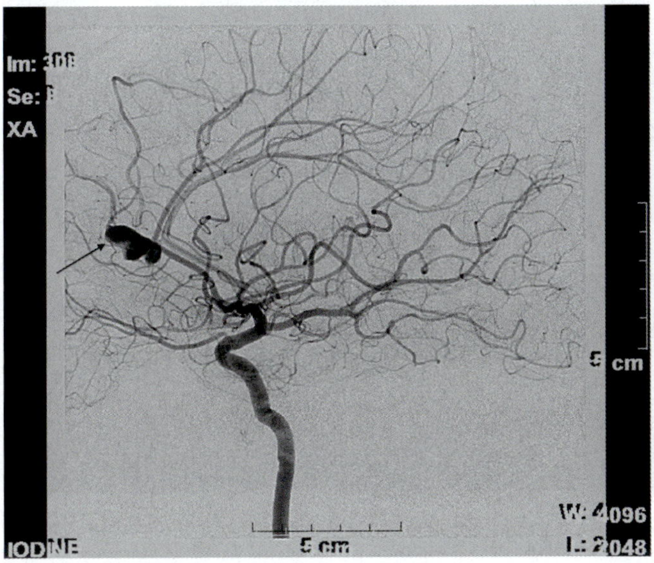

FIGURE 16-6: Lateral digital subtraction angiogram shows pericallosal artery pseudoaneurysm (*black arrow*).

Another example of imaging analysis concerns a large mass within the brain parenchyma in a 30-year-old patient. The routine MRI images reveal a large left-sided intra-axial mass with no enhancement and well-defined borders that suggest a low-grade neoplasm (Figure 16-7). A smaller, peripheral component of this mass has high diffusion (DWI) signal. This suggests more densely cellular tissue in this volume of the mass. MRS examining proton spectra shows a marked difference within the volumes inside this mass (Figure 16-8). The higher Cho/NAA

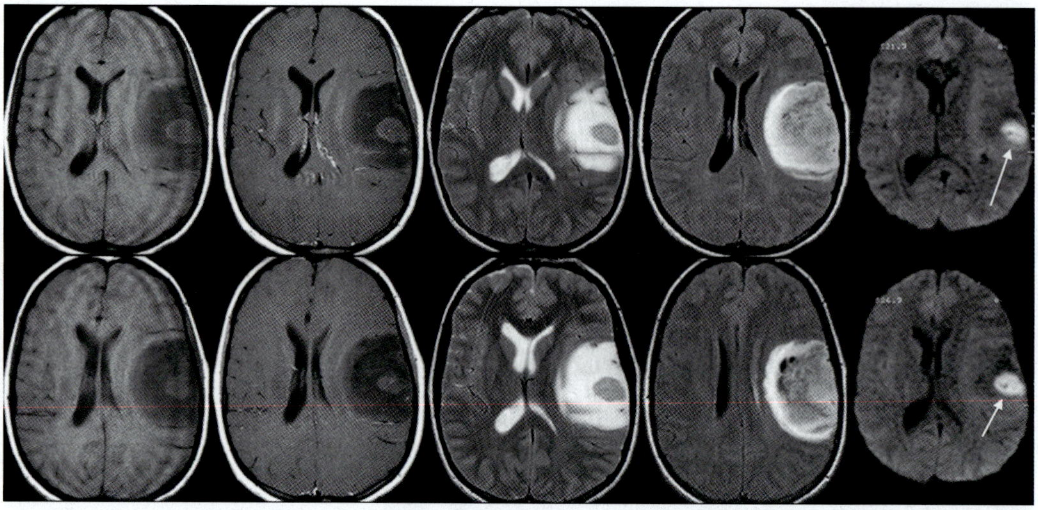

FIGURE 16-7: Axial MR images (from **left** to **right**: T1W, T1W after IV contrast, T2W, FLAIR, DWI) show a large left-sided parenchymal mass. This does not show enhancement and has well-defined margins on the FLAIR images. However, a peripheral, small part of the mass shows high DWI signal (*arrows*).

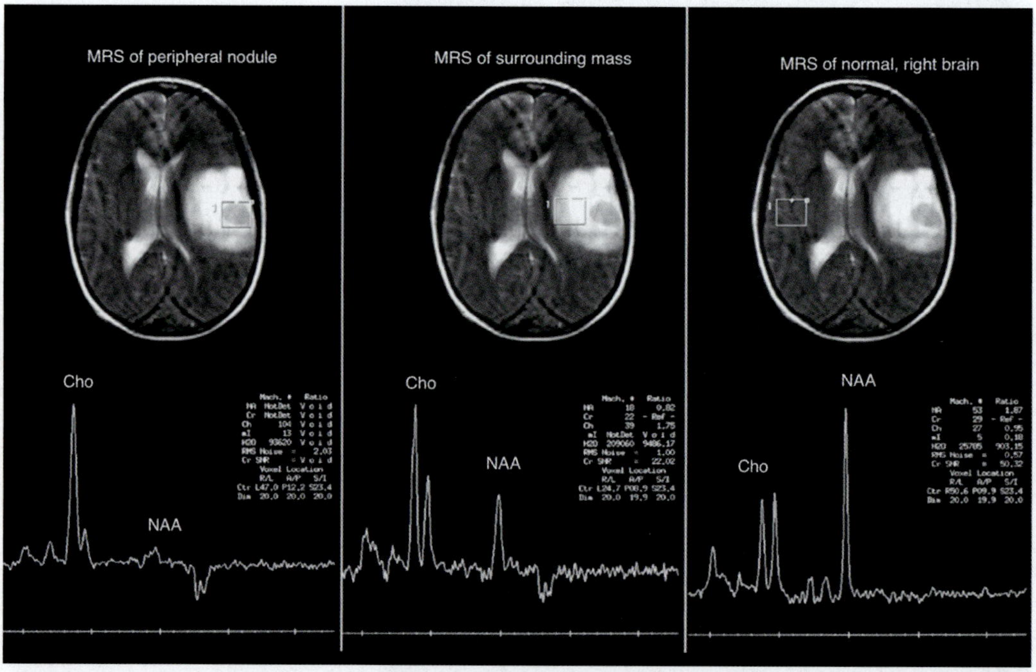

FIGURE 16-8: Proton MRS shows higher Cho/NAA ratios in the small, peripheral component of mass (spectrum on left) compared to the surrounding neoplasm (middle spectrum). Spectrum on right is from the normal, opposite brain.

ratio is within the more cellular, peripheral part of this mass. This suggests higher membrane turnover (mitoses) in this smaller volume of tumor. Tissue samples showed the most aggressive (anaplastic oligodendroglioma) part of the neoplasm to be within the small, peripheral nodule.

References

1. Gouliamos AD, Jimenez JP, Goree JA. Computed tomography and skull radiography in the diagnosis of calcified brain tumor. *AJR Am J Roentgenol* 1978;130(4):761–764.
2. Mathews VP, Caldemeyer KS, Lowe MJ, et al. Brain: gadolinium-enhanced fast fluid-attenuated inversion-recovery MR imaging. *Radiology* 1999;211:257–263.
3. Ernest FI, Kelly PJ, Scheithauer BW, et al. Cerebral astrocytomas: histopathologic correlation of MR and CT contrast enhancement with stereotactic biopsy. *Radiology* 1988;166:823–827.
4. Ginsberg LE, Fuller GN, Hashmi M, et al. The significance of lack of MR contrast enhancement of supratentorial brain tumors in adults: histopathological evaluation of a series. *Surg Neurol* 1998;49:436–440.
5. Rumboldt Z, Camacho DLA, Lake D, et al. Apparent diffusion coefficients for differentiation of cerebellar tumors in children. *AJNR Am J Neuroradiol* 2006;27:1362–1369.
6. Horska A, Barker PB. Imaging of brain tumors: MR spectroscopy and metabolic imaging. *Neuroimaging Clin N Am* 2010;20(3):293–310.

SECTION

IV

Molecular Pathology

- CHAPTER 17: Glial tumors
- CHAPTER 18: Nonglial tumors

Glial Tumors

17

Adriana Olar
Adekunle M. Adesina

Glial tumors account for approximately 30% of all brain tumors and 80% of all malignant brain tumors.[1] They are largely subdivided into diffusely infiltrative and circumscribed gliomas. In the past years, several clinically relevant molecular genetic alterations have been described in various gliomas. These advances introduced several diagnostic, prognostic, and predictive biomarkers that changed the routine practice of neuropathology. The purpose of this chapter is to familiarize the general anatomic pathologist with the most clinically relevant biomarkers and their use in the clinical practice of neuropathology.

DIFFUSE GLIOMA

Diffuse glioma tumor cells have the ability to infiltrate in between and track the normal neuropil structures (axons and dendrites) being capable of reaching distant sites (e.g., the opposite hemisphere). This property makes diffuse glioma an extremely aggressive entity. Based on histomorphologic features, diffuse glioma is subcategorized into two large subtypes: astrocytoma and oligodendroglioma. The current World Health Organization (WHO) grading system, based entirely on morphologic criteria, assigns three prognostic grades to astrocytoma (diffuse—grade II; anaplastic—grade III; and glioblastoma—grade IV) and two grades to oligodendroglioma (grades II and III).[2] The "mixed" category of diffuse glioma is problematic, because of differing diagnostic criteria and poor reproducibility among pathologists; hence its use in the primary diagnosis line is not preferred.[3,4] The WHO grade is currently the initial decision factor for therapy guidance in diffuse glioma.[5] Molecular features (summarized in Table 17-1) complement the histomorphologic information to better characterize and classify individual gliomas, providing a better prognostic and therapeutic stratification.

Isocitrate Dehydrogenase Mutations

Important molecular alterations in diffuse glioma with established role in gliomagenesis are mutations involving the isocitrate dehydrogenase (IDH) family of proteins (IDH), *IDH1* (2q33.3)[8] and *IDH2* (15q26.1),[9] which encodes Krebs cycle enzymes that catalyze the oxidative decarboxylation of isocitrate to alpha-ketoglutarate.[10] The mutated cytoplasmic isoenzymes, IDH1 and IDH2, promote accumulation of 2-hydroxyglutarate that competitively interacts with a family of enzymes, ketoglutarate-dependent dioxygenases, causing epigenetic instability with DNA hypermethylation/glioma-CpG Island methylator phenotype (G-CIMP)[11,12] and ultimately tumorigenesis.[10,11,13,14] G-CIMP describes subgroups of diffuse gliomas with high levels of DNA methylation at an increased number of CpG sites, and *IDH* mutations have been linked to this phenotype. G-CIMP tumors tend to have a better outcome.[11,12,15]

IDH1 and *IDH2* mutations are encountered in approximately 85% of supratentorial lower and intermediate-grade diffuse gliomas (grades II and III) of adolescents and younger adults

Table 17-1 Summary of Molecular Alterations in Diffuse Glioma

Astrocytoma Secondary Glioblastoma	Oligodendroglioma	Primary Glioblastoma[6,7]	Pediatric High-Grade Diffuse Glioma
IDH1/2	*IDH1/2*	LOH 10q	*H3F3A*
TP53	1p/19q LOH	*EGFR*	*ATRX*
ATRX	*CIC, FUBP1*	*p16INK4a*	*TP53*
		PTEN	*ACVR1* (DIPG)

DIPG, diffuse intrinsic pontine glioma; LOH, loss of heterozygosity.

and secondary glioblastoma.*[16–26] In contrast, *IDH* mutations are not frequent in primary glioblastoma† (~ 5%), nonsupratentorial diffuse glioma (spinal cord, cerebellum, brainstem) or pediatric patients.[21,22,26,27]

Approximately 90% of all *IDH* mutations involve *IDH1*[16,20,21] with *IDH1-R132H* (G395A) being the most common (~90% to 95%). To a much lesser extent (up to ~5%), other noncanonical *IDH1* mutations have been described, all involving codon 132. When *IDH2* is mutated, the mutation usually involves *R172K* (G515A).[16,17,20–22,28]

IDH1/2 mutations are acquired early in the pathogenesis of diffuse glioma, preceding gain of *TP53* mutations and subsequent astrocytic differentiation or 1p/19q co-deletion and subsequent oligodendroglial differentiation.[23] Recently, mutations in the alpha thalassemia/mental retardation syndrome X-linked gene (*ATRX*) have been associated with *IDH* and *TP53* mutations to define the molecular signature of astrocytoma (details in the Alpha Thalassemia/Mental Retardation Syndrome X-Linked Mutations section).[29–32] Moreover, to support the signature of secondary glioblastoma, *IDH* mutations do not usually associate with loss of chromosome 10 and *EGFR* amplification, molecular events more characteristic of primary glioblastoma.[6,7]

IDH mutations in intermediate- and high-grade glioma are independently prognostic beyond histologic grade (i.e., an *IDH* mutated glioblastoma [grade IV] might confer a better prognosis compared to an *IDH* wild-type anaplastic astrocytoma [grade III]) and beyond other associated prognostic molecular alterations (i.e., 1p/19q loss of heterozygosity [LOH] in oligodendroglioma).[17–19,33–35] The prognosis in low-grade and nonsupratentorial diffuse glioma is not clearly defined. Although the prognostic features of *IDH* mutations are strongly recognized, it is important to mention that this is not absolute, as a very small fraction of patients with *IDH* mutant tumors have a dismal prognosis (details in the "Alpha Thalassemia/Mental Retardation Syndrome X-Linked Mutations" section).[29]

A reliable mutant-specific, anti-IDH1-R132H antibody is commercially available for immunohistochemistry testing. This mutant-specific antibody can be used as a diagnostic test[20,36] in challenging small biopsy specimens (e.g., differentiating diffuse glioma from circumscribed glioma or diagnose diffuse glioma on a "biopsy-edge" of tumor with mild hypercellularity). Given its prognostic value if mutant positive, this simple test should not be denied to any adolescent and young adult with diffuse glioma. If antibody negative, *IDH1* (codon 132) and *IDH2* (codon 172) sequencing is recommended to interrogate for noncanonical *IDH* mutations.[37] *IDH* mutational status is now part of the routine neuro-oncology practice, for prognosis and treatment-decision stratification.[5]

---

*Secondary glioblastoma is defined as glioblastoma that arises following progression from a previously documented lower-grade astrocytoma (grade II or III), usually in younger adults (~40 years of age).

†Primary glioblastoma is defined as glioblastoma that arises *de novo* without prior evidence of a lower-grade astrocytoma precursor, usually in older adults (~60 years of age or greater).

1p/19q Co-Deletion

Recent evidence strongly supports combined LOH of 1p and 19q to be considered the *sine qua non* defining molecular signature of oligodendroglioma in adults. This alteration is always associated with *IDH* mutations,[38] and is mutually exclusive of *TP53* and *ATRX* mutations.[4,23,24,29,30,32,39] Similarly, *CIC* (on 19q) and *FUBP1* (on 1p) mutations tend to cluster with 1p/19q LOH and define the genetics of oligodendroglioma.[29,40,41] 1p/19q LOH is associated with the G-CIMP phenotype.[42]

Morphology can be predictive of the 1p/19q status as LOH is characteristic of diffuse glioma with classic oligodendroglial morphology (monotonous tumor cells with round dark regular nuclei).[43] It is important to emphasize that the characteristic perinuclear clear "fried-egg" halos might be missing due to tissue processing (freezing), and this feature is not a strong reliable diagnostic criterion for oligodendroglioma.

1p/19q co-deletion is both a prognostic and a predictive biomarker, associated with a better response to chemo- and radiotherapy,[44–48] and 1p/19q testing should always be performed in clinical practice on diffuse glioma with oligodendroglial or uncertain ("mixed") morphology for diagnosis, patient risk, and treatment stratification.[5] The most commonly utilized testing method is fluorescent *in situ* hybridization, but other methods might be utilized (e.g., array-CGH).[49]

Alpha Thalassemia/Mental Retardation Syndrome X-Linked Mutations

Recently, another extremely important molecular player in diffuse glioma has been recognized. Like *IDH* mutations, *ATRX* mutations have been detected in lower-grade diffuse glioma and secondary glioblastoma.[29–32]

ATRX (Xq21.1)[50] acts as a tumor suppressor gene. It encodes a switching and sucrose nonfermenting (SWI/SNF) protein family member with ATPase activity and plays a role in chromatin packaging. ATRX forms a complex with death-associated protein 6 (DAXX) that facilitates the incorporation of histone H3.3 into pericentric and telomeric heterochromatin, acting as a histone chaperone.[51–53] Briefly, its role is to bind and maintain chromatin integrity for normal DNA replication.[54] Loss or mutated ATRX may delay normal replication fork, cause DNA double-strand breaks, genome instability, and subsequent gene silencing. Double-strand breaks at telomeric sites may trigger alternative lengthening of telomeres, a telomerase-independent telomere maintenance mechanism characterized by homologous recombination, which strongly correlates with loss of normal ATRX function.[30,39,55–58]

ATRX mutations cluster with *IDH* and *TP53* mutations,[39,58,59] and are mutually exclusive from 1p/19q co-deletion, *CIC*, and *FUBP1* mutations defining the astrocytic phenotype.[29,32,39] *ATRX* mutations are present in pediatric high-grade glioma (up to ~50%)[60–62] and very rare primary adult glioblastomas (~7%).[29,32,57,58,62] *ATRX* mutations were not found in pilocytic astrocytoma.[29,32,63]

Patients with combined *IDH/ATRX* mutant anaplastic astrocytomas had a better prognosis compared to patients having *IDH* mutant and *ATRX* wild-type tumors.[29,39,59] Similarly, patients with combined *IDH/CIC and/or FUBP1* mutations *with* 1p/19q co-deletion had a better prognosis compared to patients with *IDH* mutant tumors lacking *CIC/FUBP1*/1p/19q LOH alterations.[29] The latter tumor phenotype had a worse prognosis when compared to *IDH1/ATRX* mutant tumors. Therefore, a small fraction of the *IDH* mutant tumors have a poor prognosis and behave as *IDH* wild-type tumors.[29] The prognostic impact of ATRX in low-grade gliomas is unclear.

An anti-ATRX antibody is commercially available.[32,39,57,58] Mutations in *ATRX* cause loss of nuclear protein expression in tumor cells.[29–31,39,57] The nuclear protein expression will be retained in normal cells (e.g., endothelial cells) similar to INI1 loss in atypical teratoid/rhabdoid tumor (see Figure 18-1). ATRX can be used in clinical practice as a diagnostic biomarker when faced with the difficulty of diagnosing infiltrating astrocytoma versus pilocytic astrocytoma on small biopsy samples and when faced with the subjective "mixed oligoastrocytoma" category. Loss of ATRX nuclear protein immunoexpression establishes the astrocytoma phenotype. In view of its diagnostic and its prognostic values, anti-ATRX use is encouraged in routine clinical practice.

PEDIATRIC DIFFUSE GLIOMA

Pediatric high-grade diffuse gliomas are genetically different compared to their adult counterparts.[62,64–66] Mutations in replication-independent histone 3—variant 3.3 (*H3F3A*) and variant 3.1 genes (*HIST1H3B/C*) are highly characteristic of pediatric high-grade glioma.[62,65,67] These mutations are location specific (K27M—diffuse intrinsic pontine glioma [DIPG] and thalamus and G34R/V—cerebral cortex), are mutually exclusive from *IDH* mutations, frequently accompanied by *ATRX* and *TP53* mutations, and are predictive of short survival.[60,62,64–66,68] DIPG (~20% to 30%) have mutations involving *ACVR1* encoding a type I activin receptor serine/threonine kinase. *ACVR1*-positive gliomas also have a significant number of H3.1 K27M (not H3.3 K27M) mutations and are associated with improved survival.[60,61,69,70]

CIRCUMSCRIBED GLIOMAS

Circumscribed gliomas are usually noninfiltrative and display a relatively sharp border with the surrounding neuropil.[2] Pilocytic astrocytoma, pleomorphic xanthoastrocytoma, and gangliogliomas, all share different *BRAF* genetic alterations.

BRAF (7q34) encodes a kinase with roles in MAPK/ERK cellular signaling. Most *BRAF* genetic alterations in sporadic pilocytic astrocytoma involve gene duplication with subsequent *BRAF–KIAA1549* fusion and constitutive B-RAF activation, stimulating MAPK/ERK signaling and promoting tumor cell growth.[71] However, shortly thereafter oncogene-induced senescence is activated that counteracts and slows tumor cell growth. This latter mechanism is possibly responsible for the slow growth rate of pilocytic astrocytomas.[72,73] *BRAF–KIAA1549* fusion–duplication characterizes cerebellar (~60% to 80%), brainstem, hypothalamic, and optic pathway (~60%),[74] and only about 20% of the cerebral cortical pilocytic astrocytomas,[75] and its frequency tends to decrease with increasing age.[76] It has not been reported in rosette-forming glioneuronal tumor of the fourth ventricle, a tumor that shares morphologic features with and can be easily misdiagnosed as pilocytic astrocytoma.[77,78] *BRAF–KIAA1549* fusion–duplication was reported in about 30% to 60% of cases of pilomyxoid astrocytomas.[75,79,80] Among all low-grade pediatric gliomas, the presence of the *BRAF–KIAA1549* fusion–duplication seems to be an independent predictor of favorable prognosis.[80]

In contrast to pilocytic astrocytoma, pleomorphic xanthoastrocytoma (~60% to 80%) and ganglioglioma (~30% to 50%) have different types of B-RAF activating alterations: *BRAF^{V600E}* mutations.[81–83] Pleomorphic xanthoastrocytoma of the temporal lobe seems to have a higher incidence of the mutation (>90%).[81] Interestingly, *BRAF^{V600E}* is also present in both components of the rare composite tumor pleomorphic astrocytoma–ganglioglioma suggesting a common origin and arguing against a collision tumor.[84]

BRAF^{V600E} mutations are not as common in pilocytic astrocytomas (~30% in the diencephalon, ~10% in the cerebral hemispheres and brainstem, and only ~2% in the cerebellum).[82] A mutant-specific and reliable anti-BRAF^{V600E} antibody is commercially available for immunohistochemistry testing.[81] As *BRAF* alterations should not cluster with *IDH* mutations, this antibody can be used as a tool for challenging diagnostic situations (e.g., ganglioglioma vs. diffuse glioma in small biopsy samples).[85]

Recently, in supratentorial ependymoma, a potentially significant genetic alteration has been described: *C11orf95–RELA* fusion. This fusion seems to result from chromosome 11q13.1 chromothripsis and drive NF-kB signaling. *C11orf95–RELA* fusion was associated with increased CCND1 and L1CAM protein expression, both involved in NK-kB signaling, meaning that these two proteins might be used as surrogate biomarkers to identify the fusion by immunohistochemistry.[86] A possible utility could be in the diagnosis of morphologically ambiguous cases of supratentorial cortical ependymoma.

CONCLUSIONS AND FUTURE DIRECTIONS

Several molecular signatures have proven valuable for stratification and management of glioma patients with respect to prognosis and prediction of treatment response. Molecular signatures can also act as diagnostic biomarkers and improve glioma classification (i.e., mutated *ATRX*—the astrocytoma signature and 1p/19q LOH—the oligodendroglioma signature). Based on this information, there is a rapid trend to shifting toward an integrated morphologic and molecular diagnosis (e.g., a glioma of uncertain morphology or "mixed" might be integrated in the molecular astrocytoma category if *ATRX* is mutated).

ACKNOWLEDGMENTS

Dr. Adriana Olar was supported by the National Institutes of Health/National Cancer Institute (Training Grant #5T32CA163185).

References

1. Ostrom QT, Gittleman H, Farah P, et al. CBTRUS statistical report: primary brain and central nervous system tumors diagnosed in the United States in 2006–2010. *Neuro Oncol* 2013;15(suppl 2):ii1–ii56.
2. Louis DN, Ohgaki H, Wiestler OD, et al. *WHO Classification of Tumors of the Central Nervous System.* 4th ed. Lyon, France: IARC; 2007:8–69.
3. Kros JM, Gorlia T, Kouwenhoven MC, et al. Panel review of anaplastic oligodendroglioma from European Organization for Research and Treatment of Cancer Trial 26951: assessment of consensus in diagnosis, influence of 1p/19q loss, and correlations with outcome. *J Neuropathol Exp Neurol* 2007;66(6):545–551.
4. Aldape K, Burger PC, Perry A. Clinicopathologic aspects of 1p/19q loss and the diagnosis of oligodendroglioma. *Arch Pathol Lab Med* 2007;131(2):242–251.
5. NCCN Clinical Practice Guidelines in Oncology. *Central Nervous System Cancers. Version 2*; 2014 [Updated March 11, 2014; cited April 21, 2014]; Available from: http://www.nccn.org
6. Ohgaki H, Kleihues P. Genetic pathways to primary and secondary glioblastoma. *Am J Pathol* 2007;170(5):1445–1453.
7. Bleeker FE, Molenaar RJ, Leenstra S. Recent advances in the molecular understanding of glioblastoma. *J Neurooncol* 2012;108(1):11–27.
8. Narahara K, Kimura S, Kikkawa K, et al. Probable assignment of soluble isocitrate dehydrogenase (IDH1) to 2q33.3. *Hum Genet* 1985;71(1):37–40.
9. Grzeschik KH. Assignment of a gene for human mitochondrial isocitrate dehydrogenase (ICD-M, EC 1.1.1.41) to chromosome 15. *Hum Genet* 1976;34(1):23–28.
10. Ichimura K. Molecular pathogenesis of IDH mutations in gliomas. *Brain Tumor Pathol* 2012;29:131–139.
11. Duncan CG, Barwick BG, Jin G, et al. A heterozygous IDH1r132h/WT mutation induces genome-wide alterations in DNA methylation. *Genome Res* 2012;22(12):2339–2355.
12. Turcan S, Rohle D, Goenka A, et al. IDH1 mutation is sufficient to establish the glioma hypermethylator phenotype. *Nature* 2012;483(7390):479–483.
13. Ward PS, Patel J, Wise DR, et al. The common feature of leukemia-associated IDH1 and IDH2 mutations is a neomorphic enzyme activity converting alpha-ketoglutarate to 2-hydroxyglutarate. *Cancer Cell* 2010;17(3):225–234.
14. Xu W, Yang H, Liu Y, et al. Oncometabolite 2-hydroxyglutarate is a competitive inhibitor of alpha-ketoglutarate-dependent dioxygenases. *Cancer Cell* 2011;19(1):17–30.
15. Noushmehr H, Weisenberger DJ, Diefes K, et al. Identification of a CpG Island methylator phenotype that defines a distinct subgroup of glioma. *Cancer Cell* 2010;17(5):510–522.
16. Parsons DW, Jones S, Zhang X, et al. An integrated genomic analysis of human glioblastoma multiforme. *Science* 2008;321(5897):1807–1812.
17. Yan H, Parsons DW, Jin G, et al. IDH1 and IDH2 mutations in gliomas. *N Engl J Med* 2009;360(8):765–773.
18. Sonoda Y, Kumabe T, Nakamura T, et al. Analysis of IDH1 and IDH2 mutations in Japanese glioma patients. *Cancer Sci* 2009;100(10):1996–1998.

19. Hartmann C, Hentschel B, Wick W, et al. Patients with IDH1 wild type anaplastic astrocytomas exhibit worse prognosis than IDH1-mutated glioblastomas, and IDH1 mutation status accounts for the unfavorable prognostic effect of higher age: implications for classification of gliomas. *Acta Neuropathol* 2010;120(6):707–718.
20. Horbinski C, Kofler J, Kelly LM, et al. Diagnostic use of IDH1/2 mutation analysis in routine clinical testing of formalin-fixed, paraffin-embedded glioma tissues. *J Neuropathol Exp Neurol* 2009;68(12):1319–1325.
21. Hartmann C, Meyer J, Balss J, et al. Type and frequency of IDH1 and IDH2 mutations are related to astrocytic and oligodendroglial differentiation and age: a study of 1,010 diffuse gliomas. *Acta Neuropathol* 2009;118(4):469–474.
22. Balss J, Meyer J, Mueller W, et al. Analysis of the IDH1 codon 132 mutation in brain tumors. *Acta Neuropathol* 2008;116(6):597–602.
23. Watanabe T, Nobusawa S, Kleihues P, et al. IDH1 mutations are early events in the development of astrocytomas and oligodendrogliomas. *Am J Pathol* 2009;174(4):1149–1153.
24. Ichimura K, Pearson DM, Kocialkowski S, et al. IDH1 mutations are present in the majority of common adult gliomas but rare in primary glioblastomas. *Neuro-Oncology* 2009;11(4):341–347.
25. Nobusawa S, Watanabe T, Kleihues P, et al. IDH1 mutations as molecular signature and predictive factor of secondary glioblastomas. *Clin Cancer Res* 2009;15(19):6002–6007.
26. Pollack IF, Hamilton RL, Sobol RW, et al. IDH1 mutations are common in malignant gliomas arising in adolescents: a report from the Children's Oncology Group. *Childs Nerv Syst* 2011;27(1):87–94.
27. Ellezam B, Theeler BJ, Walbert T, et al. Low rate of R132h IDH1 mutation in infratentorial and spinal cord grade II and III diffuse gliomas. *Acta Neuropathol* 2012;124(3):449–451.
28. Felsberg J, Wolter M, Seul H, et al. Rapid and sensitive assessment of the IDH1 and IDH2 mutation status in cerebral gliomas based on DNA pyrosequencing. *Acta Neuropathol* 2010;119(4):501–507.
29. Jiao Y, Killela PJ, Reitman ZJ, et al. Frequent ATRX, CIC, FUBP1 and IDH1 mutations refine the classification of malignant gliomas. *Oncotarget* 2012;3(7):709–722.
30. Kannan K, Inagaki A, Silber J, et al. Whole-exome sequencing identifies ATRX mutation as a key molecular determinant in lower-grade glioma. *Oncotarget* 2012;3(10):1194–1203.
31. Killela PJ, Pirozzi CJ, Reitman ZJ, et al. The genetic landscape of anaplastic astrocytoma. *Oncotarget* 2013;30:1452–1457.
32. Liu XY, Gerges N, Korshunov A, et al. Frequent ATRX mutations and loss of expression in adult diffuse astrocytic tumors carrying IDH1/IDH2 and TP53 mutations. *Acta Neuropathol* 2012;124(5):615–625.
33. van den Bent MJ, Dubbink HJ, Marie Y, et al. IDH1 and IDH2 mutations are prognostic but not predictive for outcome in anaplastic oligodendroglial tumors: a Report of the European Organization for Research and Treatment of Cancer Brain Tumor Group. *Clin Cancer Res* 2010;16(5):1597–1604.
34. Wick W, Hartmann C, Engel C, et al. Noa-04 randomized phase III trial of sequential radiochemotherapy of anaplastic glioma with procarbazine, lomustine, and vincristine or temozolomide. *J Clin Oncol* 2009;27(35):5874–5880.
35. Weller M, Felsberg J, Hartmann C, et al. Molecular predictors of progression-free and overall survival in patients with newly diagnosed glioblastoma: a Prospective Translational Study of the German Glioma Network. *J Clin Oncol* 2009;27(34):5743–5750.
36. Capper D, Reuss D, Schittenhelm J, et al. Mutation-specific IDH1 antibody differentiates oligodendrogliomas and oligoastrocytomas from other brain tumors with oligodendroglioma-like morphology. *Acta Neuropathol* 2011;121(2):241–252.
37. Olar A, Aldape KD. Biomarkers classification and therapeutic decision-making for malignant gliomas. *Curr Treat Options Oncol* 2012;13(4):417–436.
38. Labussiere M, Idbaih A, Wang XW, et al. All the 1p19q codeleted gliomas are mutated on IDH1 or IDH2. *Neurology* 2010;74(23):1886–1890.
39. Wiestler B, Capper D, Holland-Letz T, et al. ATRX loss refines the classification of anaplastic gliomas and identifies a subgroup of IDH mutant astrocytic tumors with better prognosis. *Acta Neuropathol* 2013;126(3):443–451.
40. Sahm F, Koelsche C, Meyer J, et al. CIC and FUBP1 mutations in oligodendrogliomas, oligoastrocytomas and astrocytomas. *Acta Neuropathol* 2012;123:853–860.
41. Yip S, Butterfield YS, Morozova O, et al. Concurrent CIC mutations, IDH mutations, and 1p/19q loss distinguish oligodendrogliomas from other cancers. *J Pathol* 2012;226(1):7–16.
42. van den Bent MJ, Gravendeel LA, Gorlia T, et al. A hypermethylated phenotype is a better predictor of survival than MGMT methylation in anaplastic oligodendroglial brain tumors: a Report from EORTC Study 26951. *Clin Cancer Res* 2011;17(22):7148–7155.

43. Scheie D, Cvancarova M, Mork S, et al. Can morphology predict 1p/19q loss in oligodendroglial tumours? *Histopathology* 2008;53(5):578–587.
44. Kaloshi G, Benouaich-Amiel A, Diakite F, et al. Temozolomide for low-grade gliomas: predictive impact of 1p/19q loss on response and outcome. *Neurology* 2007;68(21):1831–1836.
45. Cairncross G, Jenkins R. Gliomas with 1p/19q codeletion: A.K.A. oligodendroglioma. *Cancer J* 2008;14(6):352–357.
46. Cairncross JG, Ueki K, Zlatescu MC, et al. Specific genetic predictors of chemotherapeutic response and survival in patients with anaplastic oligodendrogliomas. *J Natl Cancer Inst* 1998;90(19):1473–1479.
47. van den Bent MJ, Brandes AA, Taphoorn MJ, et al. Adjuvant procarbazine, lomustine, and vincristine chemotherapy in newly diagnosed anaplastic oligodendroglioma: long-term follow-up of EORTC Brain Tumor Group Study 26951. *J Clin Oncol* 2013;31(3):344–350.
48. Cairncross G, Wang M, Shaw E, et al. Phase III trial of chemoradiotherapy for anaplastic oligodendroglioma: long-term results of RTOG 9402. *J Clin Oncol* 2013;31(3):337–343.
49. Jansen M, Yip S, Louis DN. Molecular pathology in adult gliomas: diagnostic, prognostic, and predictive markers. *Lancet Neurol* 2010;9(7):717–726.
50. Honda S, Satomura S, Hayashi S, et al. Concomitant microduplications of MECP2 and ATRX in male patients with severe mental retardation. *J Hum Genet* 2012;57(1):73–77.
51. Drane P, Ouararhni K, Depaux A, et al. The death-associated protein DAXX is a novel histone chaperone involved in the replication-independent deposition of H3.3. *Genes Dev* 2010;24(12):1253–1265.
52. Lewis PW, Elsaesser SJ, Noh KM, et al. DAXX is an H3.3-specific histone chaperone and cooperates with ATRX in replication-independent chromatin assembly at telomeres. *Proc Natl Acad Sci U S A* 2010;107(32):14075–14080.
53. Goldberg AD, Banaszynski LA, Noh KM, et al. Distinct factors control histone variant H3.3 localization at specific genomic regions. *Cell* 2010;140(5):678–691.
54. Wong LH, McGhie JD, Sim M, et al. ATRX interacts with H3.3 in maintaining telomere structural integrity in pluripotent embryonic stem cells. *Genome Res* 2010;20(3):351–360.
55. Lovejoy CA, Li W, Reisenweber S, et al. Loss of ATRX, genome instability, and an altered DNA damage response are hallmarks of the alternative lengthening of telomeres pathway. *PLoS Genet* 2012;8(7):e1002772.
56. Bower K, Napier CE, Cole SL, et al. Loss of wild-type ATRX expression in somatic cell hybrids segregates with activation of alternative lengthening of telomeres. *PLoS One* 2012;7(11):e50062.
57. Heaphy CM, de Wilde RF, Jiao Y, et al. Altered telomeres in tumors with ATRX and DAXX mutations. *Science* 2011;333(6041):425.
58. Abedalthagafi M, Phillips JJ, Kim GE, et al. The alternative lengthening of telomere phenotype is significantly associated with loss of ATRX expression in high-grade pediatric and adult astrocytomas: a Multi-Institutional Study of 214 Astrocytomas. *Mod Pathol* 2013;26(11):1425–1432.
59. Cai J, Yang P, Zhang C, et al. ATRX MRNA expression combined with IDH1/2 mutational status and Ki-67 expression refines the molecular classification of astrocytic tumors: evidence from the whole transcriptome sequencing of 169 samples samples. *Oncotarget* 2014;5:2551–2561.
60. Wu G, Diaz AK, Paugh BS, et al. The genomic landscape of diffuse intrinsic pontine glioma and pediatric non-brainstem high-grade glioma. *Nat Genet* 2014;46(5):444–450.
61. Fontebasso AM, Papillon-Cavanagh S, Schwartzentruber J, et al. Recurrent somatic mutations in ACVR1 in pediatric midline high-grade astrocytoma. *Nat Genet* 2014;46(5):462–466.
62. Schwartzentruber J, Korshunov A, Liu XY, et al. Driver mutations in histone H3.3 and chromatin remodelling genes in paediatric glioblastoma. *Nature* 2012;482(7384):226–231.
63. Zhang J, Wu G, Miller CP, et al. Whole-genome sequencing identifies genetic alterations in pediatric low-grade gliomas. *Nat Genet* 2013;45(6):602–612.
64. Jones DT, Mulholland SA, Pearson DM, et al. Adult grade II diffuse astrocytomas are genetically distinct from and more aggressive than their paediatric counterparts. *Acta Neuropathol* 2011;121(6):753–761.
65. Khuong-Quang DA, Buczkowicz P, Rakopoulos P, et al. K27m mutation in histone H3.3 defines clinically and biologically distinct subgroups of pediatric diffuse intrinsic pontine gliomas. *Acta Neuropathol* 2012;124(3):439–447.
66. Byeon SJ, Myung JK, Kim SH, et al. Distinct genetic alterations in pediatric glioblastomas. *Childs Nerv Syst* 2012;28(7):1025–1032.
67. Sturm D, Witt H, Hovestadt V, et al. Hotspot mutations in H3f3a and IDH1 define distinct epigenetic and biological subgroups of glioblastoma. *Cancer Cell* 2012;22(4):425–437.
68. Aihara K, Mukasa A, Gotoh K, et al. H3f3a K27m mutations in thalamic gliomas from young adult patients. *Neuro-Oncology* 2014;16(1):140–146.

69. Taylor KR, Mackay A, Truffaux N, et al. Recurrent activating ACVR1 mutations in diffuse intrinsic pontine glioma. *Nat Genet* 2014;46(5):457–461.
70. Buczkowicz P, Hoeman C, Rakopoulos P, et al. Genomic analysis of diffuse intrinsic pontine gliomas identifies three molecular subgroups and recurrent activating ACVR1 mutations. *Nat Genet* 2014;46(5):451–456.
71. Dhomen N, Marais R. New insight into BRAF mutations in cancer. *Curr Opin Genet Dev* 2007;17(1):31–39.
72. Raabe EH, Lim KS, Kim JM, et al. BRAF activation induces transformation and then senescence in human neural stem cells: a pilocytic astrocytoma model. *Clin Cancer Res* 2011;17(11):3590–3599.
73. Jacob K, Quang-Khuong DA, Jones DT, et al. Genetic aberrations leading to MAPK pathway activation mediate oncogene-induced senescence in sporadic pilocytic astrocytomas. *Clin Cancer Res* 2011;17(14):4650–4660.
74. Jacob K, Albrecht S, Sollier C, et al. Duplication of 7q34 is specific to juvenile pilocytic astrocytomas and a hallmark of cerebellar and optic pathway tumours. *Br J Cancer* 2009;101(4):722–733.
75. Lin A, Rodriguez FJ, Karajannis MA, et al. BRAF alterations in primary glial and glioneuronal neoplasms of the central nervous system with identification of 2 novel KIAA1549:BRAF fusion variants. *J Neuropathol Exp Neurol* 2012;71(1):66–72.
76. Hasselblatt M, Riesmeier B, Lechtape B, et al. BRAF–KIAA1549 fusion transcripts are less frequent in pilocytic astrocytomas diagnosed in adults. *Neuropathol Appl Neurobiol* 2011;37(7):803–806.
77. Gessi M, Lambert SR, Lauriola L, et al. Absence of KIAA1549–BRAF fusion in Rosette-forming glioneuronal tumors of the fourth ventricle (RGNT). *J Neurooncol* 2012;110(1):21–25.
78. Gessi M, Waha A, Setty P, et al. Analysis of KIAA1549-BRAF fusion status in a case of Rosette-forming glioneuronal tumor of the fourth ventricle (RGNT). *Neuropathology* 2011;31(6):654–657.
79. Colin C, Padovani L, Chappe C, et al. Outcome analysis of childhood pilocytic astrocytomas: a retrospective study of 148 cases at a single institution. *Neuropathol Appl Neurobiol* 2013;39(6):693–705.
80. Hawkins C, Walker E, Mohamed N, et al. BRAF–KIAA1549 fusion predicts better clinical outcome in pediatric low-grade astrocytoma. *Clin Cancer Res* 2011;17(14):4790–4798.
81. Koelsche C, Sahm F, Wohrer A, et al. BRAF-mutated pleomorphic xanthoastrocytoma is associated with temporal location, reticulin fiber deposition and Cd34 expression. *Brain Pathol* 2014;24(3):221–229.
82. Schindler G, Capper D, Meyer J, et al. Analysis of BRAF V600e mutation in 1,320 nervous system tumors reveals high mutation frequencies in pleomorphic xanthoastrocytoma, ganglioglioma and extra-cerebellar pilocytic astrocytoma. *Acta Neuropathol* 2011;121(3):397–405.
83. Dias-Santagata D, Lam Q, Vernovsky K, et al. BRAF V600e mutations are common in pleomorphic xanthoastrocytoma: diagnostic and therapeutic implications. *PLoS One* 2011;6(3):e17948.
84. Aisner DL, Newell KL, Pollack AG, et al. Composite pleomorphic xanthoastrocytoma-epithelioid glioneuronal tumor with BRAF V600e mutation—report of three cases. *Clin Neuropathol* 2014; 33(2):112–121.
85. Korshunov A, Meyer J, Capper D, et al. Combined molecular analysis of BRAF and IDH1 distinguishes pilocytic astrocytoma from diffuse astrocytoma. *Acta Neuropathol* 2009;118(3):401–405.
86. Parker M, Mohankumar KM, Punchihewa C, et al. C11orf95–RELA fusions drive oncogenic NF-Kappab signalling in ependymoma. *Nature* 2014;506(7489):451–455.

Nonglial Tumors 18

Adriana Olar
Adekunle M. Adesina

NONGLIAL TUMORS

Nonglial brain tumors comprise tumors of the meninges (e.g., meningioma), embryonal tumors, tumors of the sella and pineal region, tumors of the cranial and paraspinal nerves, lymphomas and hematopoietic neoplasms, germ cell tumors, and metastatic tumors.[1] Embryonal tumors consist of approximately 16% of all brain tumors, and their incidence is maximal in the pediatric population and decreases with age.[2] They are aggressive tumors with the tendency to disseminate through the cerebrospinal fluid.[1] In contrast, meningioma represents approximately 36% of all brain tumors and its incidence increases with age.[2] The purpose of this chapter is to familiarize the general anatomic pathologist with the newest, most clinically relevant updates on the molecular genetics of nonglial tumors with an emphasis on embryonal tumors, tumors of the meninges, and schwannomatosis.

EMBRYONAL TUMORS

Primitive neuroectodermal tumors (PNET) are subdivided into two large subgroups with distinctive molecular alterations: central PNET (cPNET), arising in the central nervous system (CNS), and peripheral PNET (pPNET), arising in the peripheral nerves, soft tissue, or bone.[1] The cPNET category is represented by medulloblastoma (cerebellar PNET), atypical teratoid/rhabdoid tumor (AT/RT), and extracerebellar PNET with its different morphologic variants (ependymoblastoma, medulloepithelioma, embryonal tumor with abundant neuropil and true rosettes [ETANTR], and cribriform neuroepithelial tumor [CRINET]).[1,3–9] The pPNET category is represented by the Ewing family group of tumors.[10,11] There are molecular differences between the cPNET and pPNET subgroups and also differences within each subgroup subcategory.[10–12] Familiarity with molecular alterations might successfully solve diagnostic dilemmas and adequately guide patient management.

Medulloblastoma

Genomic advances identified several distinct molecular subgroups of medulloblastoma with prognostic significance[13–18] that prompted a consensus defining[19] four well-characterized subgroups: the wingless-related integration site (WNT) subgroup, the sonic hedgehog (SHH) subgroup, group 3, and group 4.[20] The clinical, pathologic, and genetic alterations are summarized in Table 18-1.

The WNT medulloblastoma subgroup (~7% to 15%)[13–16] is characterized by WNT pathway activation and is associated with the best prognosis. Monosomy 6 and mutations involving *CTNNB1*, the gene encoding β-catenin, the downstream effector of the WNT pathway, seem to define this medulloblastoma subgroup. In normal cells, cytoplasmic β-catenin is degraded. WNT pathway activation in tumor cells interferes with normal protein degradation, causing rising cytoplasmic β-catenin levels, followed by its translocation to the nucleus. In the nucleus, β-catenin activates transcription factors involved in cell proliferation.[13–15,21]

Table 18-1 Molecular Subgroups in Pediatric Medulloblastoma

	WNT	SHH	Group 3	Group 4
Age at presentation	Childhood	Infant, adult	Infant, childhood	Childhood
Gender distribution	F = M	F > M	M > F	M > F
Histology	Classic, very rare LC/A	Desmoplastic/ nodular > classic > LC/A	Classic > LC/A	Classic, very rare LC/A
Genetics	Monosomy 6, *CTNNB1*	*PTCH1*, 9q loss, 10q loss	*MYC* amplification, i17	i17 +++
IHC	Nuclear β-catenin	Cytoplasmic GAB1	Cytoplasmic β-catenin/GAB1 negative	
Survival (5 years)	>90%	~75%	Frequently (~30%–40%) metastatic at presentation	
			~50%	~75%

LC/A, large cell/anaplastic.[20,22,34]

SHH medulloblastoma (~10% to 30%)[13–16] is characterized by SHH signaling pathway activation. These medulloblastomas have a bimodal age distribution with peaks in infancy (<3 years of age) and in adulthood (>18 years of age). They frequently have mutations in patched1 (*PTCH1)* (located on 9q22).[14,16]

Group 3 (~30%)[16] is characterized by *MYC* amplification and photoreceptor gene expression signatures,[14] while group 4 (~35%)[16] is characterized by isochromosome 17q and neuronal gene expression signatures.[15] Groups 3 and 4 medulloblastomas are associated with most unfavorable prognosis, frequently presenting with metastasis at diagnosis,[15,20,22] and often have anaplastic components. *TP53* mutation/p53 pathway deregulation is an independent poor prognostic marker in pediatric medulloblastoma.[23–25]

Medulloblastoma in adults is slightly different than its pediatric counterpart. In adults, the most common medulloblastoma molecular subtype is SHH whereas group C is almost missing.[20] The adult WNT medulloblastomas show WNT pathway activation and β-catenin nuclear expression; however, chromosome 6 loss and *CTNNB1* mutations are not as frequent as in children suggesting a possible different mechanism for WNT pathway activation. Also in contrast to pediatric WNT medulloblastomas, adult WNT tumors do not share the same excellent prognosis.[18,26] The most prognostic biomarkers in adult medulloblastoma seem to be 10q loss, 17p loss, 17q gain, 2 gain, and *GLI2* amplification,[26] but only when used in the context of a molecular subgroup (e.g., within SHH tumors).[22,27] Moreover, in SHH adult medulloblastoma, the desmoplastic nodular morphologic subtype is not prognostic.[27]

Syndromic medulloblastoma has been associated with mutations in patched genes (*PTCH1*, *PTCH2*) or suppressor of fused gene (*SUFU*) with subsequent deregulation of the SHH pathway in Gorlin syndrome,[28–32] mutations in the adenomatosis polyposis coli gene (*APC*) in Turcot syndrome with subsequent deregulation of the WNT pathway, and *TP53* mutations in Li-Fraumeni syndrome.[33]

In clinical practice, the use of immunohistochemistry can help subclassify medulloblastoma as belonging to WNT, SHH, or non-WNT/SHH. Nuclear β-catenin immunoexpression reliably identifies WNT medulloblastoma.[34,35] Varying patterns of β-catenin nuclear expression have been described, the most common being diffuse combined nuclear and cytoplasmic immunoexpression. A patchy pattern of nuclear immunoexpression with or without cytoplasmic immunoexpression intermixed with nuclear-immunonegative regions can also be observed. However, if only rare positive nuclei are observed (<2%), the tumors should not be classified as WNT medulloblastomas.[34,36]

GRB2-associated binding protein 1 (GAB1) has roles in intracellular signaling and cell growth, and its expression has been associated with SHH medulloblastoma. A commercially available anti-GAB1 antibody can be used to identify SHH medulloblastoma. Cytoplasmic immunoexpression, especially in the internodular regions of the desmoplastic/nodular subtype are characteristic in SHH medulloblastoma. GRB-2 immunoexpression is lacking in the rest of the medulloblastoma subtypes.[34] Alternate markers of SHH activation are downstream effectors Gli1 and Gli2.[37,38]

Atypical Teratoid/Rhabdoid Tumor

The defining molecular signature of AT/RT (~95%) is represented by *SMARCB1/hSNF5/BAF47/INI1* suppressor gene (22q11.2) inactivation due to biallelic loss, biallelic mutations, or heterozygous loss with mutations of the retained allele.[39–41] A third of patients with AT/RT have *SMARCB1* germline mutations that also predispose to schwannomatosis and multiple meningiomas.[42–46] INI1 belongs to the switching and sucrose nonfermenting (SWI/SNF) ATP-dependent protein complex with roles in chromatin remodeling. Along with BRG-1/SMARCA4 and BRG-1-associated factor (BAF), it forms the catalytic unit of the protein complex.[41] *INI1* inactivation translates into tumor cell INI1 nuclear protein loss that can be reliably identified by immunohistochemistry. The normal cells (e.g., endothelial cells, intratumoral lymphocytes) retain INI1 nuclear protein expression and serve as reliable internal positive controls[47] (Figure 18-1).

As AT/RT can mimic medulloblastoma or any type of cPNET, it is recommended to perform INI1 immunohistochemistry on any embryonal tumor to rule out the possibility of AT/RT (Figure 18-2).[41] In rare instances, *BRG-1/SMARCA4*, another gene encoding a subunit of the SWI/SNF complex is mutated and is responsible for the rhabdoid phenotype. In such instances, INI1 nuclear expression will be retained and BRG-1 nuclear protein expression will be lost on immunohistochemistry.[48] Therefore, INI1 loss is not universally diagnostic of AT/RT and in highly suspicious cases with INI1 nuclear retention, BRG-1 loss should be investigated.

CRINET is a newly described ventricular small cell tumor with striking cribriform architecture, *SMARCB1/INI1* alterations and good prognosis.[3–6] CRINET is another entity sharing INI1 nuclear loss; however, the ventricular location, prominent cribriform architectural features, and the characteristic pattern of luminal EMA immunoexpression should be helpful in establishing the diagnosis. Other entities with INI1 loss are renal rhabdoid tumor and medullary carcinoma,

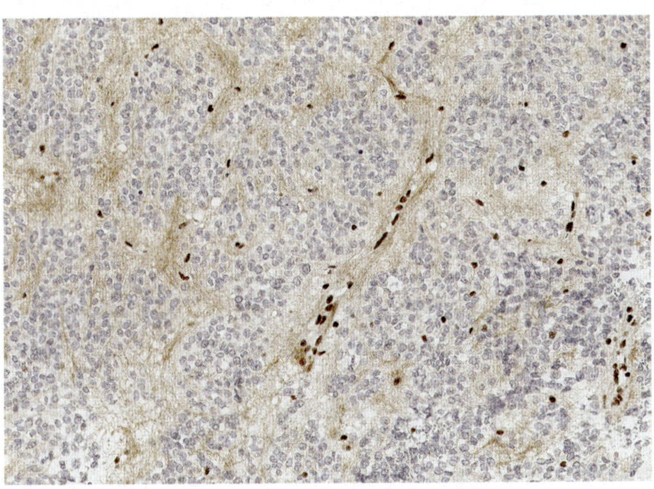

FIGURE 18-1: Diffuse INI1 nuclear protein loss in AT/RT (INI1, intermediate magnification).

FIGURE 18-2: Diffuse INI1 nuclear protein expression in a medulloblastoma (INI1, intermediate magnification).

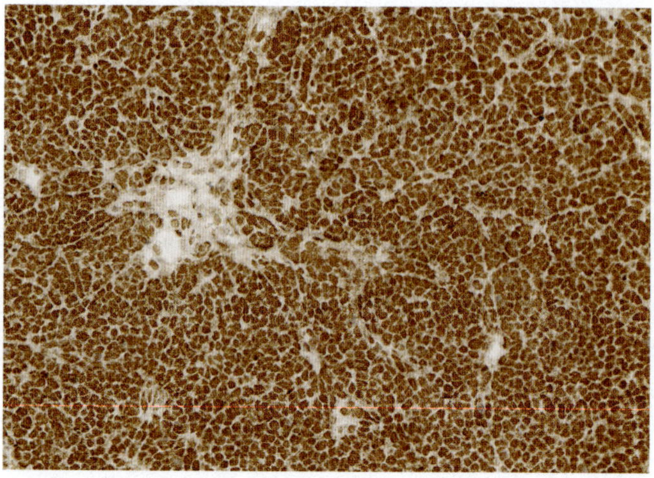

epithelioid sarcoma, epithelioid malignant peripheral nerve sheath tumor, extraskeletal myxoid chondrosarcoma,[49] myoepithelial soft tissue tumors,[49,50] small cell hepatoblastoma,[51] and poorly differentiated chordoma.[52,53] Some of these tumors have to be considered in the rare instances of CNS metastases.

Embryonal Rosette-Forming Neuroepithelial Tumors

This subgroups of embryonal tumors comprise ETANTR, ependymoblastoma, and medulloepithelioma. Recent studies indicate that these three entities share common copy number alterations and DNA methylation profiles. When compared to other CNS tumors and normal cerebellum, the patterns of DNA methylation were unique. These tumors also share clinical features including age, gender, location, and survival. All of these features suggest a possible common histogenesis with a proposal for a new label as embryonal tumor with multilayered rosettes (ETMR).[7] ETMR are characterized by amplification of 19q13.42 (over 90%)[9,54] and cytoplasmic and nuclear LIN28A immunoexpression.[7] LIN28 is a cytoplasmic RNA-binding protein with roles in miRNA modulation.[55] While exercising its function, the protein can translocate to the nucleus. LIN28 is a highly sensitive and specific biomarker for ETMR.[8]

TUMORS OF THE MENINGES

Meningioma

Meningioma is characterized by numerous chromosomal copy number aberrations, the most common of which is chromosome 22 loss (~80%), followed by 1p loss, 14q loss, and 6q loss, with the latter three aberrations being associated with more aggressive tumors. All syndromic and a significant percentage of sporadic meningiomas (~50%) have mutations involving the neurofibromatosis type 2 (*NF2)* tumor suppressor gene (22q12.2) that encodes merlin/schwannomin.[56–58]

Genomic profiles of meningioma identified three distinct molecular subgroups, the largest of which was *NF2*-associated meningioma (having chromosome 22 loss and *NF2* mutations). A second group of non-*NF2* meningioma (~25%) had TNF receptor-associated factor 7 (*TRAF7)* mutations encoding an E3 ubiquitin ligase with roles in apoptosis. *TRAF7* mutations clustered with Kruppel-like factor 4 mutations ($KLF4^{K400Q}$) encoding a transcription factor or with v-akt murine thymoma viral oncogene homolog 1 mutations ($AKT1^{E17K}$) involved in PI3K pathway activation. Smoothened frizzled family receptor (*SMO*) mutations separated a smaller subgroup (~5%) with SHH signaling activity. Non-*NF2* meningiomas were mostly grade I localized to the skull base, while *NF2* meningiomas were mostly atypical (grade II) and localized to the convexity. *TRAF7* and *KLF4* mutations characterized all secretory meningiomas.[57]

Differences in methylation have also been described by genome-wide methylation profiling that correlated hypomethylation with a more aggressive tumor grade.[59,60]

Solitary Fibrous Tumor/Hemangiopericytoma Family of Tumors

Historically, CNS hemangiopericytoma (HPC) and solitary fibrous tumor (SFT) have been regarded as distinct entities.[1] In contrast, in soft tissue pathology HPC is defined as a SFT with more aggressive behavior. This dichotomy was later removed, and the two entities became regarded as part of a spectrum of SFT tumors.[61] Although overlapping immunophenotypical and prognostic features were also observed in the CNS,[62] a strong evidence to support this concept of a spectrum was lacking, until a characteristic genetic alteration with *NAB2–STAT6* fusion was identified in SFTs of various locations, including the meninges. This finding supports the concept that the CNS HPC and SFT are part of the same biologic spectrum.[63] NAB2, a transcriptional repressor, is converted into a transcriptional activator following fusion with STAT6 with subsequent activation of mitogenic pathways that promote cell proliferation.[63] Nuclear translocation of STAT6 strongly correlates with the fusion and can be accurately detected with a commercially available antibody.[64,65] More importantly, STAT6 is not expressed in meningioma, the differential diagnosis for SFT/HPC.[66]

TUMORS OF THE CRANIAL AND PERIPHERAL NERVES—SCHWANNOMATOSIS

Schwannomatosis is a form of neurofibromatosis characterized by multiple nonvestibular schwannomas, caused by *SMARCB1/INI1* germline mutations (*SMARCB1* was described in the "Atypical Teratoid/Rhabdoid Tumor" section).[67] *SMARCB1/INI1* germline mutations contribute to 40% to 50% of familial schwannomatosis and about 10% of sporadic schwannomatosis.[67,68] In contrast to AT/RT, a four-hit model of tumorigenesis has been proposed for schwannomatosis. It starts with the *SMARCB1/INI1* germline mutation (hit 1), followed by loss of the second wild-type *SMARCB1/INI1* allele (hit 2), loss of wild-type *NF2* allele (hit 3), followed by a mutation in the retained second *NF2* allele.[67] Immunohistochemistry highlights a mosaic pattern of reactivity with admixed retained and lost nuclear INI1 expression in familial (~80% to 90%) and sporadic schwannomatosis (~50%), but not in solitary sporadic schwannomas (Figure 18-3).[45,69,70]

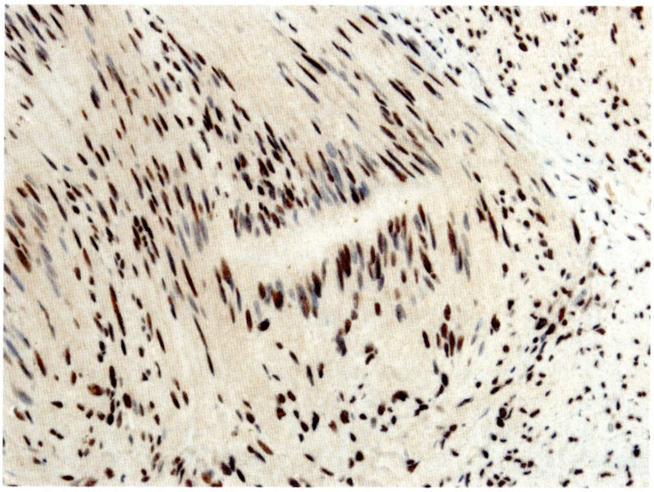

FIGURE 18-3: Mosaic INI1 pattern of immunoexpression with admixed retained and lost nuclear protein expression in familial schwannomatosis (INI1, high magnification) (Photograph courtesy of Dr. Hidehiro Takei).

ACKNOWLEDGMENTS

Dr. Adriana Olar was supported by the National Institutes of Health/National Cancer Institute (Training Grant #5T32CA163185).

References

1. Louis DN, Ohgaki H, Wiestler OD, et al. *WHO Classification of Tumors of the Central Nervous System.* 4th ed. Lyon, France: IARC; 2007:8–69.
2. Ostrom QT, Gittleman H, Farah P, et al. CBTRUS Statistical Report: primary brain and central nervous system tumors diagnosed in the United States in 2006–2010. *Neuro Oncol* 2013;15(suppl 2):ii1–ii56.
3. Arnold MA, Stallings-Archer K, Marlin E, et al. Cribriform neuroepithelial tumor arising in the lateral ventricle. *Pediatr Dev Pathol* 2013;16(4):301–307.
4. Hasselblatt M, Oyen F, Gesk S, et al. Cribriform neuroepithelial tumor (CRINET): a nonrhabdoid ventricular tumor with INI1 loss and relatively favorable prognosis. *J Neuropathol Exp Neurol* 2009;68(12):1249–1255.
5. Ibrahim GM, Huang A, Halliday W, et al. Cribriform neuroepithelial tumour: novel clinicopathological, ultrastructural and cytogenetic findings. *Acta Neuropathol* 2011;122(4):511–514.
6. Park JY, Kim E, Kim DW, et al. Cribriform neuroepithelial tumor in the third ventricle: a case report and literature review. *Neuropathology* 2012;32(5):570–576.
7. Korshunov A, Sturm D, Ryzhova M, et al. Embryonal tumor with abundant neuropil and true rosettes (ETANTR), ependymoblastoma, and medulloepithelioma share molecular similarity and comprise a single clinicopathological entity. *Acta Neuropathol* 2013;128:279–289.
8. Korshunov A, Ryzhova M, Jones DT, et al. Lin28a immunoreactivity is a potent diagnostic marker of embryonal tumor with multilayered rosettes (ETMR). *Acta Neuropathol* 2012;124(6):875–881.
9. Korshunov A, Remke M, Gessi M, et al. Focal genomic amplification at 19q13.42 comprises a powerful diagnostic marker for embryonal tumors with ependymoblastic Rosettes. *Acta Neuropathol* 2010;120(2): 253–260.
10. Antonescu C. Round cell sarcomas beyond Ewing: emerging entities. *Histopathology* 2014;64(1): 26–37.
11. Marino-Enriquez A, Fletcher CD. Round cell sarcomas—biologically important refinements in subclassification. *Int J Biochem Cell Biol* 2014;53:493–504.
12. Pomeroy SL, Tamayo P, Gaasenbeek M, et al. Prediction of central nervous system embryonal tumour outcome based on gene expression. *Nature* 2002;415(6870):436–442.
13. Thompson MC, Fuller C, Hogg TL, et al. Genomics identifies medulloblastoma subgroups that are enriched for specific genetic alterations. *J Clin Oncol* 2006;24(12):1924–1931.
14. Cho YJ, Tsherniak A, Tamayo P, et al. Integrative genomic analysis of medulloblastoma identifies a molecular subgroup that drives poor clinical outcome. *J Clin Oncol* 2011;29(11):1424–1430.
15. Kool M, Koster J, Bunt J, et al. Integrated genomics identifies five medulloblastoma subtypes with distinct genetic profiles, pathway signatures and clinicopathological features. *PLoS One* 2008;3(8):e3088.
16. Northcott PA, Korshunov A, Witt H, et al. Medulloblastoma comprises four distinct molecular variants. *J Clin Oncol* 2011;29(11):1408–1414.
17. Parsons DW, Li M, Zhang X, et al. The genetic landscape of the childhood cancer medulloblastoma. *Science* 2011;331(6016):435–439.
18. Remke M, Hielscher T, Northcott PA, et al. Adult medulloblastoma comprises three major molecular variants. *J Clin Oncol* 2011;29(19):2717–2723.
19. Taylor MD, Northcott PA, Korshunov A, et al. Molecular subgroups of medulloblastoma: the current consensus. *Acta Neuropathol* 2012;123(4):465–472.
20. Kool M, Korshunov A, Remke M, et al. Molecular subgroups of medulloblastoma: an international meta-analysis of transcriptome, genetic aberrations, and clinical data of WNT, SHH, group 3, and group 4 medulloblastomas. *Acta Neuropathol* 2012;123(4):473–484.
21. Kikuchi A. Tumor formation by genetic mutations in the components of the Wnt signaling pathway. *Cancer Sci* 2003;94(3):225–229.

22. Kool M, Korshunov A, Pfister SM. Update on molecular and genetic alterations in adult medulloblastoma. *Memo* 2012;5(3):228–232.
23. Tabori U, Baskin B, Shago M, et al. Universal poor survival in children with medulloblastoma harboring somatic TP53 mutations. *J Clin Oncol* 2010;28(8):1345–1350.
24. Gessi M, von Bueren AO, Rutkowski S, et al. P53 expression predicts dismal outcome for medulloblastoma patients with metastatic disease. *J Neurooncol* 2012;106(1):135–141.
25. Zhukova N, Ramaswamy V, Remke M, et al. Subgroup-specific prognostic implications of TP53 mutation in medulloblastoma. *J Clin Oncol* 2013;31(23):2927–2935.
26. Korshunov A, Remke M, Werft W, et al. Adult and pediatric medulloblastomas are genetically distinct and require different algorithms for molecular risk stratification. *J Clin Oncol* 2010;28(18):3054–3060.
27. Northcott PA, Hielscher T, Dubuc A, et al. Pediatric and adult sonic hedgehog medulloblastomas are clinically and molecularly distinct. *Acta Neuropathol* 2011;122(2):231–240.
28. Sasaki R, Saito K, Watanabe Y, et al. Nevoid basal cell carcinoma syndrome with cleft lip and palate associated with the novel PTCH gene mutations. *J Hum Genet* 2009;54(7):398–402.
29. Hahn H, Wicking C, Zaphiropoulous PG, et al. Mutations of the human homolog of drosophila patched in the nevoid basal cell carcinoma syndrome. *Cell* 1996;85(6):841–851.
30. Johnson RL, Rothman AL, Xie J, et al. Human homolog of patched, a candidate gene for the basal cell nevus syndrome. *Science* 1996;272(5268):1668–1671.
31. Pastorino L, Ghiorzo P, Nasti S, et al. Identification of a SUFU germline mutation in a family with Gorlin syndrome. *Am J Med Genet A* 2009;149A(7):1539–1543.
32. Smyth I, Narang MA, Evans T, et al. Isolation and characterization of human patched 2 (PTCH2), a putative tumour suppressor gene in basal cell carcinoma and medulloblastoma on chromosome 1p32. *Hum Mol Genet* 1999;8(2):291–297.
33. Hottinger AF, Khakoo Y. Neurooncology of familial cancer syndromes. *J Child Neurol* 2009;24(12):1526–1535.
34. Ellison DW, Dalton J, Kocak M, et al. Medulloblastoma: clinicopathological correlates of SHH, WNT, and non-SHH/WNT molecular subgroups. *Acta Neuropathol* 2011;121(3):381–396.
35. Fattet S, Haberler C, Legoix P, et al. Beta-catenin status in paediatric medulloblastomas: correlation of immunohistochemical expression with mutational status, genetic profiles, and clinical characteristics. *J Pathol* 2009;218(1):86–94.
36. Ellison DW, Onilude OE, Lindsey JC, et al. Beta-catenin status predicts a favorable outcome in childhood medulloblastoma: the United Kingdom Children's Cancer Study Group Brain Tumour Committee. *J Clin Oncol* 2005;23(31):7951–7957.
37. Archer TC, Weeraratne SD, Pomeroy SL. Hedgehog-GLI pathway in medulloblastoma. *J Clin Oncol* 2012;30(17):2154–2156.
38. Pizem J, Popovic M, Cor A. Expression of GLI1 and PARP1 in medulloblastoma: an immunohistochemical study of 65 cases. *J Neurooncol* 2011;103(3):459–467.
39. Versteege I, Sevenet N, Lange J, et al. Truncating mutations of HSNF5/INI1 in aggressive paediatric cancer. *Nature* 1998;394(6689):203–206.
40. Biegel JA, Zhou JY, Rorke LB, et al. Germ-line and acquired mutations of INI1 in atypical teratoid and rhabdoid tumors. *Cancer Res* 1999;59(1):74–79.
41. Biegel JA, Kalpana G, Knudsen ES, et al. The role of INI1 and the SWI/SNF complex in the development of rhabdoid tumors: meeting summary from the Workshop on Childhood Atypical Teratoid/Rhabdoid Tumors. *Cancer Res* 2002;62(1):323–328.
42. Bacci C, Sestini R, Provenzano A, et al. Schwannomatosis associated with multiple meningiomas due to a familial SMARCB1 mutation. *Neurogenetics* 2010;11(1):73–80.
43. Eaton KW, Tooke LS, Wainwright LM, et al. Spectrum of SMARCB1/INI1 mutations in familial and sporadic rhabdoid tumors. *Pediatr Blood Cancer* 2011;56(1):7–15.
44. Boyd C, Smith MJ, Kluwe L, et al. Alterations in the SMARCB1 (INI1) tumor suppressor gene in familial schwannomatosis. *Clin Genet* 2008;74(4):358–366.
45. Hulsebos TJ, Plomp AS, Wolterman RA, et al. Germline mutation of INI1/SMARCB1 in familial schwannomatosis. *Am J Hum Genet* 2007;80(4):805–810.
46. van den Munckhof P, Christiaans I, Kenter SB, et al. Germline SMARCB1 mutation predisposes to multiple meningiomas and schwannomas with preferential location of cranial meningiomas at the falx cerebri. *Neurogenetics* 2012;13(1):1–7.
47. Judkins AR, Mauger J, Ht A, et al. Immunohistochemical analysis of HSNF5/INI1 in pediatric CNS neoplasms. *Am J Surg Pathol* 2004;28(5):644–650.

48. Hasselblatt M, Gesk S, Oyen F, et al. Nonsense mutation and inactivation of SMARCA4 (BRG1) in an atypical teratoid/rhabdoid tumor showing retained SMARCB1 (INI1) expression. *Am J Surg Pathol* 2011;35(6):933–935.
49. Hollmann TJ, Hornick JL. INI1-deficient tumors: diagnostic features and molecular genetics. *Am J Surg Pathol* 2011;35(10):e47–e63.
50. Rekhi B, Sable M, Jambhekar NA. Histopathological, immunohistochemical and molecular spectrum of myoepithelial tumours of soft tissues. *Virchows Arch* 2012;461(6):687–697.
51. Trobaugh-Lotrario AD, Tomlinson GE, Finegold MJ, et al. Small cell undifferentiated variant of hepatoblastoma: adverse clinical and molecular features similar to rhabdoid tumors. *Pediatr Blood Cancer* 2009;52(3):328–334.
52. Mobley BC, McKenney JK, Bangs CD, et al. Loss of SMARCB1/INI1 expression in poorly differentiated chordomas. *Acta Neuropathol* 2010;120(6):745–753.
53. Yadav R, Sharma MC, Malgulwar PB, et al. Prognostic value of MIB-1, P53, epidermal growth factor receptor, and INI1 in childhood chordomas. *Neuro-Oncology* 2014;16(3):372–381.
54. Nobusawa S, Yokoo H, Hirato J, et al. Analysis of chromosome 19q13.42 amplification in embryonal brain tumors with ependymoblastic multilayered Rosettes. *Brain Pathol* 2012;22(5):689–697.
55. Viswanathan SR, Daley GQ, Gregory RI. Selective blockade of microRNA processing by Lin28. *Science* 2008;320(5872):97–100.
56. Riemenschneider MJ, Perry A, Reifenberger G. Histological classification and molecular genetics of meningiomas. *Lancet Neurol* 2006;5(12):1045–1054.
57. Clark VE, Erson-Omay EZ, Serin A, et al. Genomic analysis of non-NF2 meningiomas reveals mutations in TRAF7, KLF4, AKT1, and SMO. *Science* 2013;339(6123):1077–1080.
58. Ho CY, Mosier S, Safneck J, et al. Genetic profiling by single-nucleotide polymorphism-based array analysis defines three distinct subtypes of orbital meningioma. *Brain Pathol* 2014;doi: 10.1111/bpa.12150.
59. Gao F, Shi L, Russin J, et al. DNA methylation in the malignant transformation of meningiomas. *PLoS One* 2013;8(1):e54114.
60. He S, Pham MH, Pease M, et al. A review of epigenetic and gene expression alterations associated with intracranial meningiomas. *Neurosurg Focus* 2013;35(6):E5.
61. Demicco EG, Park MS, Araujo DM, et al. Solitary fibrous tumor: a clinicopathological study of 110 cases and proposed risk assessment model. *Mod Pathol* 2012;25(9):1298–1306.
62. Bouvier C, Metellus P, de Paula AM, et al. Solitary fibrous tumors and hemangiopericytomas of the meninges: overlapping pathological features and common prognostic factors suggest the same spectrum of tumors. *Brain Pathol* 2012;22(4):511–521.
63. Robinson DR, Wu YM, Kalyana-Sundaram S, et al. Identification of recurrent NAB2–STAT6 gene fusions in solitary fibrous tumor by integrative sequencing. *Nat Genet* 2013;45(2):180–185.
64. Yoshida A, Tsuta K, Ohno M, et al. STAT6 immunohistochemistry is helpful in the diagnosis of solitary fibrous tumors. *Am J Surg Pathol* 2014;38(4):552–559.
65. Koelsche C, Schweizer L, Renner M, et al. Nuclear relocation of STAT6 reliably predicts NAB2/STAT6 fusion for the diagnosis of solitary fibrous tumour. *Histopathology* 2014;65:613–622.
66. Schweizer L, Koelsche C, Sahm F, et al. Meningeal hemangiopericytoma and solitary fibrous tumors carry the NAB2–STAT6 fusion and can be diagnosed by nuclear expression of STAT6 protein. *Acta Neuropathol* 2013;125(5):651–658.
67. Plotkin SR, Blakeley JO, Evans DG, et al. Update from the 2011 International Schwannomatosis Workshop: from genetics to diagnostic criteria. *Am J Med Genet A* 2013;161A(3):405–416.
68. Rousseau G, Noguchi T, Bourdon V, et al. SMARCB1/INI1 germline mutations contribute to 10% of sporadic schwannomatosis. *BMC Neurol* 2011;11:9.
69. Patil S, Perry A, Maccollin M, et al. Immunohistochemical analysis supports a role for INI1/SMARCB1 in hereditary forms of schwannomas, but not in solitary, sporadic schwannomas. *Brain Pathol* 2008;18(4): 517–519.
70. Smith MJ, Walker JA, Shen Y, et al. Expression of SMARCB1 (INI1) mutations in familial schwannomatosis. *Hum Mol Genet* 2012;21(24):5239–5245.

SECTION

V

Current Therapy and Prognosis

▶ CHAPTER 19: Brain Cancer Treatment

Brain Cancer Treatment

19

Yvonne Kew
Qun-Fang Wan

This chapter investigates treatment of the following primary glioma and developmental brain tumors: glioblastoma (GBM), anaplastic glioma (AG), medulloblastoma, and intracranial germ cell tumors (IGCT). Beginning with a review of previous failed treatments, we summarize the current standard therapies and explore the latest advancements in treatment and cancer technology.

GLIOBLASTOMA

GBM is the most common and fatal malignancy of the central nervous system (CNS), accounting for approximately 80% of all high-grade CNS tumors.[1] It is classified as a World Health Organization (WHO) grade IV primary brain tumor that is most commonly found in adults aged 55 to 65 years old.[2] The exceptionally invasive nature of GBM and its tendency to infiltrate normal brain tissue makes it difficult to treat and explains its poor prognosis.[3]

The currently accepted standard therapy for newly diagnosed GBM is multimodal, consisting of surgical resection and possible carmustine (BCNU) wafer placement, followed by radiation plus concomitant and adjuvant temozolomide (TMZ)-based chemotherapy.[4,5] Despite the improved outcome with this standard therapy, the treatment for GBM remains a great therapeutic challenge, and the disease is associated with a very poor prognosis. In newly diagnosed GBM, mean survival is 8 to 15 months, whereas the mean survival for recurrent GBM is 3 to 9 months. Moreover, the 5-year survival rate for patients with GBM is only 5%.[6]

The inadequacy of standard therapy highlights the need to develop novel therapeutic approaches, which focus on targeting the tumor at the molecular level.[7,8] Advances in understanding the pathogenesis of GBM are critical for improving the treatment protocol and prolonging survival of GBM patients.

FDA APPROVAL TIMELINE

Standard Therapy

As stated, the currently accepted standard therapies of newly diagnosed GBM are surgical resection, followed by radiation plus adjuvant TMZ-based chemotherapy.[4,5]

Surgical Resection

Surgery is usually the first step in treating newly diagnosed GBM, with maximal safe resection and preservation of neurologic function being the main objectives.[9,10] Once the tumor is resected, carmustine (BCNU) wafers may be implanted in the cranial cavity to deliver localized chemotherapy.[11] Gross total resection (GTR) is preferred, given that it does not compromise the patient, as substantial tumor debulking has been linked to improved response to postoperative adjuvant treatments.[12,13]

Adjuvant Postoperative Radiation Therapy

Given the high recurrence rate of GBM, patients typically undergo adjuvant radiation therapy (RT) to destroy microscopic residual tumor cells. The effect of RT on survival was first shown in patients treated with whole brain radiotherapy (WBRT)[14–16] and increased median survival from 14 to 36 weeks.[17] The standard RT dose is 60 Gy given over 30 fractions, 2 Gy per fraction, 5 days/week, as recommended by the Radiation Therapy Oncology Group (RTOG).[18] However, due to the long-term adverse effects of WBRT at this dose, such as neurocognitive deficits, leukoencephalopathy, and endocrinopathy, it is no longer considered an appropriate radiation modality.[19]

Serious complications resulting from WBRT led to using limited radiation fields, called involved field radiotherapy (IFRT), as the standard therapeutic approach to minimize toxicity.[19] While the switch from WBRT to IFRT has not changed the pattern of treatment failure or reduced the percentage of patients with multifocal disease,[20] its compatibility with three-dimensional conformal radiotherapy (3D-CRT) has decreased radiation of healthy brain tissue.[21,22] Intensity-modulated radiotherapy (IMRT) has been demonstrated to be a superior technique to 3D-CRT and is considered the current standard.[23,24] MacDonald and colleagues reported improved target coverage and dose reduction to the brain, brainstem, and optic chiasm with IMRT compared to 3D-CRT.[24] IMRT can also be used to escalate RT doses to the tumor; however, there is no evidence that doses greater than 60 Gy increase treatment effectiveness.[25,26]

Other RT techniques have been evaluated in clinical trials, but their efficacy is yet to be established. These include stereotactic radiosurgery,[27,28] interstitial brachytherapy,[29,30] and heavy particle RT.[31–36]

Adjuvant Chemotherapy

Adjuvant chemotherapy using nitrosoureas, alone or in combination regimens, was first shown to have a modest impact on overall survival (OS) in patients with GBM in the 1970s and 1980s.[37,38] However, subsequent trials with the oral alkylating agent, TMZ, demonstrated superior anticancer activity in recurrent GBM[39–41] and TMZ was approved by the United States Food and Drug Administration (FDA) in 1999 (see Figure 19-1 for approved therapy timeline). Concomitant TMZ 75 mg/m^2/day is administered on days 1 to 42.[3,42] Despite its record of success in the treatment of recurrent GBM, it was not until 2005 that TMZ was FDA approved as a first-line chemotherapeutic agent for newly diagnosed disease.[43] Stupp and colleagues demonstrated that adjuvant TMZ with RT resulted in longer median progression-free survival (PFS) than RT alone

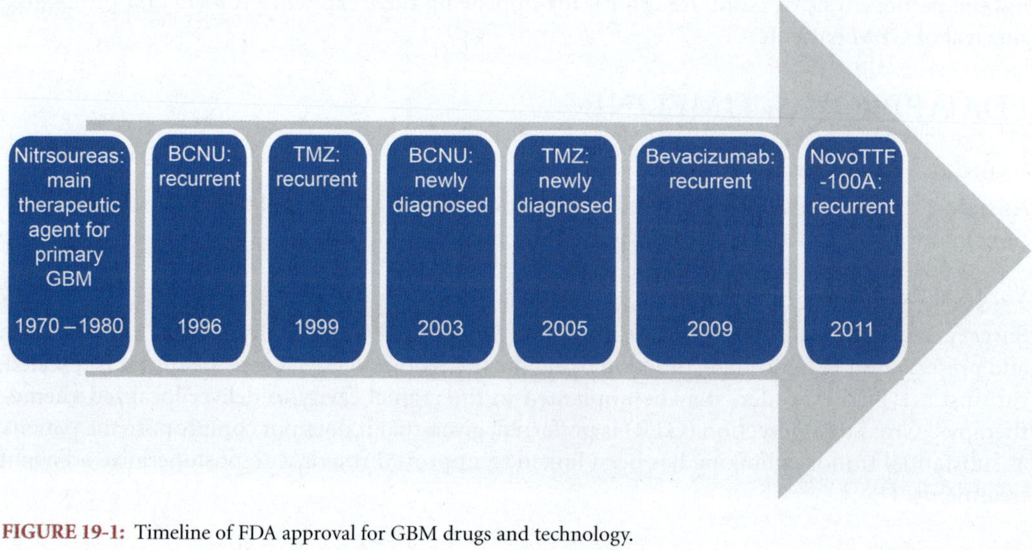

FIGURE 19-1: Timeline of FDA approval for GBM drugs and technology.

(6.9 vs. 5 months) and showed an increase in the survival rate at 2 years, from 10% with RT alone to 27% with RT plus TMZ in newly diagnosed GBM.[41] Therefore, the current standard regimen has shifted from an RT-only approach and the use of nitrosoureas, to a treatment protocol that couples TMZ-based chemotherapy with adjuvant RT. In addition to their similar abilities to cross the blood–brain barrier, TMZ has a superior bioavailability and lower toxicity than do nitrosoureas.[44,45]

Furthermore, *O*-6 methylguanine-DNA methyltransferase (*MGMT*) expression is silenced by promoter methylation that confers sensitivity to TMZ. Thus, silencing *MGMT* expression confers better OS. For those with *MGMT* methylation, the 2-year survival rates were 49% and 24% with combination therapy and with RT alone, respectively, whereas for those without *MGMT* methylation, 2-year survival rates were 15% and 2%, respectively.[46]

To date, the FDA has approved bevacizumab (Avastin) as monotherapy in recurrent GBM. However, in recent years, bevacizumab has been studied and administered for newly diagnosed GBM, along with the standard TMZ and radiotherapy protocol.[47,48] Two recent studies have investigated the use of bevacizumab as an upfront treatment: Avastin in glioblastoma (AVAglio) and RTOG 0825. Both trials demonstrated that adding bevacizumab to a standard regimen of RT and TMZ did not improve OS in newly diagnosed GBM. The AVAglio trial showed maintenance of baseline quality of life, whereas the RTOG 0825 trial showed increased adverse effects in the bevacizumab group.[49,50] Therefore, bevacizumab has limited efficacy as an upfront treatment. Nevertheless, it remains a prominent component in the therapeutic regimen for recurrent GBM.

Therapy for Recurrent Disease

Carmustine (BCNU) wafers are biodegradable polymers originally approved for use as a local chemotherapeutic agent in recurrent GBM. They are among the nitrosourea agents, DNA alkylating agents used as upfront treatments in the late 1970s and early 1980s[51]; however, these too had no significant impact on survival.[52] Nonetheless, there has been continued use of BCNU in the form of a polymer wafer, which was approved by FDA in 1996 for the treatment of recurrent GBM and in 2003 for newly diagnosed GBM.[53,54] An early placebo-controlled clinical trial demonstrated that implantation of the BCNU wafer improved survival compared to standard therapies in recurrent GBM[55]; however, the results are modest.[56,57] Although BCNU wafers have been linked to increased rates of cerebrospinal fluid leak and increased intracranial pressure secondary to edema and mass effect,[58,59] the safety and effectiveness of this new approach for treating GBM are well documented.[60,61] Currently, research is ongoing regarding the safety and efficacy of the use of BCNU wafers with other systemic chemotherapeutic agents as part of novel combination therapeutic regimens for recurrent GBM.[54]

The use of the antiangiogenic agent, bevacizumab alone was FDA approved in 2009 for the treatment of recurrent GBM,[62] although it was widely used by clinicians prior to its approval. Bevacizumab is a monoclonal antibody that binds to vascular endothelial growth factor A, essentially preventing new blood vessel formation and growth of tumor cells.[63] Thus, the use of bevacizumab should be limited to 1 month postsurgery to avoid wound healing complications.[64] Originally used to treat recurrent GBM, the antiangiogenic effect of bevacizumab is very well tolerated and linked to better outcomes and antitumoral activity in responding GBM.[65] Its use has also been shown to lengthen median survival from the time of recurrence from 4.2 to 10.6 months.[66] When combined with irinotecan, bevacizumab improved 6-month survival in recurrent high-grade glioma patients to 46% compared to 21% in patients treated with TMZ alone.[67,68] However, the combination of bevacizumab and irinotecan was not significantly superior to bevacizumab monotherapy for recurrent GBM. Friedman and colleagues demonstrated that patients who received bevacizumab alone had a very modest OS rate of 9.2 months, compared to 8.7 months for those who received a combination of bevacizumab and irinotecan.[63] Consequently, it has only been approved as a monotherapy by the FDA.

Tumor treatment fields (TTF) therapy was approved by the FDA in 2011 and is a new noninvasive technology used to treat recurrent GBM.[69] The portable, battery-operated device (NovoTTF-100A) functions by sending alternating electric fields to the tumor area using insulated electrode arrays placed on the skin surface surrounding the tumor.[70] The alternating electric fields interfere with mitosis by causing realignment of tubulin subunits, which results in abnormal mitotic spindle formation during metaphase. Subsequent polarization of organelles affects their movement in the dielectrophoretic environment during anaphase and telophase, resulting in abnormal cytokinesis and ultimately in apoptosis.[70] TTF has been shown to improve median OS by approximately 2 months compared to the standard of care.[71] Another study showed no improvement in OS with TTF; however, the efficacy and activity of the TTF device was comparable to the chemotherapy protocol for recurrent GBM, with clear advantages in terms of toxicity and quality of life.[69,72] Given the limited evidence on the long-term success of TTF, further evaluation must be conducted on its combined use with chemotherapy and as a maintenance or salvage therapy when the standard protocol is inadequate.[71] Nonetheless, TTF is an emerging novel therapy that holds great potential in the treatment of recurrent GBM.

ANAPLASTIC GLIOMA

The other common type of high-grade malignant glioma is AG, classified as WHO grade III brain tumors. AG are a diverse group of tumors that include anaplastic astrocytomas (AA), anaplastic oligodendroglioma (AO), and anaplastic oligoastrocytoma (AOA), which are differentiated on the basis of histopathologic features.[16,73] Like GBM, these tumors have an inherent capacity to infiltrate into surrounding areas of the brain, making them difficult to completely remove during surgery. These highly aggressive tumors often occur in adults, with peak incidence being in the fourth and fifth decades of life.

Treatment of AG

The treatment of AG must be individualized depending on the clinical histopathology of the tumor, molecular prognostic biomarkers, and individual patient's characteristics, including age, Karnofsky performance status, extent of tumor resection, and comorbidity. The standard therapy for AG is surgery followed by RT.[74] Maximal surgical resection is the first desirable step in treatment for all types of AG without neurologic compromise. When the mass is in an eloquent location, biopsy is typically performed to determine the glioma typing and, to some extent, grading. When possible, molecular profiling, such as 1p/19q codeletion status and isocitrate dehydrogenase 1 or 2 (*IDH1/2*) mutations should be routinely performed. The therapeutic regimens for AO, AOA, or AA are determined based on the status of three molecular prognostic biomarkers: *IDH1/2* mutations,[75] 1p/19q codeletion,[76–78] and *MGMT* promoter methylation.[79,80]

A German study (NOA-04) compared the efficacy and safety of RT followed by chemotherapy at the time of progression with the reverse order in patients with newly diagnosed AG. Patients (n = 318), the majority having AA, were randomly assigned to three arms of upfront treatments: arm A received conventional RT; arm B1 received procarbazine, lomustine (CCNU), and vincristine (PCV); and arm B2 received TMZ. When maximum toxicity was reached, patients in arm A were treated with either PCV or TMZ, while patients in arms B1 and B2 received RT. Initial RT or chemotherapy yielded comparable results (Table 19-1)[74] so that delaying either treatment option provides no significant difference in patient outcome.

Another study examined the efficacy of combining α-difluoromethyl ornithine (DFMO), a suicide enzyme inhibitor of ornithine decarboxylase, with nitrosourea-based PCV chemotherapy in the treatment of AG. There were 114 patients in the DFMO–PCV arm: 78.1% AA, 3.5% AOA, 14% AO, and 4.4% other malignant gliomas. These tumor-type groupings were comparable with those of the 114 patients in the PCV-only arm: 69.3% AA, 7% AOA, 21.1% AO, and 2.6% other malignant gliomas. Researchers found that DFMO increased the efficacy of PCV when administered 14 days before and after each cycle of chemotherapy. The median PFS for the two treatment groups was 71.1 months for the DFMO–PCV arm and 37.5 months for the PCV-only arm. Median OS was 75.8 and 61.1 months for the DFMO–PCV and PCV arms, respectively.

Table 19-1 OS and PFS by Genotype and Treatment

Trial	Patients	Molecular Biomarker		Treatment	PFS (Years)	OS (Years)
EORTC 26951	368 AO/AOA	1p/19q status	Codeleted	RT ($n = 37$)	4.2	9.3
				RT → PCV ($n = 43$)	13.1	Not reached
			Noncodeleted	RT ($n = 122$)	0.75	1.75
				RT → PCV ($n = 114$)	1.25	2.1
		IDH status	Mutated	RT ($n = 36$)	3	5.4
				RT → PCV ($n = 45$)	5.9	Not reached
			Wild type	RT ($n = 50$)	0.6	1.2
				RT → PCV ($n = 47$)	0.8	1.6
		MGMT promoter	Methylated	RT ($n = 62$)	1.3	3.6
				RT → PCV ($n = 74$)	4.6	5.9
			Unmethylated	RT ($n = 24$)	0.6	1.3
				RT → PCV ($n = 23$)	0.8	1.4
RTOG 9402	291 AO/AOA	1p/19q status	Codeleted	RT ($n = 67$)	2.9	7.3
				PCV → RT ($n = 59$)	8.4	14.7
			Noncodeleted	RT ($n = 61$)	1	2.7
				PCV → RT ($n = 76$)	1.2	2.6
		IDH status	Mutated	RT ($n = 76$)	—	5.7
				PCV → RT ($n = 80$)	—	9.4
			Wild-type	RT ($n = 23$)	—	1.8
				PCV → RT ($n = 31$)	—	1.3
		1p/19q + *IDH* status	Codeleted mutated	RT ($n = 46$)	—	6.8
				PCV → RT ($n = 42$)	—	14.7
			Noncodeleted mutated	RT ($n = 29$)	—	3.3
				PCV → RT ($n = 37$)	—	5.5
			Noncodeleted nonmutated	RT ($n = 18$)	—	1.3
				PCV → RT ($n = 26$)	—	1
NOA-04	318 AG	None		RT ($n = 160$)	2.6	6
				PCV/TMZ ($n = 158$)	2.7	6.9

Although DFMO is an easily tolerated drug with clear benefits in a combination treatment regimen, it has not yet been approved by the FDA as a cancer therapy.[81]

More recently, *IDH1* and *IDH2* gene mutations have been recognized as important independent markers for glial tumors. In fact, regardless of histology, *IDH1/2* mutation status is the strongest prognostic marker for improved OS.[82] *IDH1/2* are mutated in 50% to 80% of AG and secondary GBM, but are rarely mutated in primary GBM.[83] Randomized clinical trials and larger series have demonstrated a prolonged survival for participants with *IDH1/2*-mutant AG.[74,77,84] Overall, *IDH1/2* mutations appear to be very promising factors in the diagnosis and treatment of AG patients.

Treatment of AO/AOA

Two prospective randomized phase III trials have examined the use of PCV in AO, yielding similar improvements in survival rates, particularly in patients with 1p/19q codeletion. One study utilized sequential chemotherapy followed by RT, while the other employed adjuvant PCV. It appears that 1p/19q codeletion confers greater sensitivity to treatment than does the absence of codeletion.[85]

Cairncross et al. evaluated the efficacy of administering neoadjuvant PCV plus RT versus RT alone in AO patients with 1p/19q codeletion. They found that OS and PFS were markedly longer after combined therapy (Table 19-1). In this study (RTOG 9402), the median OS for this group was 14.7 years in the PCV plus RT arm versus 7.3 years after RT, whereas the median PFS was 8.4 years after PCV plus RT versus 2.9 years after RT alone.[76] Similar survival rates were shown in the European Organization for Research and Treatment of Cancer (EORTC) 26951 trial, in which PCV was used after RT for AO patients with the codeletion. They found that adjuvant PCV following RT increased both OS (not reached vs. 9.3 years) and PFS (13.1 vs. 4.2 years) in AO with 1p/19q codeletion.[77] In short, upfront chemoradiotherapy administered in tandem (PCV plus RT or RT plus PCV) conferred a strikingly improved clinical response in AO/AOA patients with 1p/19q codeletion than did upfront RT alone.

Conversely, patients without 1p/19q codeletion had poorer outcomes than did the group with the codeletion (Table 19-1). In the RTOG 9402 study, the addition of adjuvant PCV had no significant impact on PFS and OS, which were strikingly lower than in the codeletion group. The PFS for the RT-alone group and the RT plus PCV group was 1 and 1.2 years, respectively. Meanwhile, the OS for the RT-alone group and the RT plus PCV group was 2.7 and 2.6 years, respectively.[76] The EORTC 26951 study yielded similar poor survival rates, with upfront PCV having no significant benefit. The PFS for the RT-alone group and the RT plus PCV group was 0.75 and 1.25 years, respectively. Meanwhile, the OS for the RT-alone group and the RT plus PCV group was 1.75 and 2.1 years, respectively.[77] Overall, in AO/AOA without 1p/19q codeletion, treating patients with upfront chemotherapy with RT can confer greater toxicity than improved survival benefits.

Following the conclusion of enrollment for the EORTC study, researchers identified two other markers that affect outcome in diffuse glioma: *MGMT* promoter methylation and *IDH* mutations. In general, patients with *MGMT* promoter methylation and *IDH* mutation derived more benefit from PCV with prolonged OS and PFS (Table 19-1).[77] *IDH* mutation is also a significant prognostic factor in AO for OS; however, it has not been shown to be a significant marker for outcome to PCV chemotherapy.[86] Overall, the EORTC study yields no definitive conclusions regarding the predictive value of *MGMT* promoter methylation or of *IDH* mutations in the absence of 1p/19q codeletion.

Despite the efficacy of PCV in tumors with particular biomarkers, in both trials, PCV was associated with high levels of toxicity. In the RTOG study, patients who were randomly assigned to PCV plus RT had more acute toxicities, such as myelosuppression, cognitive or mood changes, peripheral or autonomic neuropathy, vomiting, hepatic dysfunction, and allergic rash.[76] Similar adverse reactions were noted in the EORTC study, as only 30% of patients were able to complete the six cycles of adjuvant chemotherapy as originally prescribed.[77] Therefore, additional studies have evaluated the efficacy of TMZ as a replacement for PCV in the treatment of AO/AOA. Gwak et al. found that RT plus TMZ had an efficacy equal to PCV chemotherapy at first relapse. For patients previously treated with PCV, TMZ was a good second-line salvage treatment with an acceptable toxicity rate.[87] Currently, two major ongoing clinical trials are investigating the efficacy of the combination of RT with or without TMZ at different time points for AG patients: CATNON (Concurrent and Adjuvant Temozolomide Chemotherapy in Non-1p/19q Deleted Anaplastic Glioma) and CODEL (Codeleted Tumors).[88]

Treatment of AA

The mainstay treatment for primary AA is surgery followed by RT; however, there is no standard of care regimen for recurrent AA. The molecular biomarkers that are associated with a dramatic improvement in outcome for AO/AOA play less of a prognostic role in AA. The NOA-04 study found that 1p/19q codeletion was more common in AO/AOA than in AA and there are no prospective data to delineate the role of 1p/19q codeletion in AA. Wick and colleagues also demonstrated that *MGMT* promoter methylation was more common and linked to 1p/19q codeletion in AO/AOA than in AA (71% vs. 50%).[74]

Furthermore, the potential benefit of adding chemotherapy has not yet been established, although TMZ has been granted accelerated approval by the FDA based on its efficacy in recurrent AA.[89] One retrospective analysis evaluated the difference in survival rates following adjuvant PCV and TMZ for newly diagnosed AA. Among 109 AA patients, 49 were treated with PCV and 60 with TMZ. Researchers found no significant difference in median PFS between adjuvant PCV and TMZ (34.4 vs. 36.1 months). Nonetheless, TMZ is preferred because of its greater tolerability in patients.[90]

However, a recent study noted an additional risk of TMZ chemotherapy: TMZ-induced hypermutation, which triggers the evolution of recurrent low-grade gliomas to secondary GBM. Six of the 10 patients who received TMZ displayed a TMZ mutational signature: 31.9 to 90.9 transition mutations (C > T/G > A) per megabase, predominantly occurring at CpC and CpT dinucleotides, a signature of TMZ-induced mutagenesis. This signature was associated with the transformation from low-grade gliomas to high-grade gliomas. Therefore, further research must be conducted to examine the antitumor effects of TMZ versus the potential risk of TMZ-induced tumor progression or anaplastic conversion.[91]

MEDULLOBLASTOMA

Introduction

Medulloblastoma is a highly malignant, WHO grade IV, primitive neuroectodermal tumor. It is the most common embryonal tumor in children, accounting for approximately 20% of all pediatric brain tumors, with peak incidence occurring in patients between 3 and 9 years of age.[92] In comparison, medulloblastoma is extremely rare in adults and accounts for only 1% of their intracranial tumors.[93]

Medulloblastomas originate in the cerebellar ventricular zone and arise in the midline in the roof of the fourth ventricle, causing blockage of normal cerebral spinal fluid (CSF) flow as the tumor grows; therefore, medulloblastoma patients usually present with impaired motor control and increased intracranial pressure due to obstructive hydrocephalus.[94]

The outcome for children with medulloblastoma has improved greatly during the last few decades, with current therapies including surgery, followed by adjuvant radiation and chemotherapy. However, the outcome for infants is much poorer due to the toxicity of RT on the developing CNS.[95] Despite improvements in long-term survival, quality of life for survivors is of major concern, as the toxicity of treatments may lead to irreversible neurocognitive deficits.[96] Therefore, further research must be conducted to determine the optimal methods and parameters of therapy to maximize survival, while minimizing late effects.

Subgroups of Medulloblastoma

Four subgroups of medulloblastoma have been identified: wingless (WNT), sonic hedgehog (SHH), group C, and group D.[97] These disparate subgroups exhibit activation mutations in certain molecular signaling pathways, resulting in clinically and anatomically unique tumors with varied clinical outcomes.[98] The WNT subgroup is named after the disruption of the wingless signaling pathway and constitutes approximately 10% of medulloblastoma, mostly in older children. Tumors of the WNT subgroup have a classic histology and are highly curable, with a 5-year PFS of 80%.[92] The SHH subgroup refers to mutations in the sonic hedgehog signaling pathway and accounts for approximately 30% of medulloblastoma, mostly in infants and young adults.[99,100] Tumors of the SHH subgroup display a nodular/desmoplastic histology and are often associated with intermediate outcome.[100] The group C subtype displays *Myc* amplification and appears as large cell/anaplastic tumors with poor prognosis. However, the biologic indications and mechanisms of the group D subtype are less well understood, and this subgroup is associated with intermediate outcome.[101]

This stratification of patients based on the biologic markers of the four medulloblastoma subgroups is preferred over clinical risk stratification. This method permits the greater individualization of treatment and offers a better prediction of outcome at the time of diagnosis, with potential for future targeted therapy.[102]

Treatment of Medulloblastoma

Craniotomy

Surgery is often the first step in the treatment of medulloblastoma, with the main focus being maximum safe resection and reduction of intracranial pressure through the placement of a ventriculoperitoneal shunt (VPS) or an endoscopic third ventriculostomy (ETV). With 10% to 40% of patients requiring permanent CSF diversion after tumor resection, ETV has been shown to be the preferred method of treatment for medulloblastoma-induced hydrocephalus due to the shorter duration of surgery, lower morbidity and mortality rates, and most importantly, the absence of shunt dependence.[103,104]

Adjuvant Chemoradiotherapy

Despite the inevitable neuropsychological deficits, craniospinal radiotherapy (CSRT) is an integral component of the therapeutic regimen for medulloblastoma as it targets microscopic residual tumor cells. When treated with radiotherapy alone, the standard CSRT protocol uses a dose of 36 Gy to the entire brain and spinal cord and a supplemental local boost radiation of 54 Gy.[105] However, this full-dose CSRT is associated with approximately 50% mortality rate from early recurrence, and almost all patients experience debilitating sequelae.[94,105,106] The toxicity of CSRT is devastating to neurologic, cognitive, and endocrine function, which ultimately affects quality of life. Patients may experience growth retardation and hypothyroidism as a result of endocrine dysfunction, whereas neurocognitive deficits are marked by impaired attention, learning, memory, and executive or social function.[107]

Therefore, the current standard protocol utilizes reduced-dose RT: patients receive 23.4 Gy to the craniospinal axis with a posterior fossa boost of 55.8 Gy with weekly concurrent vincristine. Four hundred twenty-one patients with nondisseminated disease were randomly assigned to treatment with this reduced-dose CSRT, plus one of two chemotherapy regimens: (a) CCNU, CDDP, and VCR or (b) CMP, CDDP, and VCR (see Table 19-2, COG A9961). Chemotherapy comprises eight, 4-week cycles of maintenance chemotherapy initiated 6 weeks after RT (COG A9961). Filgrastim (G-CSF) is also added to the therapeutic regimen to rescue postchemotherapy neutropenia. The 5-year event-free survival (EFS) was 83% ± 2.2% in the WNT group versus 73% ± 5.8% in the SHH group versus 75% ± 13% in group C (*Myc* positive) versus 36% ± 15% in group D.[108] A long-term follow-up study by Packer and colleagues evaluated survival rates and pattern of relapse in 379 eligible patients from the COG A9961 study. The 5- and 10-year EFS rates

Table 19-2 Standard Maintenance Chemotherapy Regimens for Average-Risk Medulloblastoma (COG A9961)

	Regimen	Drug	Route	Dosage
A	Day 0	Lomustine (CCNU)	Orally	75 mg/m^2
	Day 1	Cisplatin (CDDP)	IV over 6 hours	75 mg/m^2
	Days 1, 7, 14	Vincristine (VCR)	IV bolus	1.5 mg/m^2, max. 2 mg, max. eight doses
B	Day 0	Cisplatin (CDDP)	IV over 6 hours	75 mg/m^2
	Days 1, 7, 14	Vincristine (VCR)	IV bolus	1.5 mg/m^2
	Days 21, 22	Cyclophosphamide (CPM)	IV over 60 minutes	1,000 mg/m^2
	Start on day 4 and continue for at least 10 days until postnadir ANC > 1,500 μL	Filgrastim (G-CSF)	SubQ (preferred) or IV	5 mg/kg daily

Note: Concomitant vincristine is administered weekly during RT.

were 81% ± 2% and 75.8% ± 2.3%, respectively, and OS were 87% ± 1.8% and 81.3% ± 2.1%, respectively. In addition, EFS was not impacted by chemotherapeutic regimen, sex, race, age at diagnosis, or gender.[109]

A more recent phase III double-randomized trial (ACNS0331) is evaluating the efficacy of further reducing the CSRT dosage to 18 Gy with a boost of 54 Gy to the tumor bed, rather than the entire posterior fossa. The study consists of children 3 to 7 years of age with newly diagnosed average-risk medulloblastoma. Radiation begins 4 weeks after surgery and is administered 5 days a week for 6 weeks with weekly concomitant vincristine. Four weeks after the completion of radiation, adjuvant chemotherapy will begin (Tables 19-3 and 19-4). Chemotherapy is identical for all patients: beginning 4 weeks after completion of chemoradiotherapy, patients receive two alternating regimens of maintenance chemotherapy for a total of nine courses. Each cycle in regimen A (six cycles) is 6 weeks in duration, consisting of lomustine, cisplatin, and vincristine. Each cycle in regimen B (three cycles) is 4 weeks in duration and consists of vincristine and cyclophosphamide with concurrent MESNA, a drug administered 15 to 30 minutes starting 15 minutes prior to or at the same time as cyclophosphamide for the prevention of cyclophosphamide-induced hemorrhagic cystitis.[110]

Therapy for High-Risk Patients

Despite the reduced toxicity of CSRT and increased survival, the current protocol is unsuitable for high-risk patients younger than 3 years old due to the radiation damage to the primitive CNS caused by the treatment.[94] Therefore, CSRT should be replaced with proton beam therapy[111,112] or chemotherapy alone for infants with GTR and nonmetastatic medulloblastoma.[94,113] A study by von Bueren and colleagues demonstrated that chemotherapy alone enabled sustained control of desmoplastic/nodular medulloblastoma types, given nondissemination at the time of diagnosis.[114] Although similar clinical trials reported the success of an exclusive chemotherapy regimen for at least 12 months,[115] in most cases of medulloblastoma in infants, adjuvant chemotherapy merely delays the delivery of radiation until the patient is older, as a chemotherapy-only regimen is inadequate.[116] For these high-risk patients, the CSRT dosage is 36 Gy, rather than 23.4 Gy for the average-risk group.[117] Notably, some prospective studies have linked preradiation chemotherapy to worse outcome than administrating chemotherapy following radiation in high-risk patients.[118–120]

Table 19-3 Current Clinical Trial Chemoradiotherapy Regimen for Average-Risk Medulloblastoma (COG ACNS 0331)

Surgery		Chemoradiotherapy								Maintenance							
	31 days			Radiation therapy: CSRT (18 Gy) + tumor bed (55.8 Gy)					4 weeks								
	Cycle									1	2	3	4	5	7	8	9
	Week	0	1	2	3	4	5	6		11	17	23	27	33	43	49	55
	Day	1	8	15	22	29	36	43									
			Chemotherapy							Maintenance Chemotherapy							
			VCR	VCR	VCR	VCR	VCR	VCR		A	A	B	A	A	A	A	B

Table 19-4 Current Clinical Trial Maintenance Chemotherapy Regimens for Average-Risk Medulloblastoma (COG ACNS 0331)

	Regimen	Drug	Route	Dosage
A	Day 1	Cisplatin (CDDP)	IV over 6 hours	75 mg/m^2
	Day 1	Lomustine (CCNU)	Orally	75 mg/m^2
	Days 1, 8, 15	Vincristine (VCR)	IV push/infusion	1.5 mg/m^2, max. 2 mg
B	Days 1, 2	MESNA	IV over 0.5 hours	360 mg/m^2/dose
	Days 1, 2	Cyclophosphamide (CPM)	IV over 1 hour	1,000 mg/m^2
	Days 1, 8	Vincristine (VCR)	IV push/infusion	1.5 mg/m^2, max. 2 mg

An ongoing COG phase III double-randomized, four-arm trial (COG ACNS0332) evaluates the efficacy of adding carboplatin to radiation as a radiosensitizer and/or isotretinoin to maintenance chemotherapy in patients 3 to 21 years of age with newly diagnosed high-risk medulloblastoma. CSR is 36 Gy with a posterior fossa boost of 55.8 Gy with weekly vincristine injection with or without carboplatin (35 mg/m^2/day) daily before RT for a total of 30 doses. For maintenance chemotherapy, patients were given regimen B in COG A9961 trial with CMP, CCNU, and VCR (see Table 19-2) with or without isotretinoin (80 mg/m^2/dose twice daily for a total of 160 mg/m^2/day on day 1 and days 16 to 28). The maintenance treatment repeats every 28 days and given in up to six cycles in the absence of disease progression or unacceptable toxicity. Patients in arms 3 and 4 (who will receive standard chemoradiation plus or minus carboplatin and isotretinoin with maintenance chemotherapy) will also undergo continuation therapy of oral isotretinoin twice daily on days 15 to 28, every 28 days in the absence of disease progression or unacceptable toxicity. Upon treatment completion, the patients are followed periodically for up to 10 years (http://www.cancer.gov/clinicaltrials/search/view?version=healthprofessional&cdrid=511991).

INTRACRANIAL GERM CELL TUMORS

Introduction

IGCT are heterogeneous neoplasms that generally constitute for fewer than 5% of primary brain tumors in children and young adults.[121] However, IGCTs are much more common in Japan and other East Asian countries, which have reported up to an 11% incidence rate.[122] Approximately 90% of IGCT cases occur in patients less than 20 years old, with peak incidence at 10 to 12 years.[123] The IGCTs are located in the pineal and suprasellar regions of the brain,[123] although 5% to 10% of IGCTs may present as synchronous lesions in both of these areas.[124] Interestingly, there is a large difference in the incidence of pineal IGCTs between males and females, with a male-to-female incidence ratio of 15:1.[125,126]

Neuroimaging studies such as computerized tomography and magnetic resonance imaging (MRI) cannot differentiate IGCTs from other tumors and a biopsy is usually required to confirm histology.[123] Serum and CSF studies measuring elevated tumor markers should include alpha-fetoprotein and/or beta-human chorionic gonadotropin, which suggest secretion by a subgroup of IGCT. Imaging findings in conjunction with tumor marker elevation are diagnostic of IGCT.[123,127]

The clinical presentation of IGCT varies by tumor size and location, with common symptoms including signs of hydrocephalus and endocrinopathy.[123] Pineal IGCTs often present with neurologic symptoms[128] due to their tendency to obstruct CSF flow and increasing intracranial pressure (ICP). Surgeons lower ICP by redirecting CSF flow through the placement of a VPS. However, this procedure increases the risk of metastasis and infection.[129] Moreover, suprasellar IGCTs are often associated with endocrinopathies such as diabetes insipidus or growth retardation, which may present prior to imaging verification of a brain tumor.[128,130]

Subtypes of IGCT

IGCTs are a very rare and diverse group of tumors classified as *germinomatous germ cell tumors* (GGCT) or *nongerminomatous germ cell tumors* (NGGCTs). NGGCTs are further divided into the following groups: teratoma, embryonal carcinoma, choriocarcinoma, endodermal sinus tumor (yolk sac tumor), and mixed cell tumor.[131] Histology of the tumor is an indicator of treatment protocol and prognosis. GGCTs lack histologic differentiation and are associated with good outcome. In contrast, NGGCTs are histologically heterogeneous and are much less sensitive to therapy, resulting in much poorer outcomes.[132]

Treatment

Germinomatous Germ Cell Tumor

GGCTs are very chemoradiosensitive and therefore, respond well to treatment. This good prognosis obviates the need for surgery, which has been shown to have no impact on the survival of patients with GGCT.[127,133] The standard treatment has been WBRT or CSRT with a local boost of up to 40 to 55 Gy.[134] Surgical intervention is undertaken only to relieve ICP or perform a tumor biopsy. Despite the excellent prognosis for GGCT with RT alone, the high doses of radiation are toxic to the developing CNS and may severely affect quality of life.[135] Tumor location and radiation field and dosage are two main factors that can affect neurocognitive, emotional, and behavioral dysfunction in long-term survivors after RT.[136] Therefore, further research is being conducted to determine the safest and most effective dosage of radiation.[137,138]

Historically, a radiation dose of 36 Gy was delivered to the craniospinal axis, followed by a 14 Gy local boost to the tumor region for a total dose of 50 Gy.[139] However, substantial late effects can occur after using this large dose and many studies have investigated the efficacy of reduced-dose radiation to the primary site. Multiple studies found that a reduced dose of 45 Gy yielded the same survival rates of greater than 90% as the full dose.[139–141] Nonetheless, craniospinal irradiation (CSI) is no longer the gold standard in the treatment of localized germinoma and has been replaced with whole ventricle irradiation (WVI) of 23.4 Gy, followed by a local boost of 45 to 50 Gy.[142] Once again, the efficacy of WVI is comparable with CSI, as there is no increase in recurrence rates.[143] In addition, WVI is associated with better neurocognitive performance than is CSI.[144]

It has been suggested that radiation dose can be further lowered by supplementing WVI with neoadjuvant chemotherapy.[140,145,146] However, the management of patients receiving chemotherapy drugs that require hyperhydration is difficult due to the high prevalence of diabetes insipidus in this particular population.[147] Pure germinomas are treated with preradiation chemotherapy (EP regimen) consisting of cisplatin and etoposide, 5 consecutive days per week every 4 weeks, followed by 24 Gy local RT. Patients with gross total or subtotal resection underwent three cycles, while those with partial resection or biopsy had four cycles of chemotherapy (Table 19-5).[134]

Treatment regimens consisting only of chemotherapy have also been investigated but have proved to be less effective than are treatments involving radiation.[148] In the largest germinoma study using chemotherapy alone, 22 of 45 patients relapsed, which is considerably higher than studies including RT.[127] Therefore, chemotherapy is an effective method to lower the dose of radiation, but chemotherapy alone is not an effective treatment for GGCT.

Table 19-5 Maintenance Chemotherapy (EP Regimen) for Pure Germinomas

Drug	Route	Dosage	Days
Cisplatin	IV	100 mg/m^2	1, 2, 3, 4, 5
Etoposide	IV	20 mg/m^2	1, 2, 3, 4, 5

Schedule: Every 4 weeks, followed by 24 Gy local RT.

Nongerminomatous Germ Cell Tumor

The therapeutic regimen is multimodal, composed of surgery, radiotherapy, and chemotherapy. However, the outcomes from the standard protocol are suboptimal for most cases of NGGCT and patients are often exposed to dangerous levels of toxicity, resulting in neurologic deficits and other adverse effects. The low quality of life, combined with the very poor prognosis, warrants further research to find the optimal treatment protocol for NGGCT.

Because of the heterogeneity of its subgroups, treating of NGGCTs poses a great therapeutic challenge for clinicians.[149] Histologic confirmation of mixed tumor subtype is essential for selecting the best treatment protocol, including optimal dose, timing, and volume of radiation. Matsutani et al. developed a grading system in which NGGCTs were divided into three subgroups: good prognosis, intermediate prognosis, and poor prognosis. Tumors with good prognosis included pure germinoma and mature teratoma, which can often be treated with surgery alone to yield a 3-year OS rate of 94.1%. Intermediate prognosis tumors include immature teratoma, embryonal carcinoma, and mixed tumors composed mainly of germinomas or teratomas. This group had a 3-year OS rate of 70% following surgery and adjuvant therapies. The poor prognosis group consisted of yolk sac tumor and mixed tumors, choriocarcinoma. This group had a 3-year OS rate of only 9.3% after surgery and adjuvant therapies.[137] The classification of NGGCT subtypes enables clinicians to administer an appropriate treatment protocol in accordance with the prognostic profile of the various tumor subtypes.

Unlike GGCTs, surgical resection is essential in the treatment of patients with NGGCTs.[150] Some patients may also receive gamma-knife surgery after the initial resection.[151] However, the value of GTRs over partial resection has not been proven and the validity of radical resection in NGGCTs is unclear.[121,127,152] Usually, mature teratomas (good prognosis) can be treated with surgery alone with a 100% 5-year survival rate,[153] while the other subtypes of NGGCTs require further adjuvant therapy according to their histology.[154,155]

A preradiation chemotherapy regimen has been shown to improve OS in the intermediate and poor prognosis groups.[156] However, an international study demonstrated that the use of chemotherapy alone is ineffectual, as 50% of patients either relapsed or progressed despite high-dose chemotherapy.[157] Similarly, the intermediate and poor prognosis groups are refractory to RT alone[132] and CSI (30 Gy) followed by a local boost (20 Gy) resulted in disease control in only 40% to 60% of patients,[158] with the majority having disease progression within 18 months.[132,159] These results emphasize the need to administer aggressive chemotherapy to the therapeutic regimen for NGGCTs of intermediate and poor prognosis, followed by RT. The standard chemotherapy regimen for nongerminomas (ICE regimen) consists of ifosfamide, cisplatin, and etoposide, 5 consecutive days per week every 4 weeks, followed by 40 to 54 Gy local RT (Table 19-6). Patients with gross total or subtotal surgical resection and normalized serum HCG levels receive three cycles, while those with partial resection and elevated serum HCG have four cycles of chemotherapy.[160]

Several studies of the intermediate prognosis group indicated that surgery, followed by combined chemotherapy and RT led to much more favorable outcomes than did surgery and RT without chemotherapy.[161,162] In fact, Matsutani et al. reported a 5-year survival rate of 62%

Table 19-6 Maintenance Chemotherapy (ICE Regimen) for Nongerminomas

Drug	Route	Dosage	Days
ifosfamide	IV	900 mg/m^2	1, 2, 3, 4, 5
Cisplatin	IV	20 mg/m^2	1, 2, 3, 4, 5
Etoposide	IV	60 mg/m^2	1, 2, 3, 4, 5

Schedule: Every 4 weeks, followed by 40–54 Gy local RT and possible second-look surgery if tumor markers remain elevated with negative radiographic imaging.

for patients who did not receive adjuvant chemotherapy, compared to 92.9% for patients who received additional chemotherapy.[163] Similarly, in a study of 14 patients in the poor prognosis group, those who underwent surgery with adjuvant radiation and chemotherapy had a 5-year survival rate of 18%, whereas 100% of patients who did not receive chemotherapy experienced intracranial recurrence.[164] Overall, patients who responded well to neoadjuvant chemotherapy were able to receive significantly reduced-dose radiation to lessen toxicity without compromising OS.[146]

Nonetheless, the results for the poor prognosis group remain dismal and the only treatment option available is the same multimodal approach used for the intermediate prognosis group.[151,165] Clearly, further research must be conducted to delineate the optimal parameters of therapy for the most malignant group of NGGCT.

Recurrent IGCT

Seventy percent of tumor recurrences occur at the primary site and are associated with very poor outcomes, especially for NGCCTs.[166,167] Salvage therapies include additional surgery, focal or craniospinal radiation, chemotherapy with re-irradiation, and myeloablative chemotherapy with autologous stem cell rescue.[123] GGCT patients who were initially treated with chemotherapy alone were shown to benefit from chemotherapy followed by RT.[166,168] High-dose chemotherapy and autologous stem cell rescue have demonstrated limited benefits in relapsed NGGCT, especially in chemosensitive patients, however, their outlook remains poor.[169,170]

Growing Teratoma Syndrome

During or following chemotherapy, NGGCT patients may experience a rare phenomenon in which there is an enlarging lesion, despite normal tumor marker levels.[171] This is known as growing tumor syndrome (GTS), and clinicians must take great care not to mistake this event for tumor recurrence.[172] If possible, second-look surgery is necessary to determine whether the mass is GTS or residual NGGCT.[173] GTS is best treated with early surgical excision following histologic confirmation.[174]

ACKNOWLEDGMENT

The author would like to acknowledge Stephanie Nguyen, of Rice University, for her contributions to this chapter.

References

1. Wrensch M, et al. Epidemiology of primary brain tumors: current concepts and review of the literature. *Neuro Oncol* 2002;4(4):278–299.
2. Kleihues P, et al. The WHO classification of tumors of the nervous system. *J Neuropathol Exp Neurol* 2002;61(3):215–225; discussion 226–229.
3. Clarke J, Butowski N, Chang S. Recent advances in therapy for glioblastoma. *Arch Neurol* 2010; 67(3):279–283.
4. Ohka F, Natsume A, Wakabayashi T. Current trends in targeted therapies for glioblastoma multiforme. *Neurol Res Int* 2012;2012:878425.
5. Weller M, et al. Standards of care for treatment of recurrent glioblastoma—are we there yet? *Neuro Oncol* 2013;15(1):4–27.
6. Vredenburgh JJ, et al. Phase II trial of bevacizumab and irinotecan in recurrent malignant glioma. *Clin Cancer Res* 2007;13(4):1253–1259.
7. Mischel PS, Cloughesy TF, Nelson SF. DNA-microarray analysis of brain cancer: molecular classification for therapy. *Nat Rev Neurosci* 2004;5(10):782–792.

8. Rich JN, Bigner DD. Development of novel targeted therapies in the treatment of malignant glioma. *Nat Rev Drug Discov* 2004;3(5):430–446.
9. Kreth FW, et al. Surgical resection and radiation therapy versus biopsy and radiation therapy in the treatment of glioblastoma multiforme. *J Neurosurg* 1993;78(5):762–766.
10. Quigley MR, Maroon JC. The relationship between survival and the extent of the resection in patients with supratentorial malignant gliomas. *Neurosurgery* 1991;29(3):385–388; discussion 388–389.
11. Pan E, Mitchell SB, Tsai JS. A retrospective study of the safety of BCNU wafers with concurrent temozolomide and radiotherapy and adjuvant temozolomide for newly diagnosed glioblastoma patients. *J Neurooncol* 2008;88(3):353–357.
12. Salcman M. Surgical resection of malignant brain tumors: who benefits? *Oncology (Williston Park)* 1988;2(8):47–56, 59, 60, 63.
13. Glantz MJ, et al. Influence of the type of surgery on the histologic diagnosis in patients with anaplastic gliomas. *Neurology* 1991;41(11):1741–1744.
14. Walker MD, et al. Evaluation of BCNU and/or radiotherapy in the treatment of anaplastic gliomas. A cooperative clinical trial. *J Neurosurg* 1978;49(3):333–343.
15. Andersen AP. Postoperative irradiation of glioblastomas. Results in a randomized series. *Acta Radiol Oncol Radiat Phys Biol* 1978;17(6):475–484.
16. Walker MD, et al. Randomized comparisons of radiotherapy and nitrosoureas for the treatment of malignant glioma after surgery. *N Engl J Med* 1980;303(23):1323–1329.
17. Green SB, et al. Comparisons of carmustine, procarbazine, and high-dose methylprednisolone as additions to surgery and radiotherapy for the treatment of malignant glioma. *Cancer Treat Rep* 1983;67(2):121–132.
18. Pashaki AS, et al. Efficacy of high dose radiotherapy in post-operative treatment of glioblastoma multiform—a single institution report. *Asian Pac J Cancer Prev* 2014;15(6):2793–2796.
19. Choucair AK, et al. Development of multiple lesions during radiation therapy and chemotherapy in patients with gliomas. *J Neurosurg* 1986;65(5):654–658.
20. Thornton AF Jr, et al. Three-dimensional treatment planning of astrocytomas: a dosimetric study of cerebral irradiation. *Int J Radiat Oncol Biol Phys* 1991;20(6):1309–1315.
21. Glatstein E, et al. The imaging revolution and radiation oncology: use of CT, ultrasound, and NMR for localization, treatment planning and treatment delivery. *Int J Radiat Oncol Biol Phys* 1985;11(2):299–314.
22. Gross MW, et al. The value of F-18-fluorodeoxyglucose PET for the 3-D radiation treatment planning of malignant gliomas. *Int J Radiat Oncol Biol Phys* 1998;41(5):989–995.
23. Lorentini S, et al. IMRT or 3D-CRT in glioblastoma? A dosimetric criterion for patient selection. *Technol Cancer Res Treat* 2013;12(5):411–420.
24. MacDonald SM, et al. Intensity modulated radiation therapy versus three-dimensional conformal radiation therapy for the treatment of high grade glioma: a dosimetric comparison. *J Appl Clin Med Phys* 2007;8(2):47–60.
25. Paulino AC, et al. Radiation-induced malignant gliomas: is there a role for reirradiation? *Int J Radiat Oncol Biol Phys* 2008;71(5):1381–1387.
26. Shrieve DC, et al. Treatment of patients with primary glioblastoma multiforme with standard postoperative radiotherapy and radiosurgical boost: prognostic factors and long-term outcome. *J Neurosurg* 1999;90(1):72–77.
27. Tsao MN, et al. The American Society for Therapeutic Radiology and Oncology (ASTRO) evidence-based review of the role of radiosurgery for malignant glioma. *Int J Radiat Oncol Biol Phys* 2005;63(1):47–55.
28. Cardinale R, et al. A phase II trial of accelerated radiotherapy using weekly stereotactic conformal boost for supratentorial glioblastoma multiforme: RTOG 0023. *Int J Radiat Oncol Biol Phys* 2006;65(5):1422–1428.
29. Sneed PK, et al. Demonstration of brachytherapy boost dose–response relationships in glioblastoma multiforme. *Int J Radiat Oncol Biol Phys* 1996;35(1):37–44.
30. Marin LA, et al. Response of glioblastoma cell lines to low dose rate irradiation. *Int J Radiat Oncol Biol Phys* 1991;21(2):397–402.
31. Fitzek MM, et al. Accelerated fractionated proton/photon irradiation to 90 cobalt gray equivalent for glioblastoma multiforme: results of a phase II prospective trial. *J Neurosurg* 1999;91(2):251–260.
32. Castro JR, et al. Neon heavy charged particle radiotherapy of glioblastoma of the brain. *Int J Radiat Oncol Biol Phys* 1997;38(2):257–261.

33. Castro JR, et al. A phase I–II trial of heavy charged particle irradiation of malignant glioma of the brain: a Northern California Oncology Group Study. *Int J Radiat Oncol Biol Phys* 1985;11(10):1795–1800.
34. Griffin TW, et al. Fast neutron radiation therapy for glioblastoma multiforme. Results of an RTOG study. *Am J Clin Oncol* 1983;6(6):661–667.
35. Cohen L, et al. Clinical evaluation of neutron beam therapy. Current results and prospects 1983. *Cancer* 1985;55(1):10–17.
36. Cohen L, Awschalom M. Fast neutron radiation therapy. *Annu Rev Biophys Bioeng* 1982;11:359–390.
37. Huncharek M, Muscat J, Geschwind JF. Multi-drug versus single agent chemotherapy for high grade astrocytoma; results of a meta-analysis. *Anticancer Res* 1998;18(6B):4693–4697.
38. Stewart LA. Chemotherapy in adult high-grade glioma: a systematic review and meta-analysis of individual patient data from 12 randomised trials. *Lancet* 2002;359(9311):1011–1018.
39. Plowman J, et al. Preclinical antitumor activity of temozolomide in mice: efficacy against human brain tumor xenografts and synergism with 1,3-*bis*(2-chloroethyl)-1-nitrosourea. *Cancer Res* 1994;54(14): 3793–3799.
40. O'Reilly SM, et al. Temozolomide: a new oral cytotoxic chemotherapeutic agent with promising activity against primary brain tumours. *Eur J Cancer* 1993;29A(7):940–942.
41. Stupp R, et al. Radiotherapy plus concomitant and adjuvant temozolomide for glioblastoma. *N Engl J Med* 2005;352(10):987–996.
42. Stupp R, et al. High-grade malignant glioma: ESMO clinical practice guidelines for diagnosis, treatment and follow-up. *Ann Oncol* 2010;21(suppl 5):v190–v193.
43. Cohen MH, Pazdur R. Food and Drug Administration Drug approval summary: temozolomide plus radiation therapy for the treatment of newly diagnosed glioblastoma multiforme. *Clin Cancer Res* 2005;11(19 Pt 1):6767–6771.
44. Patel M, et al. Plasma and cerebrospinal fluid pharmacokinetics of intravenous temozolomide in nonhuman primates. *J Neurooncol* 2003;61(3):203–207.
45. Friedman HS, Kerby T, Calvert H. Temozolomide and treatment of malignant glioma. *Clin Cancer Res* 2000;6(7):2585–2597.
46. Stupp R, et al. Effects of radiotherapy with concomitant and adjuvant temozolomide versus radiotherapy alone on survival in glioblastoma in a randomised phase III study: 5-year analysis of the EORTC-NCIC trial. *Lancet Oncol* 2009;10(5):459–466.
47. Lai A, et al. Phase II study of bevacizumab plus temozolomide during and after radiation therapy for patients with newly diagnosed glioblastoma multiforme. *J Clin Oncol* 2011;29(2):142–148.
48. Vredenburgh JJ, et al. Addition of bevacizumab to standard radiation therapy and daily temozolomide is associated with minimal toxicity in newly diagnosed glioblastoma multiforme. *Int J Radiat Oncol Biol Phys* 2012;82(1):58–66.
49. Chinot OL, et al. Bevacizumab plus radiotherapy-temozolomide for newly diagnosed glioblastoma. *N Engl J Med* 2014;370(8):709–722.
50. Gilbert MR, et al. A randomized trial of bevacizumab for newly diagnosed glioblastoma. *N Engl J Med* 2014;370(8):699–708.
51. Burton E, Prados M. New chemotherapy options for the treatment of malignant gliomas. *Curr Opin Oncol* 1999;11(3):157–161.
52. Cokgor I, Friedman HS, Friedman AH. Chemotherapy for adults with malignant glioma. *Cancer Invest* 1999;17(4):264–272.
53. Bota DA, et al. Interstitial chemotherapy with biodegradable BCNU (Gliadel) wafers in the treatment of malignant gliomas. *Ther Clin Risk Manag* 2007;3(5):707–715.
54. Ashby LS, Ryken TC. Management of malignant glioma: steady progress with multimodal approaches. *Neurosurg Focus* 2006;20(4):E3.
55. Brem H, et al. Placebo-controlled trial of safety and efficacy of intraoperative controlled delivery by biodegradable polymers of chemotherapy for recurrent gliomas. The Polymer-brain Tumor Treatment Group. *Lancet* 1995;345(8956):1008–1012.
56. Gilbert MR. Establishing the standard of care for patients with newly diagnosed and recurrent glioblastoma. *Am Soc Clin Oncol Educ Book* 2012; 112–117.
57. Perry J, et al. Gliadel wafers in the treatment of malignant glioma: a systematic review. *Curr Oncol* 2007;14(5):189–194.
58. Gutenberg A, et al. MGMT promoter methylation status and prognosis of patients with primary or recurrent glioblastoma treated with carmustine wafers. *Br J Neurosurg* 2013;27(6):772–778.

59. Shapiro WR, et al. Randomized trial of three chemotherapy regimens and two radiotherapy regimens and two radiotherapy regimens in postoperative treatment of malignant glioma. Brain Tumor Cooperative Group Trial 8001. *J Neurosurg* 1989;71(1):1–9.
60. Lombardi G, et al. The combination of carmustine wafers and fotemustine in recurrent glioblastoma patients: a monoinstitutional experience. *Biomed Res Int* 2014;2014:4.
61. Reithmeier T, et al. BCNU for recurrent glioblastoma multiforme: efficacy, toxicity and prognostic factors. *BMC Cancer* 2010;10:30.
62. Cohen MH, et al. FDA drug approval summary: bevacizumab (Avastin) as treatment of recurrent glioblastoma multiforme. *Oncologist* 2009;14(11):1131–1138.
63. Friedman HS, et al. Bevacizumab alone and in combination with irinotecan in recurrent glioblastoma. *J Clin Oncol* 2009;27(28):4733–4740.
64. Lu Y, et al. [Preliminary clinical evaluations of bevacizumab for recurrent malignant glioma in Chinese patients]. *Zhonghua Yi Xue Za Zhi* 2014;94(15):1165–1168.
65. Hattingen E, et al. Bevacizumab impairs oxidative energy metabolism and shows antitumoral effects in recurrent glioblastomas: a 31P/1H MRSI and quantitative magnetic resonance imaging study. *Neuro Oncol* 2011;13(12):1349–1363.
66. Nagpal S, Harsh G, Recht L. Bevacizumab improves quality of life in patients with recurrent glioblastoma. *Chemother Res Pract* 2011;2011:602812.
67. Vredenburgh JJ, et al. Phase II trial of bevacizumab and irinotecan in recurrent malignant glioma. *Clin Cancer Res* 2007;13(4):1253–1259.
68. Vredenburgh JJ, et al. Bevacizumab plus irinotecan in recurrent glioblastoma multiforme. *J Clin Oncol* 2007;25(30):4722–4729.
69. Stupp R, et al. NovoTTF-100A versus physician's choice chemotherapy in recurrent glioblastoma: a randomised phase III trial of a novel treatment modality. *Eur J Cancer* 2012;48(14):2192–2202.
70. Gutin PH, Wong ET. Noninvasive application of alternating electric fields in glioblastoma: a fourth cancer treatment modality. *Am Soc Clin Oncol Educ Book* 2012; 126–131.
71. Pless M, Weinberg U. Tumor treating fields: concept, evidence and future. *Expert Opin Investig Drugs* 2011;20(8):1099–1106.
72. Turner SG, et al. The effect of field strength on glioblastoma multiforme response in patients treated with the NovoTTF-100A system. *World J Surg Oncol* 2014;12(1):162.
73. DeAngelis LM. Anaplastic glioma: how to prognosticate outcome and choose a treatment strategy [corrected]. *J Clin Oncol* 2009;27(35):5861–5862.
74. Wick W, et al. NOA-04 randomized phase III trial of sequential radiochemotherapy of anaplastic glioma with procarbazine, lomustine, and vincristine or temozolomide. *J Clin Oncol* 2009;27(35):5874–5880.
75. Parsons DW, et al. An integrated genomic analysis of human glioblastoma multiforme. *Science* 2008;321(5897):1807–1812.
76. Cairncross G, et al. Phase III trial of chemoradiotherapy for anaplastic oligodendroglioma: long-term results of RTOG 9402. *J Clin Oncol* 2013;31(3):337–343.
77. van den Bent MJ, et al. Adjuvant procarbazine, lomustine, and vincristine chemotherapy in newly diagnosed anaplastic oligodendroglioma: long-term follow-up of EORTC brain tumor group study 26951. *J Clin Oncol* 2013;31(3):344–350.
78. Smith JS, et al. Alterations of chromosome arms 1p and 19q as predictors of survival in oligodendrogliomas, astrocytomas, and mixed oligoastrocytomas. *J Clin Oncol* 2000;18(3):636–645.
79. Wick W, et al. Temozolomide chemotherapy alone versus radiotherapy alone for malignant astrocytoma in the elderly: the NOA-08 randomised, phase 3 trial. *Lancet Oncol* 2012;13(7):707–715.
80. Hegi ME, et al. MGMT gene silencing and benefit from temozolomide in glioblastoma. *N Engl J Med* 2005;352(10):997–1003.
81. Levin VA, et al. Phase III randomized study of postradiotherapy chemotherapy with combination α-difluoromethylornithine-PCV versus PCV for anaplastic gliomas. *Clin Cancer Res* 2003;9(3): 981–990.
82. Hartmann C, et al. Molecular markers in low-grade gliomas: predictive or prognostic? *Clin Cancer Res* 2011;17(13):4588–4599.
83. Zhang C, et al. IDH1/2 mutations target a key hallmark of cancer by deregulating cellular metabolism in glioma. *Neuro Oncol* 2013;15(9):1114–1126.
84. Sanson M, et al. Isocitrate dehydrogenase 1 codon 132 mutation is an important prognostic biomarker in gliomas. *J Clin Oncol* 2009;27(25):4150–4154.

85. Kros JM, et al. Panel review of anaplastic oligodendroglioma from European Organization For Research and Treatment of Cancer Trial 26951: assessment of consensus in diagnosis, influence of 1p/19q loss, and correlations with outcome. *J Neuropathol Exp Neurol* 2007;66(6):545–551.
86. van den Bent MJ, et al. IDH1 and IDH2 mutations are prognostic but not predictive for outcome in anaplastic oligodendroglial tumors: a report of the European Organization for Research and Treatment of Cancer Brain Tumor Group. *Clin Cancer Res* 2010;16(5):1597–1604.
87. Gwak HS, et al. Temozolomide salvage chemotherapy for recurrent anaplastic oligodendroglioma and oligo-astrocytoma. *J Korean Neurosurg Soc* 2013;54(6):489–495.
88. Lassman AB, et al. International retrospective study of over 1000 adults with anaplastic oligodendroglial tumors. *Neuro Oncol* 2011;13(6):649–659.
89. DeAngelis LM. Anaplastic glioma: how to prognosticate outcome and choose a treatment strategy. *J Clin Oncol* 2009;27(35):5861–5862.
90. Brandes AA, et al. Survival following adjuvant PCV or temozolomide for anaplastic astrocytoma. *Neuro Oncol* 2006;8(3):253–260.
91. Johnson BE, et al. Mutational analysis reveals the origin and therapy-driven evolution of recurrent glioma. *Science* 2014;343(6167):189–193.
92. Packer RJ, Vezina G. Management of and prognosis with medulloblastoma: therapy at a crossroads. *Arch Neurol* 2008;65(11):1419–1424.
93. Sant M, et al. Survival of European patients with central nervous system tumors. *Int J Cancer* 2012;131(1):173–185.
94. Raffel C. Medulloblastoma: molecular genetics and animal models. *Neoplasia* 2004;6(4):310–322.
95. Babcock MA, et al. Tumors of the central nervous system: clinical aspects, molecular mechanisms, unanswered questions, and future research directions. *J Child Neurol* 2008;23(10):1103–1121.
96. Walter AW, et al. Survival and neurodevelopmental outcome of young children with medulloblastoma at St Jude Children's Research Hospital. *J Clin Oncol* 1999;17(12):3720–3728.
97. Northcott PA, et al. Medulloblastoma comprises four distinct molecular variants. *J Clin Oncol* 2011;29(11):1408–1414.
98. Gibson P, et al. Subtypes of medulloblastoma have distinct developmental origins. *Nature* 2010;468(7327):1095–1099.
99. Kool M, et al. Integrated genomics identifies five medulloblastoma subtypes with distinct genetic profiles, pathway signatures and clinicopathological features. *PLoS One* 2008;3(8):e3088.
100. Thompson MC, et al. Genomics identifies medulloblastoma subgroups that are enriched for specific genetic alterations. *J Clin Oncol* 2006;24(12):1924–1931.
101. Taylor MD, et al. Molecular subgroups of medulloblastoma: the current consensus. *Acta Neuropathol* 2012;123(4):465–472.
102. Kool M, et al. Molecular subgroups of medulloblastoma: an international meta-analysis of transcriptome, genetic aberrations, and clinical data of WNT, SHH, group 3, and group 4 medulloblastomas. *Acta Neuropathol* 2012;123(4):473–484.
103. El-Ghandour NM. Endoscopic third ventriculostomy versus ventriculoperitoneal shunt in the treatment of obstructive hydrocephalus due to posterior fossa tumors in children. *Childs Nerv Syst* 2011;27(1):117–126.
104. Tamburrini G, et al. Endoscopic third ventriculostomy: the best option in the treatment of persistent hydrocephalus after posterior cranial fossa tumour removal? *Childs Nerv Syst* 2008;24(12): 1405–1412.
105. Paulino AC. Radiotherapeutic management of medulloblastoma *Oncology (Williston Park)* 1997;11(6): 813–823; discussion 823, 827–828, 831.
106. Gilbertson RJ. Medulloblastoma: signalling a change in treatment. *Lancet Oncol* 2004;5(4):209–218.
107. Ribi K, et al. Outcome of medulloblastoma in children: long-term complications and quality of life. *Neuropediatrics* 2005;36(6):357–365.
108. Packer RJ, et al. Phase III study of craniospinal radiation therapy followed by adjuvant chemotherapy for newly diagnosed average-risk medulloblastoma. *J Clin Oncol* 2006;24(25):4202–4208.
109. Packer RJ, et al. Survival and secondary tumors in children with medulloblastoma receiving radiotherapy and adjuvant chemotherapy: results of Children's Oncology Group Trial A9961. *Neuro Oncol* 2013;15(1):97–103.
110. Khaw SL, et al. Adverse hypersensitivity reactions to mesna as adjunctive therapy for cyclophosphamide. *Pediatr Blood Cancer* 2007;49(3):341–343.

111. Jimenez RB, et al. Proton radiation therapy for pediatric medulloblastoma and supratentorial primitive neuroectodermal tumors: outcomes for very young children treated with upfront chemotherapy. *Int J Radiat Oncol Biol Phys* 2013;87(1):120–126.
112. Gibbs IC, Tuamokumo N, Yock TI. Role of radiation therapy in pediatric cancer. *Hematol Oncol Clin North Am* 2006;20(2):455–470.
113. Grill J, et al. Treatment of medulloblastoma with postoperative chemotherapy alone: an SFOP prospective trial in young children. *Lancet Oncol* 2005;6(8):573–580.
114. von Bueren AO, et al. Treatment of young children with localized medulloblastoma by chemotherapy alone: results of the prospective, multicenter trial HIT 2000 confirming the prognostic impact of histology. *Neuro Oncol* 2011;13(6):669–679.
115. Rutkowski S, et al. Treatment of early childhood medulloblastoma by postoperative chemotherapy alone. *N Engl J Med* 2005;352(10):978–986.
116. Duffner PK, et al. Postoperative chemotherapy and delayed radiation in children less than three years of age with malignant brain tumors. *N Engl J Med* 1993;328(24):1725–1731.
117. Jakacki RI, et al. Outcome of children with metastatic medulloblastoma treated with carboplatin during craniospinal radiotherapy: a Children's Oncology Group Phase I/II study. *J Clin Oncol* 2012;30(21):2648–2653.
118. Bailey CC, et al. Prospective randomised trial of chemotherapy given before radiotherapy in childhood medulloblastoma. International Society of Paediatric Oncology (SIOP) and the (German) Society of Paediatric Oncology (GPO): SIOP II. *Med Pediatr Oncol* 1995;25(3):166–178.
119. Taylor RE, et al. Impact of radiotherapy parameters on outcome in the International Society of Paediatric Oncology/United Kingdom Children's Cancer Study Group PNET-3 study of preradiotherapy chemotherapy for M0–M1 medulloblastoma. *Int J Radiat Oncol Biol Phys* 2004;58(4):1184–1193.
120. von Hoff K, et al. Long-term outcome and clinical prognostic factors in children with medulloblastoma treated in the prospective randomised multicentre trial HIT'91. *Eur J Cancer* 2009;45(7):1209–1217.
121. Balmaceda C, Finlay J. Current advances in the diagnosis and management of intracranial germ cell tumors. *Curr Neurol Neurosci Rep* 2004;4(3):253–262.
122. Lin IJ, et al. Primary intracranial germ-cell tumor in children. *Zhonghua Yi Xue Za Zhi (Taipei)* 1997;60(5):259–264.
123. Echevarria ME, Fangusaro J, Goldman S. Pediatric central nervous system germ cell tumors: a review. *Oncologist* 2008;13(6):690–699.
124. Haque F, et al. Synchronous germinomas in the pineal and suprasellar region. *Indian Pediatr* 2005;42(4):376–379.
125. Thakkar JP, Chew L, Villano JL. Primary CNS germ cell tumors: current epidemiology and update on treatment. *Med Oncol* 2013;30(2):496.
126. Villano JL, et al. Malignant pineal germ-cell tumors: an analysis of cases from three tumor registries. *Neuro Oncol* 2008;10(2):121–130.
127. Packer RJ, Cohen BH, Cooney K. Intracranial germ cell tumors. *Oncologist* 2000;5(4):312–320.
128. Jorsal T, Rorth M. Intracranial germ cell tumours. A review with special reference to endocrine manifestations. *Acta Oncol* 2012;51(1):3–9.
129. Matsumoto J, et al. A long-term ventricular drainage for patients with germ cell tumors or medulloblastoma. *Surg Neurol* 2006;65(1):74–80; discussion 80.
130. Kreutz J, et al. Intracranial germ cell tumor. *JBR-BTR* 2010;93(4):196–197.
131. Sato K, Takeuchi H, Kubota T. Pathology of intracranial germ cell tumors. *Prog Neurol Surg* 2009;23:59–75.
132. Jennings MT, Gelman R, Hochberg F. Intracranial germ-cell tumors: natural history and pathogenesis. *J Neurosurg* 1985;63(2):155–167.
133. Weiner HL, Finlay JL. Surgery in the management of primary intracranial germ cell tumors. *Childs Nerv Syst* 1999;15(11–12):770–773.
134. Aoyama H, et al. Induction chemotherapy followed by low-dose involved-field radiotherapy for intracranial germ cell tumors. *J Clin Oncol* 2002;20(3):857–865.
135. Matsutani M. Pineal germ cell tumors. *Prog Neurol Surg* 2009;23:76–85.
136. Liang SY, et al. Neuropsychological functions and quality of life in survived patients with intracranial germ cell tumors after treatment. *Neuro-Oncology* 2013;15(11):1543–1551.
137. Matsutani M, et al. Primary intracranial germ cell tumors: a clinical analysis of 153 histologically verified cases. *J Neurosurg* 1997;86(3):446–455.

138. Sawamura Y, et al. Germ cell tumours of the central nervous system: treatment consideration based on 111 cases and their long-term clinical outcomes. *Eur J Cancer* 1998;34(1):104–110.
139. Bamberg M, et al. Radiation therapy for intracranial germinoma: results of the German cooperative prospective trials MAKEI 83/86/89. *J Clin Oncol* 1999;17(8):2585–2592.
140. Aoyama H, et al. Pathologically-proven intracranial germinoma treated with radiation therapy. *Radiother Oncol* 1998;47(2):201–205.
141. Shibamoto Y, Takahashi M, Abe M. Reduction of the radiation dose for intracranial germinoma: a prospective study. *Br J Cancer* 1994;70(5):984–989.
142. Rogers SJ, Mosleh-Shirazi MA, Saran FH. Radiotherapy of localised intracranial germinoma: time to sever historical ties? *Lancet Oncol* 2005;6(7):509–519.
143. Haas-Kogan DA, et al. Radiation therapy for intracranial germ cell tumors. *Int J Radiat Oncol Biol Phys* 2003;56(2):511–518.
144. Mabbott DJ, et al. Longitudinal evaluation of neurocognitive function after treatment for central nervous system germ cell tumors in childhood. *Cancer* 2011;117(23):5402–5411.
145. Calaminus G, et al. Intracranial germ cell tumors: a comprehensive update of the European data. *Neuropediatrics* 1994;25(1):26–32.
146. Allen JC, Kim JH, Packer RJ. Neoadjuvant chemotherapy for newly diagnosed germ-cell tumors of the central nervous system. *J Neurosurg* 1987;67(1):65–70.
147. Afzal S, et al. Challenges in management of patients with intracranial germ cell tumor and diabetes insipidus treated with cisplatin and/or ifosfamide based chemotherapy. *J Neurooncol* 2010;97(3):393–399.
148. da Silva NS, et al. Primary chemotherapy for intracranial germ cell tumors: results of the third international CNS germ cell tumor study. *Pediatr Blood Cancer* 2010;54(3):377–383.
149. Allen JC. Management of primary intracranial germ cell tumors of childhood. *Pediatr Neurosci* 1987;13(3):152–157.
150. Somma AD, et al. The "extended" endoscopic endonasal approach for the removal of a mixed intrasuprasellar germinoma: technical case report. *Surg Neurol Int* 2014;5:14.
151. Huang X, et al. Modified grading system for clinical outcome of intracranial non-germinomatous malignant germ cell tumors. *Oncol Lett* 2010;1(4):627–631.
152. Sawamura Y, et al. Management of primary intracranial germinomas: diagnostic surgery or radical resection? *J Neurosurg* 1997;87(2):262–266.
153. Aoyama H, et al. Retrospective multi-institutional study of radiotherapy for intracranial non-germinomatous germ cell tumors. *Radiother Oncol* 1998;49(1):55–59.
154. Glezer A, Paraiba DB, Bronstein MD. Rare sellar lesions. *Endocrinol Metab Clin North Am* 2008;37(1):195–211, x.
155. Muzumdar D, et al. Mature teratoma arising from the sella—case report. *Neurol Med Chir (Tokyo)* 2001;41(7):356–359.
156. Ji S, et al. Responses and adverse effects of carboplatin-based chemotherapy for pediatric intracranial germ cell tumors. *Korean J Pediatr* 2011;54(3):128–132.
157. Balmaceda C, et al. Chemotherapy without irradiation—a novel approach for newly diagnosed CNS germ cell tumors: results of an international cooperative trial. The First International Central Nervous System Germ Cell Tumor Study. *J Clin Oncol* 1996;14(11):2908–2915.
158. Calaminus G, et al. AFP/beta-HCG secreting CNS germ cell tumors: long-term outcome with respect to initial symptoms and primary tumor resection. Results of the cooperative trial MAKEI 89. *Neuropediatrics* 2005;36(2):71–77.
159. Allen JC. Controversies in the management of intracranial germ cell tumors. *Neurol Clin* 1991;9(2): 441–452.
160. Sawamura Y, et al. Induction chemotherapy followed by reduced-volume radiation therapy for newly diagnosed central nervous system germinoma. *J Neurosurg* 1998;88(1):66–72.
161. Schild SE, et al. Histologically confirmed pineal tumors and other germ cell tumors of the brain. *Cancer* 1996;78(12):2564–2571.
162. Robertson PL, DaRosso RC, Allen JC. Improved prognosis of intracranial non-germinoma germ cell tumors with multimodality therapy. *J Neurooncol* 1997;32(1):71–80.
163. Matsutani M. Combined chemotherapy and radiation therapy for CNS germ cell tumors—the Japanese experience. *J Neurooncol* 2001;54(3):311–316.
164. Ogawa K, et al. Treatment and prognosis of patients with intracranial nongerminomatous malignant germ cell tumors: a multiinstitutional retrospective analysis of 41 patients. *Cancer* 2003;98(2):369–376.

165. Kanamori M, et al. Optimal treatment strategy for intracranial germ cell tumors: a single institution analysis. *J Neurosurg Pediatr* 2009;4(6):506–514.
166. Merchant TE, et al. CNS germinoma: disease control and long-term functional outcome for 12 children treated with craniospinal irradiation. *Int J Radiat Oncol Biol Phys* 2000;46(5):1171–1176.
167. Modak S, et al. Thiotepa-based high-dose chemotherapy with autologous stem-cell rescue in patients with recurrent or progressive CNS germ cell tumors. *J Clin Oncol* 2004;22(10):1934–1943.
168. Sawamura Y, et al. Salvage therapy for recurrent germinomas in the central nervous system. *Br J Neurosurg* 1999;13(4):376–381.
169. Beyer J, et al. High-dose chemotherapy as salvage treatment in germ cell tumors: a multivariate analysis of prognostic variables. *J Clin Oncol* 1996;14(10):2638–2645.
170. Motzer RJ, et al. High-dose carboplatin, etoposide, and cyclophosphamide for patients with refractory germ cell tumors: treatment results and prognostic factors for survival and toxicity. *J Clin Oncol* 1996;14(4):1098–1105.
171. Gorbatiy V, Spiess PE, Pisters LL. The growing teratoma syndrome: current review of the literature. *Indian J Urol* 2009;25(2):186–189.
172. Kong DS, et al. Intracranial growing teratoma syndrome mimicking tumor relapse: a diagnostic dilemma. *J Neurosurg Pediatr* 2009;3(5):392–396.
173. Bi WL, Bannykh SI, Baehring J. The growing teratoma syndrome after subtotal resection of an intracranial nongerminomatous germ cell tumor in an adult: case report. *Neurosurgery* 2005;56(1):188.
174. Kim CY, et al. Intracranial growing teratoma syndrome: clinical characteristics and treatment strategy. *J Neurooncol* 2011;101(1):109–115.

Index

Note: Page numbers followed by *f* indicate figures; those followed by *t* indicate tables.

A

Adenomatous polyposis coli (APC) gene, 152
Alpha thalassemia/mental retardation syndrome X-linked mutations, 213–214
Anaplastic astrocytoma. *See* Diffuse astrocytoma and anaplastic astrocytoma
Anaplastic ependymoma
  genetics, 47
  histologic features, 45–46, 45*f*, 46*f*
  prognostic factors, 46–47
Anaplastic glioma (AG), 232, 233*t*, 234
  anaplastic astrocytomas (AA), 235
  anaplastic oligoastrocytoma (AOA), 234–235
  anaplastic oligodendroglioma (AO), 234–235
    (*See also* Oligodendroglioma and anaplastic oligodendroglioma)
Angiocentric glioma, 53–56, 55*f*
Angiomatous meningiomas, 127, 127*f*
Astroblastoma, 53, 54*f*
Atypical choroid plexus papilloma (APP), 91–94, 92*f*, 93*f*, 95–96. *See also* Choroid plexus papilloma (CPP)
Atypical teratoid/rhabdoid tumor (AT/RT), 221–222, 221*f*, 222*f*
  clinical symptoms, 81
  cytology, 81–82
  differential diagnosis, 84
  histologic features, 81, 82*f*
  histologic variability, 82
  immunohistochemically, 83, 83*f*, 84*f*
  treatment options, 81

B

Bilateral inherited retinoblastomas, 104
Brain cancer treatment
  anaplastic glioma (AG), 232, 233*t*, 234
    anaplastic astrocytomas (AA), 235
    anaplastic oligodendroglioma (AO) and anaplastic oligoastrocytoma (AOA), 234–235
  FDA approval timeline
    adjuvant chemotherapy, 230–231, 230*f*
    adjuvant postoperative radiation therapy, 230
    recurrent disease, therapy for, 231–232
    surgical resection, 229
  glioblastoma (GBM), 229
  intracranial germ cell tumors (IGCT)
    germinomatous germ cell tumor (GGCTs), 240, 240*t*
    growing teratoma syndrome (GTS), 242
    nongerminomatous germ cell tumor (NGGCT), 241–242, 241*t*
    overview, 239
    recurrent IGCT, 242
    subtypes of, 240
  medulloblastoma
    adjuvant chemoradiotherapy, 236–237, 237*t*, 238*t*, 239*t*
    craniotomy, 236
    high-risk patients, 237, 239
    subgroups of, 236
Brain tumors, anatomy and histology
  cerebellum, 6–7, 7*f*
  cerebral cortex, 3, 4*f*
  gray matter, 3, 4*f*, 5*f*, 6
  gray–white junction, 5*f*
  leptomeninges, 3, 4*f*
  meninges, 3, 4*f*
  pituitary and pineal glands, 7–8, 7*f*, 8*f*
  ventricles, 6, 6*f*
  white matter, 3, 5*f*, 6

C

Carney complex (CNC), 154
Central Brain Tumor Registry of the United States (CBTRUS), 123
Central nervous system (CNS), embryonal tumors of, 74
Central nervous system (CNS) metastasis
  clinical features, 188
  pathologic features
    gross findings, 190*f*, 191
    microscopic and immunohistochemical findings, 190*f*, 191, 192*t*
  pathologic forms
    leptomeningeal carcinomatosis (LC), 193–193, 194*f*
    prognosis and treatment, 190*f*, 193–194
    tumor-to-tumor metastasis, 192, 193*f*, 194*f*
  radiologic features, 189–191, 190*f*
Central nervous system primitive neuroectodermal tumors (CNS PNETs), 84–86, 85*f*, 87*f*
  differential diagnosis of, 86
  embryonal tumor with abundant neuropil and true rosettes (ETANTR), 86–87, 88*f*
  embryonal tumor with multilayered rosettes, 86–88, 88*f*, 89*f*
  ependymoblastoma (EBL), 85, 86–87, 88*f*
  ganglioneuroblastoma, 85, 86
  medulloepithelioma (MEPL), 85, 86–87, 89*f*
  neuroblastoma, 85, 85*f*, 86
  WHO classification, 84–85
Central neurocytomas, 65–67, 66*f*
Cerebellar liponeurocytomas, 65–67, 66*f*
Chordoid glioma, 51–52, 52*f*
Chordoid meningioma, 129
Choriocarcinoma, 110
Choroid plexus carcinoma (CPC)
  vs. atypical teratoid rhabdoid tumor (ATRT), 95–96
  cytology, 95, 95*f*
  differential diagnosis, 95
  MRI, 94, 94*f*
  WHO classification, 94
Choroid plexus papilloma (CPP)
  cytology, 91, 92*f*
  immunohistochemistry, 93
  magnetic resonance imaging (MRI), 91, 92*f*
  WHO classification, 91
Choroid plexus tumors
  atypical choroid plexus papilloma (APP), 91–94, 92*f*, 93*f*
  choroid plexus carcinoma (CPC), 94–96, 94*f*–96*f*
  choroid plexus papilloma (CPP), 91–94, 92*f*, 93*f*

Choroid plexus tumors (*Continued*)
  metastasis, 97, 98*f*
  xanthogranuloma, 96–97, 97*f*
Clear cell meningioma, 128, 129*f*
CNC. *See* Carney complex (CNC)
Conventional ependymomas
  ependymoma variants, 42–45, 43*f*, 44*f*
  histologic features, 42
  macroscopic features, 42
  radiologic features, 41, 41*f*, 42*f*
Costello syndrome, 142
Cowden syndrome (CS), 153
CP. *See* Craniopharyngioma (CP)
CPC. *See* Choroid plexus carcinoma (CPC)
CPP. *See* Choroid plexus papilloma (CPP)
Cranial nerve MPNSTs, 166
Craniopharyngioma (CP)
  adamantinomatous craniopharyngioma, 113
  clinical features and imaging, 114, 115*f*
  differential diagnosis, 115
  histopathology, 114–115, 115*f*
Cribriform neuroepithelial tumor (CRINET), 84
CS. *See* Cowden syndrome (CS)
Cytokeratin (CK)-7, 93, 93*f*

D

Desmoplastic infantile astrocytoma (DIA), 62–64, 63*f*
Desmoplastic infantile ganglioglioma (DIG), 62–64, 63*f*
Desmoplastic/nodular medulloblastoma, 77, 79*f*
DIA. *See* Desmoplastic infantile astrocytoma (DIA)
Differential diagnosis
  atypical teratoid/rhabdoid tumor (AT/RT), 84
  of central nervous system primitive neuroectodermal tumors (CNS PNETs), 86
  choroid plexus carcinoma (CPC), 95
  craniopharyngioma (CP), 115
  diffuse astrocytoma and anaplastic astrocytoma, 21
  gliomatosis cerebri, 27–28
  granular cell tumor (GCT), of infundibulum, 118*f*, 120
  malignant peripheral nerve sheath tumors (MPNSTs), 167–168
  neurofibromatosis type 2 (NF2), from NF1, 144–145
  oligodendroglioma and anaplastic oligodendroglioma, 18–19
  papillary craniopharyngioma (Papillary CP), 116, 116*f*
  papillary tumor of the pineal region (PTPR), 106
  of pineal parenchymal tumor of intermediate differentiation (PPTID), 103
  pituicytoma, 117
  Rathke cleft cyst (RCC), 113
  spindle cell oncocytoma (SCO), 117, 118*t*, 119
Diffuse astrocytoma and anaplastic astrocytoma
  clinical and radiologic features, 19
  differential diagnosis, 21
  grading, 21
  histologic and immunohistochemical features, 20, 20*f*
Diffuse glioma
  alpha thalassemia/mental retardation syndrome X-linked mutations, 213–214
  isocitrate dehydrogenase mutations, 211–212
  molecular alterations in, 211, 212*t*
  1p/19q co-deletion, 213
Diffuse (infiltrating) gliomas
  diffuse astrocytoma and anaplastic astrocytoma
    clinical and radiologic features, 19
    differential diagnosis, 21
    grading, 21
    histologic and immunohistochemical features, 20, 20*f*
  gemistocytic astrocytoma, 21, 22*f*
  glioblastoma
    clinical and radiologic features, 23, 23*f*
    GBM, with primitive neuroectodermal tumor-like foci, 25–26
    grading, 26
    histologic features, 23–24, 24*f*
    histologic types and variants, 24–25, 25*f*, 26*f*
    molecular features, 26
  gliomatosis cerebri
    clinical and radiologic features, 27, 27*f*
    differential diagnosis, 27–28
    histologic features and grading, 27
    molecular features and prognosis, 27
  oligoastrocytoma/"mixed" glioma, 22
  oligodendroglioma and anaplastic oligodendroglioma
    clinical and radiologic features, 14, 15*f*
    differential diagnosis, 18–19
    grading, 16–17, 17*f*
    histologic and immunohistochemical features, 15–16, 15*f*
    molecular features and prognosis, 17–18
Diffuse large B-cell lymphomas (DLBCL), 173
DIG. *See* Desmoplastic infantile ganglioglioma (DIG)
DLBCL. *See* Diffuse large B-cell lymphomas (DLBCL)
DNT. *See* Dysembryoplastic neuroepithelial tumor (DNT)
Dysembryoplastic neuroepithelial tumor (DNT), 69–71, 70*f*
Dysplastic gangliocytoma of cerebellum, 64, 153

E

Embryonal carcinoma, 110
Embryonal tumor with abundant neuropil and true rosettes (ETANTR), 86–87, 88*f*
Embryonal tumors
  atypical teratoid/rhabdoid tumor, 81–82, 82*f*–84*f*, 84
  atypical teratoid/rhabdoid tumor (AT/RT), 221–222, 221*f*, 222*f*
  central nervous system primitive neuroectodermal tumors, 84–86, 85*f*, 87*f*
    with abundant neuropil and true rosettes (ETANTR), 86–88, 88*f*
    with multilayered rosettes, 86–88, 88*f*, 89*f*
    neuroblastoma and ganglioneuroblastoma, 86
  medulloblastoma, 74–78, 76*f*–80*f*, 81, 219–221, 220*t*
Endodermal sinus tumor, 109
Ependymoblastoma (EBL), 85, 86–87, 88*f*
Ependymomas
  anaplastic ependymoma
    genetics, 47
    histologic features, 45–46, 45*f*, 46*f*
    prognostic factors, 46–47
  conventional
    ependymoma variants, 42–45, 43*f*, 44*f*
    histologic features, 42
    macroscopic features, 42
    radiologic features, 41, 41*f*, 42*f*
  ependymal tumors, epidemiology of, 37
  myxopapillary ependymoma
    genetics, 40
    histologic features, 39–40, 40*f*
    macroscopic features, 39
    prognosis, 40–41
    radiologic features, 39, 39*f*
  subependymoma
    histologic features, 37–38, 38*f*
    prognosis, 38
    radiologic features, 37, 38*f*

ETANTR. *See* Embryonal tumor with abundant neuropil and true rosettes (ETANTR)
Extraventricular neurocytomas, 65–67, 66*f*

F

Fibrous (fibroblastic) meningioma, 125, 126*f*
FLAIR. *See* Fluid attenuated inversion recovery (FLAIR)
Flexner–Wintersteiner rosettes, 105
Fluid attenuated inversion recovery (FLAIR), 201, 202*f*

G

Gangliocytoma, 60–62, 61*f*
Ganglioglioma, 60–62, 61*f*
Ganglioneuroblastoma, 85, 86
Gemistocytic astrocytoma, 21, 22*f*
Germ cell tumors (GCTs)
- choriocarcinoma, 110
- clinical presentation, 108
- embryonal carcinoma, 110
- germinoma, 109
- radiology, 108, 108*f*
- teratoma, 109
- WHO classification, 107
- yolk sac tumor, 109

Germinoma, 109
Glial fibrillary acidic protein (GFAP), 76, 93, 93*f*
Glial tumors
- circumscribed gliomas, 214
- diffuse glioma
  - alpha thalassemia/mental retardation syndrome X-linked mutations, 213–214
  - isocitrate dehydrogenase mutations, 211–212
  - molecular alterations in, 211, 212*t*
  - 1p/19q co-deletion, 213
- molecular signatures, 215
- pediatric diffuse glioma, 214

Glioblastoma (GBM)
- clinical and radiologic features, 23, 23*f*
- GBM, with primitive neuroectodermal tumor-like foci, 25–26
- grading, 26
- histologic features, 23–24, 24*f*
- histologic types and variants, 24–25, 25*f*, 26*f*
- molecular features, 26
- therapy for, 229

Gliomatosis cerebri
- clinical and radiologic features, 27, 27*f*
- differential diagnosis, 27–28
- histologic features and grading, 27
- molecular features and prognosis, 27

Gorlin syndrome, 152–153. *See also* Nevoid basal cell carcinoma syndrome (NBCCS)
Granular cell tumor (GCT), 165–166
- of infundibulum
  - clinical features and imaging, 120
  - differential diagnosis, 118*f*, 120
  - histopathology, 120, 120*f*

H

Hemangiopericytoma (HPC)
- grading, 137, 138*t*
- histology, 136, 137*f*
- immunohistochemistry, 137–138, 138*f*
- incidence, 136
- macroscopic findings, 136
- meninges, 223
- molecular genetic characteristics, 137–138, 138*f*
- prognostic factors, 137
- solitary fibrous tumor (SFT), 135, 136

Hematolymphoid and histiocytic tumors
- Langerhans cell histiocytosis (LCH)
  - clinical features, 184
  - definition, 183
  - histologic background, 184
  - neuroimaging findings, 184
  - pathologic features, 184–185, 185*f*
  - treatment and prognosis, 185
- lymphomas
  - intravascular lymphomatosis (IVL), 179–180
  - lymphomatoid granulomatosis (LYG), 178–179
- myeloid sarcoma (MS), 179*f*, 182
- plasmacytoma, 181–182, 181*f*
- primary central nervous system lymphoma (PCNSL)
  - clinical features, 173
  - corticosteroids, 176–177, 177*f*
  - definition, 173
  - historical background, 173
  - neuroimaging findings, 173, 174*f*
  - pathologic features, 174–176, 175*f*–177*f*
  - prognosis, 177
  - prognostic and diagnostic biomarkers, 177–178
  - treatment, 177
- primary dural lymphoma (PDL)
  - clinical features, 180
  - definition, 180
  - neuroimaging findings, 180
  - pathologic features, 180–181
  - treatment and prognosis, 181
- Rosai–Dorfman disease
  - definition, 181
  - histologic background and clinical features, 182
  - neuroimaging findings, 181*f*, 182
  - pathologic features, 182–183, 183*f*
  - treatment and prognosis, 183
- secondary hematolymphoid tumors
  - secondary leukemia, 180
  - secondary lymphoma, 180

Hereditary syndromes
- Carney complex (CNC), 154
- Cowden syndrome (CS), 153
- Li-Fraumeni syndrome (LFS), 153
- neurofibromatosis type 1 (NF1), 142–143
- neurofibromatosis type 2 (NF2), 143–145, 144*t*, 145*f*
- nevoid basal cell carcinoma syndrome (NBCCS), 152–153
- rhabdoid tumor predisposition syndromes (RTPSs), 153–154
- schwannomatosis, 145–146, 146*t*
- tuberous sclerosis complex (TSC), 146–148, 147*t*
- von Hippel–Lindau disease (VHL), 149–151, 150*f*, 150*t*, 151*f*, 152*t*

HPC. *See* Hemangiopericytoma (HPC)
Hybrid peripheral nerve sheath tumors, 163–165

I

Imaging with pathology
- cases, 203, 204*f*–206*f*, 205, 206
- computed tomography (CT), 200, 200*f*, 201*f*
- magnetic resonance imaging (MRI), 200, 201, 202*f*, 202*t*, 203, 203*f*

Immature teratoma, 109
Intracranial germ cell tumors (IGCT)
- germinomatous germ cell tumor (GGCTs), 240, 240*t*
- growing teratoma syndrome (GTS), 242
- nongerminomatous germ cell tumor (NGGCT), 241–242, 241*t*
- overview, 239
- recurrent IGCT, 242
- subtypes of, 240

Intracranial granular cell tumor, 165. *See also* Granular cell tumor (GCT)
Intracranial schwannomas, 157. *See also* Schwannomas
Intravascular lymphomatosis (IVL), 179–180

L

Langerhans cell histiocytosis (LCH)
- clinical features, 184
- definition, 183
- histologic background, 184
- neuroimaging findings, 184
- pathologic features, 184–185, 185*f*
- treatment and prognosis, 185

LC. *See* Leptomeningeal carcinomatosis (LC)
LDD. *See* Lhermitte–Duclos disease (LDD)
Legius syndrome, 142
LEOPARD syndrome, 142
Leptomeningeal carcinomatosis (LC), 193–193, 194*f*
LFS. *See* Li–Fraumeni syndrome (LFS)
Lhermitte–Duclos disease (LDD), 64, 153
Li–Fraumeni syndrome (LFS), 153
Lymphomas
- intravascular lymphomatosis (IVL), 179–180
- lymphomatoid granulomatosis (LYG), 178–179

Lymphomatoid granulomatosis (LYG), 178–179
Lymphoplasmacyte-rich meningioma, 128, 129*f*

M

Malignant peripheral nerve sheath tumors (MPNSTs)
- conventional type
  - clinical findings, 166
  - differential diagnosis, 167–168
  - pathologic findings, 167, 167*f*
- definition, WHO, 166
- epithelioid MPNST, 168, 169*f*
- genetics, 166
- with glandular differentiation, 168
- with rhabdomyoblastic differentiation, 168, 168*f*

Malignant triton tumor (MTT), 168
Mature teratoma, 109, 110*f*
Medulloblastoma (MB)
- adjuvant chemoradiotherapy, 75, 236–237, 237*t*, 238*t*, 239*t*
- anaplastic, 77–78, 80*f*
- craniotomy, 236
- desmoplastic/nodular, 77, 79*f*
- embryonal tumors, 219–221, 220*t*
- with extensive nodularity, 77, 79*f*
- high-risk patients, 237, 239
- immunohistochemistry, 76, 77*f*
- large cell, 78, 80*f*
- sonic hedgehog (SHH) subgroup, 75
- subgroups of, 236
- symptoms, 74–75
- WHO classification, 77
- WNT subgroup, 75

Medulloepithelioma (MEPL), 85, 86–87, 89*f*
Meningeal tumors
- hemangiopericytoma/solitary fibrous tumor
  - grading, 137, 138*t*
  - histology, 136, 137*f*
  - immunohistochemistry, 137–138, 138*f*
  - incidence, 136
  - macroscopic findings, 136
  - molecular genetic characteristics, 137–138, 138*f*
  - prognostic factors, 137
- meningiomas
  - arachnoid membrane, 123, 124*f*
  - cytologic preparations, 130, 131*t*
  - embolized meningioma, 133–134, 134*f*
  - histologic subtypes, 125–130, 126*t*, 127*f*–130*f*
  - hormones, 124
  - immunohistochemistry, 126*f*, 128*f*, 130, 131*t*
  - incidence and epidemiology, 123
  - location, 125
  - macroscopic features, 125
  - microscopic features, 125
  - molecular genetics of, 134–135f
  - neurofibromatosis type 2 (NF2), 123–124
  - prognostic factors, 134
  - proliferation, 131, 131*f*
  - radiation, 124
  - radiologic findings, 125
  - risk factors, 123–124
  - WHO grading system, 132, 132*f*, 133*f*

Meninges
- meningioma, 222–223
- solitary fibrous tumor (SFT)/hemangiopericytoma (HPC), 223

Meningiomas
- arachnoid membrane, 123, 124*f*
- definition, 123
- embolized meningioma, 133–134, 134*f*
- histologic subtypes
  - angiomatous meningiomas, 127, 127*f*
  - chordoid meningioma, 129
  - clear cell meningioma, 128, 129*f*
  - fibrous (fibroblastic) meningioma, 125, 126*f*
  - lymphoplasmacyte-rich meningioma, 128, 129*f*
  - meningothelial meningioma, 125, 126*f*
  - metaplastic meningioma, 128, 129*f*
  - microcystic meningioma, 127, 128*f*
  - papillary meningioma, 129, 130*f*
  - psammomatous meningiomas, 127, 127*f*
  - rhabdoid meningioma, 129, 130*f*
  - secretory meningioma, 127, 128*f*
  - transitional meningioma, 127
- immunohistochemistry, 126*f*, 128*f*, 130, 131*t*
- incidence and epidemiology, 123
- location, 125
- macroscopic features, 125
- microscopic features, 125
- molecular genetics of, 134–135f
- prognostic factors, 134
- proliferation, 131, 131*f*
- radiologic findings, 125
- risk factors
  - hormones, 124
  - neurofibromatosis type 2 (NF2), 123–124
  - radiation, 124
- WHO grading system, 132, 132*f*, 133*f*

Meningothelial meningioma, 125, 126*f*
MEPL. *See* Medulloepithelioma (MEPL)
Metaplastic meningioma, 128, 129*f*
Metastasis
- choroid plexus tumors, 97, 98*f*
- sellar and suprasellar region tumors, 121

Microcystic meningioma, 127, 128*f*
MS. *See* Myeloid sarcoma (MS)
Multiple hamartoma syndrome, 153. *See also* Cowden syndrome (CS)
Myeloid sarcoma (MS), 179*f*, 182
Myxopapillary ependymoma
- genetics, 40
- histologic features, 39–40, 40*f*
- macroscopic features, 39
- prognosis, 40–41
- radiologic features, 39, 39*f*

N

Nerve sheath myxoma, 165, 166*f*
Neurilemmomas. *See* Schwannomas
Neurinomas. *See* Schwannomas
Neuroblastoma, 85, 85*f*, 86
Neurocytomas, 65–67, 66*f*
Neurofibroma
  clinical and pathologic findings, 161, 162*f*
  definition, 160–161
  genetics, 161
  malignant change in, 161–162
  variants, 161, 162*f*
Neurofibromatosis type 1 (NF1)
  clinical and radiologic findings, 142
  peripheral and central nervous system neoplasms, 143
Neurofibromatosis type 2 (NF2)
  brain tumors, 143, 145*f*
  clinical features and diagnosis, 143, 144*t*
  differential diagnosis from NF1, 144–145
  meningiomas, 123–124
Neurofibromatosis type 3 (NF3), 145. *See also* Schwannomatosis
Neurofilament proteins (NFPs), 60
Neuromas. *See* Schwannomas
Neuronal/mixed glioneuronal tumors
  desmoplastic infantile astrocytoma (DIA), 62–64, 63*f*
  desmoplastic infantile ganglioglioma (DIG), 62–64, 63*f*
  dysembryoplastic neuroepithelial tumor (DNT), 69–71, 70*f*
  gangliocytoma and ganglioglioma, 60–62, 61*f*
  Lhermitte–Duclos disease (LDD), 64
  neurocytomas, 65–67, 66*f*
  overview, 58–60, 59*t*
  papillary glioneuronal tumor (PGNT), 67, 68*f*
  rosette-forming glioneuronal tumor (RGNT), 68–69, 69*f*
Nevoid basal cell carcinoma syndrome (NBCCS), 152–153
NF1. *See* Neurofibromatosis type 1 (NF1)
NF2. *See* Neurofibromatosis type 2 (NF2)
Nonglial tumors, 219
Noonan syndrome, 142

O

Oligoastrocytoma/“mixed” glioma, 22
Oligodendroglioma and anaplastic oligodendroglioma
  clinical and radiologic features, 14, 15*f*
  differential diagnosis, 18–19
  grading, 16–17, 17*f*
  histologic and immunohistochemical features, 15–16, 15*f*
  molecular features and prognosis, 17–18

P

Papillary craniopharyngioma (Papillary CP)
  clinical features and imaging, 115
  differential diagnosis, 116, 116*f*
  histopathology, 116, 116*f*
Papillary glioneuronal tumor (PGNT), 67, 68*f*
Papillary meningioma, 129, 130*f*
Papillary thyroid carcinoma (PTC), 97, 98*f*
Papillary tumor of the pineal region (PTPR)
  differential diagnosis, 106
  histology, 106, 107*f*
  molecular genetic analysis, 106
  MRI, 106
  WHO classification, 106
Parinaud syndrome, 104
PAS. *See* Periodic acid Schiff (PAS)
PAs. *See* Pilocytic astrocytomas (PAs)
PB. *See* Pineoblastoma (PB)
PC. *See* Pineocytoma (PC)
PCNSL. *See* Primary central nervous system lymphoma (PCNSL)
PDL. *See* Primary dural lymphoma (PDL)
Perineurioma
  genetics, 163
  intraneural perineurioma, 163
  soft tissue perineurioma, 163, 164*f*
Periodic acid Schiff (PAS), 127
Perivascular mononuclear inflammatory cells, 21, 22*f*
PGNT. *See* Papillary glioneuronal tumor (PGNT)
Pilocytic astrocytomas, 143
Pilocytic astrocytomas (PAs), 30–31, 31*f*, 31*t*
Pilomyxoid astrocytomas (PMAs), 31–33, 32*f*
Pineal parenchymal tumor of intermediate differentiation (PPTID)
  differential diagnosis of, 103
  histology, 103*f*, 104
  immunohistochemistry, 104
  MRI, 103, 103*f*
  real-time RT-PCR, 103
  WHO classification, 104
Pineal region tumors
  germ cell tumors (GCTs)
    choriocarcinoma, 110
    clinical presentation, 108
    embryonal carcinoma, 110
    germinoma, 109
    radiology, 108, 108*f*
    teratoma, 109
    WHO classification, 107
    yolk sac tumor, 109
  papillary tumor of the pineal region (PTPR)
    differential diagnosis, 106
    histology, 106, 107*f*
    molecular genetic analysis, 106
    MRI, 106
    WHO classification, 106
  pineal parenchymal tumor of intermediate differentiation (PPTID)
    differential diagnosis of, 103
    histology, 103*f*, 104
    immunohistochemistry, 104
    MRI, 103, 103*f*
    real-time RT-PCR, 103
    WHO classification, 104
  pineoblastoma (PB)
    bilateral inherited retinoblastomas, 104
    calcification, 104
    Flexner-Wintersteiner rosettes, 105
    histology, 104
    immunohistochemistry, 105–106
    Parinaud syndrome, 104
    WHO classification, 105
  pineocytoma (PC)
    clinical symptoms, 101
    histology, 102, 102*f*
    immunohistochemistry, 102, 103
    molecular pathologic features, 102
    MRI, 102, 102*f*
Pineoblastoma (PB)
  bilateral inherited retinoblastomas, 104
  calcification, 104
  Flexner–Wintersteiner rosettes, 105
  histology, 104
  immunohistochemistry, 105–106
  Parinaud syndrome, 104
  WHO classification, 105

Pineocytoma (PC)
clinical symptoms, 101
histology, 102, 102*f*
immunohistochemistry, 102, 103
molecular pathologic features, 102
MRI, 102, 102*f*
Pituicytoma
clinical presentation and imaging, 117
differential diagnosis, 117
histopathology, 117, 118*f*
Plasmacytoma, 181–182, 181*f*
Pleomorphic xanthoastrocytoma (PXA), 33, 34*f*
PMAs. *See* Pilomyxoid astrocytomas (PMAs)
PPTID. *See* Pineal parenchymal tumor of intermediate differentiation (PPTID)
Primary central nervous system lymphoma (PCNSL)
clinical features, 173
corticosteroids, 176–177, 177*f*
definition, 173
historical background, 173
neuroimaging findings, 173, 174*f*
pathologic features
histology, permanent section, 175–176, 176*f*, 177*f*
intraoperative consultation, 174, 175*f*
prognosis, 177
prognostic and diagnostic biomarkers, 177–178
treatment, 177
Primary dural lymphoma (PDL)
clinical features, 180
definition, 180
neuroimaging findings, 180
pathologic features, 180–181
treatment and prognosis, 181
Psammomatous meningiomas, 127, 127*f*
PTC. *See* Papillary thyroid carcinoma (PTC)
PTEN hamartoma tumor syndrome (PTHS), 153
PTHS. *See* PTEN hamartoma tumor syndrome (PTHS)
PTPR. *See* Papillary tumor of the pineal region (PTPR)
PXA. *See* Pleomorphic xanthoastrocytoma (PXA)

R

Rathke cleft cyst (RCC)
clinical and radiologic features, 112, 114*f*
differential diagnosis, 113
histopathology, 112, 114*f*
RGNT. *See* Rosette-forming glioneuronal tumor (RGNT)
Rhabdoid meningioma, 129, 130*f*
Rhabdoid tumor (RT), 81–82, 82*f*–84*f*, 84
Rhabdoid tumor predisposition syndromes (RTPSs), 153–154
Rosai–Dorfman disease
definition, 181
histologic background and clinical features, 182
neuroimaging findings, 181*f*, 182
pathologic features, 182–183, 183*f*
treatment and prognosis, 183
Rosette-forming glioneuronal tumor (RGNT), 68–69, 69*f*
RTPSs. *See* Rhabdoid tumor predisposition syndromes (RTPSs)

S

S100 protein, 93, 93*f*
Schwannomas
cellular schwannoma, 158, 159*f*
clinical findings, 157
genetics, 157
melanotic schwannoma (MS), 159–160
pathologic findings, 158, 158*f*
plexiform schwannoma (PS), 159, 160*f*
schwannomatosis, 160
Schwannomatosis
clinical features and diagnosis, 145–146, 146*t*
overview, 145
SMARCB1/INI1 germline mutations, 223, 223*f*
SCO. *See* Spindle cell oncocytoma (SCO)
Secondary leukemia, 180
Secondary lymphoma, 180
Secretory meningioma, 127, 128*f*
SEGAs. *See* Subependymal giant cell astrocytomas (SEGAs)
Sellar and suprasellar region tumors
craniopharyngioma (CP)
adamantinomatous craniopharyngioma, 113
clinical features and imaging, 114, 115*f*
differential diagnosis, 115
histopathology, 114–115, 115*f*
granular cell tumor (GCT), of infundibulum
clinical features and imaging, 120
differential diagnosis, 118*f*, 120
histopathology, 120, 120*f*
lesions, 112, 113*t*
metastasis, 121
papillary craniopharyngioma (Papillary CP)
clinical features and imaging, 115
differential diagnosis, 116, 116*f*
histopathology, 116, 116*f*
pituicytoma
clinical presentation and imaging, 117
differential diagnosis, 117
histopathology, 117, 118*f*
Rathke cleft cyst (RCC)
clinical and radiologic features, 112, 114*f*
differential diagnosis, 113
histopathology, 112, 114*f*
spindle cell oncocytoma (SCO)
clinical presentation and imaging, 117
differential diagnosis, 117, 118*t*, 119
histopathology, 119, 119*f*
SENs. *See* Subependymal nodules (SENs)
SFT. *See* Solitary fibrous tumor (SFT)
Sinus histiocytosis, 182. *See also* Rosai–Dorfman Disease
SMARCB1/INI1 germline mutations, 221, 223, 223*f*
Solitary fibrous tumor (SFT)
grading, 137, 138*t*
hemangiopericytoma (HPC), 135, 136
histology, 136, 137*f*
immunohistochemistry, 137–138, 138*f*
incidence, 136
macroscopic findings, 136
meninges, 223
molecular genetic characteristics, 137–138, 138*f*
prognostic factors, 137
Spindle cell oncocytoma (SCO)
clinical presentation and imaging, 117
differential diagnosis, 117, 118*t*, 119
histopathology, 119, 119*f*
Stereotactic radiosurgery, 194
Subependymal giant cell astrocytomas (SEGAs), 34–35, 34*f*
Subependymal nodules (SENs), 34–35, 34*f*
Subependymoma
histologic features, 37–38, 38*f*
prognosis, 38
radiologic features, 37, 38*f*
Synaptophysin, 93, 93*f*

T
Transitional meningioma, 127
Transthyretin (prealbumin), 93, 93*f*
TS. *See* Turcot syndrome (TS)
Tuberous sclerosis complex (TSC)
  clinical features and diagnosis, 147–148, 147*t*
  neuropathologic manifestations and pathologic features
    cortical dysplasias, 148
    subependymal nodule and subependymal giant cell astrocytoma, 148
  overview, 146–148
Tumor-to-tumor metastasis, 192, 193*f*, 194*f*
Turcot syndrome (TS), 151–152

V
von Hippel–Lindau disease (VHL)
  clinical features and diagnosis, 149
  endolymphatic sac tumor, 151, 151*f*, 152*t*
  hemangioblastoma, 149–150, 150*f*, 510*t*
von Recklinghausen disease, 142. *See also* Neurofibromatosis type 1 (NF1)

W
Whole-brain radiation therapy (WBRT), 194
World Health Organization (WHO) classification
  central nervous system primitive neuroectodermal tumors (CNS PNETs), 84–85
  choroid plexus carcinoma (CPC), 94
  choroid plexus papilloma (CPP), 91
  germ cell tumors (GCTs), 107
  medulloblastoma (MB), 77
  meningeal tumors, 132, 132*f*, 133*f*
  papillary tumor of the pineal region (PTPR), 106
  pineal parenchymal tumor of intermediate differentiation (PPTID), 104
  pineoblastoma (PB), 105

X
Xanthogranuloma, of choroid plexus, 96–97, 97*f*

Y
Yolk sac tumor, 109